Churchill's
Clinical Pharmacy
Survival Guide

For Churchill Livingstone:

Commissioning editor: Ellen Green
Project editor: Jim Killgore
Project controller: Derek Robertson
Design direction: Judith Wright

Churchill's Clinical Pharmacy Survival Guide

Edited by

Nick Barber BPharm PhD MRPharmS FRSM

Professor of the Practice of Pharmacy,
The School of Pharmacy,
University of London, London

Alan Willson BPharm MSc MRPharmS

Director of Patient Care, Iechyd Morgannwg Health,
Swansea

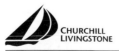

CHURCHILL
LIVINGSTONE

EDINBURGH LONDON NEW YORK PHILADELPHIA SYDNEY
TORONTO 1999

Churchill Livingstone
An imprint of Harcourt Brace and Company Limited

© Harcourt Brace and Company Limited 1999

⚓ is a registered trademark of Harcourt Brace and
Company Limited

First published 1999

ISBN 0443 06477 6

British Library Cataloguing in Publication Data
A catalogue record for this book is available from the
British Library

Library of Congress Cataloging in Publication Data
A catalog record for this book is available from the
Library of Congress

Note
Medical knowledge is constantly changing. As new
information becomes available, changes in treatment,
procedures, equipment and the use of drugs become
necessary. The editors, contributors and the publishers have,
as far as it is possible, taken care to ensure that the
information given in this text is accurate and up-to-date.
However, readers are strongly advised to confirm that the
information, especially with regard to drug usage, complies
with the latest legislation and standards of practice.

The
publisher's
policy is to use
paper manufactured
from sustainable forests

Printed in China

Contents

Contributors

Nick Barber BPharm PhD MRPharmS FRSM
Professor of the Practice of Pharmacy,
Centre for Pharmacy Practice,
The School of Pharmacy,
University of London, London
1 Philosophy of clinical pharmacy

Erica Barrie MSc MRPharmS
Secretary to the Welsh Executive,
Royal Pharmaceutical Society of Great Britain,
formerly Consultant in Pharmaceutical Public Health,
Iechyd Morgannwg Health Authority, Swansea
2 Supporting prescribing in general practice

Ros Batty BPharm MSc MRPharmS
Principal Pharmacist, North Thames Pharmacy Services,
Clinical Pharmacy Unit,
Northwick Park and St Mark's NHS Trust, Harrow
13 Prescription monitoring

Anne C Boyter BSc MSc MRPharmS
Lecturer in Clinical Practice,
Department of Pharmaceutical Sciences,
University of Strathclyde, Glasgow
10 Anti-infectives

Kim Brackley DipPharm(Dist) MSc MRPharmS
Principal Pharmacist, North Thames Pharmacy Services,
Chelsea and Westminster Health Care Trust, London
13 Prescription monitoring

Graham Davies BPharm MSc PhD MRPharmS
Academic Director of Clinical Studies,
School of Pharmacy and Biomolecular Sciences,
University of Brighton, Brighton
18 Drug removal by continuous renal replacement therapies

Soraya Dhillon BPharm PhD MRPharmS
Postgraduate Course Director,
Centre for Pharmacy Practice,
The School of Pharmacy, University of London, London

Rachel Elliot BPharm PhD MRPharmS
Clinical Lecturer,
School of Pharmacy and Pharmaceutical Sciences,
University of Manchester, Manchester

Steve Hudson BPharm MPharm FRPharmS
Professor of Pharmaceutical Care,
School of Pharmacy,
University of Strathclyde, Glasgow

Bryn Hughes BPharm PhD MRPharmS
Consultant Pharmacist,
formerly Chief Pharmacist and
Clinical Director of Medical Support Services
Royal Brompton Hospital, London

Jeremy Hyde BPharm PhD MRPharmS
Chief Executive Officer,
ClinPharm International, Maidenhead

Ann Jacklin BPharm CHSM MRPharmS
Chief Pharmacist,
Hammersmith Hospitals NHS Trust, London

Nicola John BPharm MPhil DMS MRPharmS
Consultant in Pharmaceutical Public Health,
Iechyd Morgannwg Health Authority, Swansea,
formerly Chief Pharmacist,
Glan-y-Mor NHS Trust, Neath

Wendy K Kingdom BSc PhD MRPharmS
Clinical Project Manager,
ClinPharm Ltd, Maidenhead
5 Clinical trial design

Andrzej J Kostrzewski BSc MSc MMedEd MRPharmS
Principal Pharmacist, Education,
Guy's and St Thomas' NHS Trust, London
and Clinical Lecturer, The School of Pharmacy,
University of London, London
23 Laboratory tests

Beryl Langfield BPharm MRPharmS
Principal Pharmacist, Clinical Services,
Hammersmith Hospitals NHS Trust, London
21 Intravenous drug administration
22 Sodium content of injectable drugs

Martin Lee BSc MBA MRPharmS
Assistant Head of Pharmacy,
Derby Royal Infirmary, Derby
12 Parenteral nutrition in adults

Ronan Lyons MD MPH FFPHMI FFPHM
Clinical Senior Lecturer,
Welsh Combined Centres for Public Health,
University of Wales College of Medicine
4 Evidence based practice

Adele Mackeller BPharm MRPharmS
Staff Pharmacist,
Hammersmith Hospitals NHS Trust, London
21 Intravenous drug administration

Clare A Mackie BSc MSc MCPP MRPharmS
Professor and Head of School of Pharmacy,
The Robert Gordon University,
Aberdeen
8 Over-the-counter prescribing

Deborah J Scholey PhD
Director of Regulatory Affairs,
Cerebrus, Wokingham
6 Drug licensing

Amanda Scott BSc PhD MRPharmS
Senior Pharmacist,
Derby Royal Infirmary, Derby
12 Parenteral nutrition in adults

Janie Sheridan BPharm PhD MRPharmS
Senior Research Pharmacist,
National Addiction Centre, London
15 Substance misuse

Katja Taxis Apothekerin MSc MRPharmS
Research Pharmacist,
Centre for Pharmacy Practice,
The School of Pharmacy,
University of London, London
11 Insulins

Roger Walker BPharm PhD MRPharmS
Professor of Pharmacy Practice,
Welsh School of Pharmacy,
Cardiff University, Cardiff
and Director of Pharmaceutical Public Health,
Gwent Health Authority, Wales
14 Medication adherence

Catherine Walsh BSc MRPharmS
Staff Pharmacist,
Hammersmith Hospitals NHS Trust, London
22 Sodium content of injectable drugs

Alan Willson BPharm MSc MRPharmS
Director of Patient Care,
Iechyd Morgannwg Health, Swansea
23 Laboratory tests

Preface

The aim of this book is to be a quick prompt for practising pharmacists, pre-registration trainees and students in the latter half of their course. Like other survival guides it is designed as a book to help you in your every day practice. It should support hospital and community pharmacists alike and will be of use when dealing with individual patients or when providing other services such as advising doctors, be they GPs or consultants, on their prescribing.

The book starts with a fundamental chapter on the philosophy of clinical pharmacy and is then split into four sections:

Policy
A large part of clinical pharmacist's influence has come from setting and influencing policy – deciding and getting agreement on what is the right thing to do. To do that effectively you require an idea of what clinical pharmacy is, how to deliver advice to doctors, and a thorough knowledge of the evidence on which you are basing your recommendations.

Choice
Pharmacists influence the choice of drugs either by advising others on which drug or regime to use for a particular patient, or by choosing the appropriate drug themselves. These chapters deal with some common situations.

Monitoring
Once a drug has been prescribed it is only the beginning of what is often a long process of taking the drug. The patient's condition and what they want from drug treatment can vary over time and some form of monitoring and feedback is required. Some common situations and patient groups are included in this section.

Reference
A repository of useful information you may not be able to summon to the forefront of your mind just when you need it!

When preparing this book we have kept in mind the excellence of the British National Formulary; we have tried not to duplicate any of its functions, so that the two books complement each other rather than compete.

The information in this book is as up to date and accurate as the authors can make it, but we hope you won't just look up a chapter for a quick fix – we want you to *evaluate* information and apply it dependent on the circumstances. If you have any doubts, check with other reference sources or another colleague.

Acknowledgement

We would like to thank SafeScript Limited (Ch. 16) for permission to reproduce their copyright material.

1999   Nick Barber
                                                        Alan Willson

A PHILOSOPHY OF CLINICAL PHARMACY

N Barber

What is clinical pharmacy trying to achieve? Unless we can answer this question we will have difficulty delivering and developing a service and convincing others of its value. In this chapter I will present you with a philosophy of clinical pharmacy; the rest of the book will help you achieve it.

The key point about clinical pharmacy is that it suggests what is *right* about therapy, so it involves *values* as well as *facts*. This is why clinical pharmacy has been so important in the development of pharmacy as a whole — it moves beyond our knowledge of facts and into the arena of how we should use that knowledge.

In tracing the development of clinical pharmacy in the UK, one sees parallels with the development of a religious sect as much as the development of a new way of practice. The early prophets developed clinical services in hospitals, educated prolifically to spread the gospel and pushed back the boundaries of pharmacy. Most of us were fired by the belief that we could use our knowledge of drugs to help patients be better treated; what is more we used our skills to minimise the use of inappropriately expensive drugs. We were so successful that a whole series of clinical pharmacy services grew over a few years. But were they any good?

In the USA clinical pharmacy had developed earlier than in the UK and researchers Heppler and Strand (1990) pointed out that clinical pharmacy was just a name for a series of services. There was no ideal against which we could measure it so we could not really assess clinical pharmacy. Unless we knew where we wanted to be, how could we know how close we were to our goal? And, if we didn't know how far we were from our goal, how could we assess clinical pharmacy services or, most importantly for our future, persuade others of their value? The solution Heppler and Strand suggested was pharmaceutical care — a *philosophy* on which clinical pharmacy should be based. The essence of this philosophy (usually ignored in UK interpretations of it) was the morality (the definition of what is right) of the relationship between the pharmacist and the patient — it suggested that the pharmacist effectively contracted herself to the patient to serve the patient's needs.

While pharmaceutical care is a significant step in the development of clinical pharmacy, and is an attractive 'sound bite' to use when explaining a service to others, I tend not to use it. The difficulty of applying it in UK hospitals is that it could lead to escalating expenditure on drugs and it ignores the moral case that saving money on one patient provides more for the treatment of others. However, the creation of pharmaceutical care is a significant first step in defining the 'patient orientation' that is at the heart of clinical pharmacy and it may well be more of a reality in community pharmacy. In the rest of this chapter I'll explain what I think is the philosophy of clinical pharmacy and how its aims should be applied to your practice.

WHAT ARE WE TRYING TO ACHIEVE?

Clinical pharmacy services aim to improve prescribing, either through influencing what others do or by doing the prescribing ourselves, something already done in community pharmacy and likely to expand in hospital pharmacy. Our philosophy should therefore be rooted in a philosophy of good prescribing, a subject with a curiously sparse literature. I think our philosophy, the philosophy of clinical pharmacy, is to improve the quality of prescribing. To do this I have suggested four aims of prescribing that doctors and pharmacists should be trying to achieve:

- maximising clinical effect
- minimising risk of treatment induced adverse events
- minimising cost of treatment to the NHS
- respecting the patient's choices.

I have explained these in more depth elsewhere (Barber 1996), but, briefly, these are rooted in four principles of medical ethics. The first is *beneficence* — doing good — and we aim to achieve this by making the drug have the clinical effect desired. The second is *nonmaleficence* — not doing harm — where we aim to reduce the chance and extent of harm by minimising adverse events resulting from drug treatment. The third is *justice*, and in this case I'm taking the theory of distributive justice on which the NHS was founded — utilitarianism — which is often defined as providing the greatest good for the greatest number. Given there is a fixed budget, we can treat more people if we keep costs down. The fourth principle recognises *patient autonomy*, which means that patients can choose what their ends are and how they should be met. Patients always have a choice in what happens to them (even if that choice is to let the doctor do what she wants) and we should recognise this and be responsive to it.

These are the four aims on which clinical pharmacy should be founded. It will not be possible to achieve all the aims completely on all occasions, and debate is needed about situations in which conflicts occur; however they give a foundation to our practice and a way for us to explain our service to others.

GETTING AIMS INTO PRACTICE

Aims are all very well but we needed processes — pharmacy services — to make them happen. There are three points at which clinical pharmacy services are delivered to meet the aims of clinical pharmacy; they are before, during and after the prescription is written.

• *Before*. Through the creation and influence of policy — deciding what is the right thing to be done by whom. This starts with licensing the drug and includes formularies, prescribing policies, guidelines and so on.

• *During*. Influencing the prescriber by affecting their knowledge, attitudes and priorities in prescribing. This may be done by feedback of their prescribing practice in comparison to others, for example through PACT data or by education, such as 'academic detailing'. An alternative is to be present at the time of prescribing and contributing to the decision-making process. Finally, the pharmacist may actually make the prescribing decision, as in prescribing over the counter in community pharmacy or running an anticoagulant clinic in a hospital.

• *After*. This involves correcting or improving the quality of prescribing. It can happen just after the prescription is written or as part of a regular medicines management process that goes on for years. Communication with the patient is essential — checking how they are getting on with their drugs, what their needs are, offering help and advice to improve adherence, and working towards accurate recording and transmission of information on their drug therapy (for example when transferring across the primary-secondary interface).

BEING A GOOD CLINICAL PHARMACIST

What do you need to contribute to the above? First, you need to believe in a philosophy of clinical pharmacy and accept your professional and moral responsibility to deliver it. This is easier said than done and may make you unpopular at times — one needs to strike a balance between moral responsibility and professional suicide. Having said that, pharmacists have the power to influence drug therapy, and with that power comes responsibility; sometimes your responsibility is to argue against company or hospital policy. Second, you need the background knowledge to judge whether a prescribing decision is appropriate or not. This knowledge increasingly focuses around the relative weights of evidence, so you have to understand the strengths and weaknesses of the methods through which the evidence is obtained. These are, predominantly, clinical trials to assess effectiveness; pharmacoepidemiology to assess risk and pharmacoeconomics to understand costs and their relationships to outcomes. These three disciplines underpin the knowledge base required for three of the aims of prescribing; they must be accompanied by background knowledge of the ways by which we assess the disease and its progress, the characteristics of medicines, their mode of action, formulation, pharmacokinetics and method of delivery.

This leaves us one area to discuss, which is respecting the patient's choice. The key to this is establishing what the patient wants — the things they think important — and using your knowledge and communication skills to ensure, as much as possible, that they get them. One should also anticipate future choices the patient may want to make — what if they feel worse on the medication? What if they can't fit the dosing interval into their lives? Information, guidance and the encouragement to come back for further advice are the keys to this.

Finally, one needs to develop the skills necessary to deliver many of these services. Skills are learned through repetition and feedback; in learning to ride a bicycle you wobble frequently and occasionally fall off before mastering the skill. Pharmacists need to have the space and support to do this and develop the skills through which they can deliver their service.

The contents of this book are there to provide some support for the philosophy of clinical pharmacy laid out in this chapter. We hope they help you become a better clinical pharmacist, You must keep developing your skills, a process which will involve some unpleasant wobbles; this book alone will not be enough.

FURTHER READING

Hepler CD, Strand LM 1990 Opportunities and responsibilities in pharmaceutical care. American Journal of Hospital Pharmacy 47:533–543

Barber N 1995 What constitutes good prescribing? British Medical Journal 310:293–295

Barber N 1996 Towards a philosophy of clinical pharmacy. Pharmaceutical Journal 257:289–291

Policy

SUPPORTING PRESCRIBING IN GENERAL PRACTICE

2

E Barrie, N John

AIMS OF INTERACTION WITH GENERAL PRACTITIONERS

Support effective and efficient prescribing

We are all aware that the costs of prescribing are rising year on year. There are many reasons for this, including:

- an ageing population
- new drugs becoming available, sometimes for conditions that were previously untreatable
- increasing patient knowledge and expectations.

General practitioners (GPs) are keen to meet the needs of their patients, and recognise that in order for cost pressures to be afforded, resources available for prescribing need to be used optimally. However, busy doctors often find it difficult to find the time to apply evidence-based principles to prescribing decisions to ensure that both clinical and cost effectiveness are achieved. They value input of another professional who is able to identify and assist the practice to implement prescribing changes relevant to their own practice.

Facilitate a common approach to prescribing across primary and secondary care

Hospital prescribing accounts for a small proportion of the overall cost, but is thought to have a major impact on the trends for long-term GP prescribing which makes up the bulk of the cost.

Joint working of pharmacists and prescribers from the primary and secondary care sectors to develop mutually agreed prescribing guidelines, which take into account the quality and cost of individual medicines, will help to promote a global rational approach to prescribing.

One way of facilitating this has been developed through the establishment of local prescribing groups. These have many different names, but in general they are made up of representatives of doctors and pharmacists from hospitals, general practice and the health authority/board, with a remit to promote understanding of the issues surrounding prescribing in the local area. The advice offered to an individual practice should be complementary to this strategic approach.

Integrate local community pharmacists into the primary care team

Rationalising prescribing will only be effective and sustained when all those with an interest are willing to cooperate to achieve the preferred outcome. This means that the prescribers and the general practice teams who organise the production of prescriptions, community pharmacists who interact with patients on a regular basis to advise on medicines' management, and the patients, need to work closely as a team.

Make use of all available information

A prescribing adviser needs to have a good background knowledge of therapeutics and new trends in prescribing. This is acquired from formal education, and also from reading journals and other sources of drug information. Where specific advice is being offered, it is useful to back this up with reference to national publications such as the *Drugs and Therapeutics Bulletin* or the material produced by national prescribing or medicines resource centres in the UK.

Each practice now has access to comprehensive information on their prescribing, obtained from the pricing of all prescriptions that have been presented for dispensing, collated and produced by the national prescription pricing authorities. This information consists of:

• a limited report sent to the practice which shows the total spend in each British National Formulary (BNF) chapter, and gives an indication of the drugs which are prescribed most frequently and those upon which the most money is spent, giving comparisons with health authority/board averages

• a prescribing catalogue which details all prescriptions from the practice which have been dispensed in a given period, in BNF order. This is available, on request, to the practice or the health authority/board prescribing adviser

• graphical representations of trends in prescribing, and comparisons between practices. Health authority/board and national averages are now being made available from software developed by the national prescription pricing authorities.

Remember also to refer to local hospital and practice formularies, and national or locally produced guidelines. For specific patients, general practice computer records or patient notes and pharmacy patient medication records (PMRs) can be useful.

ACHIEVING AND MONITORING CHANGE

Preparation

• Contact the pharmaceutical or medical adviser at your health authority/board to explore possibilities of working with local general practices.

• Approach practice to discuss ways of working together.

• Agree format, time, service to be provided, and reimbursement. In some health authorities/boards funding will be available to support pharmacists working with practices. If not, fundholders may be willing to pay pharmacists for the advisory services. If non-fundholders have received payments through successful participation in a local non-fundholder prescribing incentive scheme, they may be able to make a case to purchase pharmaceutical advice. New opportunities to reward cost effective prescribing will replace these when the White Paper on the future of the NHS in England, Scotland and Wales published in 1997 is implemented.

Suggested joint working approaches

• Approach the practice in a friendly and supportive manner.

• Obtain permission from the practice to study their prescribing reports and catalogue to prioritise therapeutic areas for discussion at practice meetings.

• Suggest prescribing targets for change.

• Do not expect the practice to implement too many changes at the same time. It is best to concentrate initially on those which will have the most impact.

• Suggest developing/amending the practice's repeat prescribing system to take account of the needs of the practice patients and community pharmacists. Suggest involving all practice staff and use any local repeat prescribing guidelines.

• Facilitate practice meetings to develop and update the practice formulary. This can be a short list of medicines used in conjunction with the BNF. Provide practice specific information on the cost impact of prescribing changes.

• Suggest involving local community pharmacists to assist practices to adhere to their formulary and to communicate consistent messages to patients.

• Assist in auditing change by reviewing the prescribing data a year later. Suggest new targets to repeat the audit cycle.

• Make the most of your time by delegating word processing and data handling tasks to clerical staff if you have access to this resource.

EXAMPLES OF METHODS EMPLOYED

There are many different models for collaborative working. Although this list is in no way exhaustive, a few of the methods used are described below.

• Most health authorities/boards have in place a mechanism for at least an annual visit by a prescribing adviser (pharmacist or doctor) to all practices to provide advice and agree prescribing targets from a range of ideas. This may be an employed adviser or a sessional trust employed/self employed adviser contracted to provide the service.

• As part of the Welsh Prescribing Support Project, community pharmacists monitored GP compliance with their own formularies by identifying repeat prescriptions falling outside the formulary and completing intervention forms to report this to the practice.

• The NHS Executive in England made available £1 million in 1995–96 to fund 17 projects to evaluate different models for the development of the community pharmacist's wider role to advise GPs on prescribing. A summary report of these projects will be published as a resource to help choose the types of services to purchase locally in order to achieve effective partnerships to implement rational and cost-effective use of medicines.

The projects fell broadly into the following types:

— joint development of practice repeat prescribing policies with pharmacists suggesting appropriate changes to patients' routine prescriptions using referral forms

— pharmacists facilitating regular practice meetings to discuss prescribing issues

— pharmacists reviewing prescriptions for residential and nursing homes and making recommendations to prescribers

— pharmacists operating 'brown bag' schemes where patients bring all their medicines in for a review with the pharmacist, and thereafter a practice meeting is held to discuss possible changes with the prescribers.

• The IMPACT (Independent monitoring of prescribing analysis, costs and trends) model developed at Keele University uses traditional pharmaceutical industry marketing techniques to put good prescribing messages across to GPs using trained local community pharmacists to present a researched clinical case for a specific prescribing change.

• The 'practice' pharmacist is directly employed by the general practice to undertake a variety of tasks concerning prescribing, for example anticoagulant clinics, *Helicobacter pylori* eradication programmes or pain clinics.

• Another approach involves the GP practice identifying particular patients on more than five medicines and a visiting clinical pharmacist works with the GP to review the prescription from the patient's notes.

• Repeat dispensing by community pharmacists has been piloted extensively in Scotland, as a means of controlling the issue of repeat prescriptions to avoid waste.

• The NHS Executive in England supported projects in 1997 to evaluate different methods for community pharmacists to provide repeat dispensing, assistance for patients with compliance problems, and pharmaceutical care for medicines' management.

Key points:

• Support on prescribing is valued by general practitioners.
• Work within the framework of the health authority strategy.
• Involve all local community pharmacists to facilitate consistent messages.
• Make use of all available information sources.
• Work with practices to identify and implement appropriate change.
• Learn from the approaches used by others.
• Share experience gained.

CLINICAL DIRECTORATES AND THE ROLE OF THE PHARMACIST

3

A Jacklin

Clinical Directorates were widely introduced into the NHS during the mid to late 1980s in response to two major initiatives.

The Resource Management Initiative

This was a joint DoH and BMA project to involve doctors in managing information and resources.

The White Paper 'Working for Patients'

This introduced the purchaser–provider model of health care commissioning by which all hospital work would be paid for via contracts. Contracts were to be based on clinical activity.

Common to both of these changes was the need to involve doctors in management and to provide doctors with improved information and business support to enable them to manage their 'clinical' business.

Prior to the introduction of clinical directorates doctors were already grouped together in clinical specialties but were not always integrated into other disciplines particularly nursing and management. Directorates in many places were hence a strengthening of existing medical structures with the introduction of multidisciplinary working in directorate teams. A common initial structure for a clinical directorate (also known as Care Groups, Clinical Teams and various other names) is shown in Figure 3.1.

As directorates have developed, this structure has been further

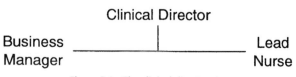

Clinical Director

Business Manager ———————— Lead Nurse

Figure 3.1   The clinical directorate.

strengthened by the identification by directorate groupings of other health care professionals including pharmacists so that commonly directorates will have a support team including:

- directorate pharmacist
- directorate finance officer
- directorate contracts/information manager.

The Clinical Director will be the budget holder for a number of budgets which will include medical staff, nursing staff, drugs and equipment. He will be responsible for ensuring that expenditure within these budgets is managed and contained and he will need support and information to enable him to do this. Advising on drug budgets is hence an important role for directorate pharmacists but is not the only role clinical pharmacists have in supporting the directorate.

HC(88)54, 'The Way Forward', in advocating clinical pharmacy described the developing role of pharmacists in which skills are applied to medicine usage both at the 'policy making level' and in the treatment of individual patients.

Prior to the introduction of clinical directorates 'policy making' contributions were often confined to only one or two senior pharmacists in each hospital. A hospital with multiple clinical directorates each with an allocated directorate pharmacist provides an increased number of opportunities for involvement in business decision-making.

WHAT IS A DIRECTORATE PHARMACIST?

Directorate pharmacists' roles can be described as having four key elements:

- *Being a clinical specialist*

   — know the literature relating to your directorate
   — have a working knowledge of current practice and protocols.

- *Supporting the directorate*

   — not only in providing drug budget support but also supporting clinical audit, new drug evaluations, protocol preparation, drug security and training for other directorate staff.

- *Monitoring drug expenditure*

   — provide regular information and interpretation of drug expenditure, advice on how to best manage expenditure
   — predict and advise on changes.

- *Supporting pharmacy*
  - be a service ambassador for all pharmacy services
  - advise pharmacy of directorate service plans
  - train and educate other pharmacy staff in specialist area.

To perform well at a directorate level pharmacists need to have knowledge and skills in a number of areas:

- clinical knowledge appropriate to directorate
- data handling/presentation/interpretation skills
- knowledge of local pharmacy systems, including computers
- knowledge of hospital organisation structure and management style
- knowledge of local purchasers and understanding of relevance of contracting round
- interpersonal skills appropriate for dealing with senior doctors, nurses and business managers
- knowledge of procurement practices locally and how best prices are obtained.

BUDGET MANAGEMENT

Whilst a directorate pharmacist will be involved in many of the roles outlined above, most will be regularly involved in drugs budget support which is described here in more detail. In managing a budget a budget holder compares budget to expenditure and aims to spend less than the budgeted allowance. The basic questions to be answered when monitoring a budget are:

Q1 What is my budget position this month?
Am I underspent, overspent or balanced?

Q2 By how much?

Q3 How does this affect my position year to date?
Am I better off, worse off or the same?

Q4 By how much?

Q5 How different was this month to previous months this year/last year?

Q6 What is my predicted position at the end of the financial year?

Q7 How does this compare to last year?

The answers to these basic questions will establish whether a budget is a 'problem' or not and dictate the amount of further information and interpretation required.

A directorate pharmacist having answered all the above questions might be fulfilling a role similar to an accountant or manager. The skills of the specialist pharmacist will then be required to provide interpretation which could include answering the following questions.

Q8 What are the reasons for my under/over spend or balanced position?

Q9 Is this what we expected or is it a surprise?

Q10 Which drugs, patients, doctors, therapeutic class (e.g. antibiotics), patient group, disease state, are responsible for my over/under spend? (This is the biggest question to answer).

Q11 Do we think these were clinically appropriate?

Q12 What actions could or should we take? (e.g. restrict availability, define guidelines).

Q13 How many of the problems are recurring/non-recurring?

Q14 What does the year end position look like after we take out the non-recurring elements?

Q15 What else are we aware of that will improve or worsen our position? (e.g. new drugs or change in use of existing drugs).

Q16 How can you/pharmacy help me?

By asking these questions when preparing a report, which can be either verbal or written, for a clinical director a directorate pharmacist will be able to target the requirements of the recipient.

The following section describes data which are likely to be available to a directorate pharmacist to help answer these questions. Before using any data it is imperative to have a full understanding of the systems (human, procedural and technological) used to capture data in order to be able to provide interpretation.

By understanding how the pharmacy computer system works and, more importantly, how your pharmacy uses the computer, you will know how best to make use of data available to you. You will also be able to interpret any apparent quirks by understanding the potential for errors or anomalies.

DATA AVAILABLE FOR EXPENDITURE INTERPRETATION

Pharmacy computer systems provide us with a large amount of data which need to be sorted and manipulated to suit the needs of a clinical director. Thought needs to be given to the relative advantages and disadvantages of presenting all of the data available.

> ⚠️ Do not give data for the sake of it; just give that information which is going to result in action essential for decision-making.

In preparing reports a directorate pharmacist should consider the relevance and importance of showing:

data to:
- consultant
- specialty
- directorate

data by:
- inpatient
- outpatient
- daycase.

Unless showing data by any of these groupings is relevant to the management of expenditure, then conciseness is lost and interpretation may be clouded — so don't subdivide into too many categories.

Merge pack size/formulations
Occasionally different formulations/strengths will be used in different clinical indications and hence be relevant to report separately; more often this data should be merged.

Top N
Showing doctors their 'top of the pops' is interesting, but unless targeted to show relative change can be of limited repeated value. Often this is best saved for once or twice yearly snapshot reviews.

Level of detail
How many decimal points you report to will depend on the scale of expenditure; too much detail can be irrelevant and impair concise interpretation.

Similarly, grouping drugs by therapeutic class may be more meaningful than reporting individual drugs where there are no particularly high cost drugs.

Other hospital data
The amount and quality of data available from the Trust's Patient Information Administration System will depend very much on local circumstances.

Before commencing to use any PAS data it is always worth establishing how the directorate view the data. In many hospitals clinical directors have often expressed concerns about the:

— reliability
— accuracy
— interpretation
— timeliness
— usefulness of data.

If this is the case it may be best to avoid the use of such data. If the data are well supported locally then activity and case mix data may be useful to include in drug reports, for example to provide figures on average drug cost per outpatient attendance or average drug cost per finished consultant episode.

> It is always necessary to clarify the definitions of inpatient stays compared to day case or regular day attenders to ensure interpretability of data. If in any doubt it is better to not use such data.

INFORMATION TO SUPPORT A BROADER ROLE

Other information both generated within pharmacy and available externally can be used to facilitate activity in some of the broader roles described earlier.

Examples of such information are:

- *Clinical interventions*

    — either statistics to show volume and nature of these or grouped into topics these will act as audit data and highlight protocol changes or educational requirements.

- *Clinical trials*

    — depending on the number and size of trials this may or may not be relevant or interesting.

- *Drug Information queries*

    — a review of these may form the basis of future clinical audit initiatives or individual patient reviews.

- *Unlicensed drugs or indications*

    — clinical directors may be interested in reviewing unlicensed use of medicines within the directorate.

- *'Policy Compliance' data*
  — for example a review of outpatient 'scripts will reveal compliance (or not) with outpatient policies in addition to formulary compliance.
  — a review of inpatient 'scripts will similarly review compliance with formulary and locally agreed protocols.

Information should be relevant, accurate, timely, concise, comparative, consistent, unbiased, unambiguous and most important of all practical/economic to produce and directed to action.

It is important with such a mass of data which can be presented in many ways that a focus is kept on the key issue: to sort, manage and present only data that is 'directed to action'.

EVIDENCE BASED PRACTICE

4

R Lyons

The phrases 'evidence based medicine' (EBM) and 'evidence based practice' (EBP) (not all health care is medicine) became popular in the 1990s following a movement to increase the scientific basis of health care. Those practising evidence based health care aim to maximise the percentage of interventions used by them which have been scientifically shown to be effective.

EVIDENCE OF EFFECTIVENESS

There is a hierarchy of evidence used to judge the strength of evidence on the effectiveness of health care interventions which is generally graded from top down as follows:

1. Systematic reviews.
2. Randomised controlled trials (RCTs).
3. Non-randomised experimental studies.
4. Observational studies.
5. Expert opinion.

A systematic review is a summary of the literature (generally from a groups of RCTs) in which evidence is systematically identified, appraised and summarised.

A randomised controlled trial is an experimental study whereby people with a certain condition are randomly allocated to one or more intervention or control groups. Properly performed it allows an unbiased estimate of an intervention's effectiveness.

Non-randomised experimental studies include those where people are allocated to treatment groups sequentially or by other methods known to the investigator. These studies have a possibility of being biased if the investigator favours one treatment.

Observational studies include cohort studies (before and after studies), and case control studies (comparison of a treated group with a non-treated group).

Expert opinion relies on the teaching and experience of clinicians. This may be reliable or biased due to a clinician having experienced an atypical group of cases.

Whilst it is generally accepted that systematic reviews of randomised controlled trials are more accurate than single randomised controlled trials, very large trials (mega trials) which give precise results are the best source of evidence as meta analyses of trials may be prone to publication bias if a number of negative result trials have not been published, e.g. use of magnesium after myocardial infarction was advocated in a meta analysis, but found to be useless in the ISIS-4 mega trial (Egger & Smith 1995).

It must also be borne in mind that randomised controlled trials can only be ethically carried out if the investigators are in equipoise (believe both treatments to be equally effective). As a result many interventions with large effects, e.g. the introduction of penicillin which massively reduced mortality, have never been formally scientifically tested in trials and are never likely to be.

However, such major effects are rare and all new drugs (but not all surgical procedures) are now tested for effectiveness using randomised controlled trials. Unfortunately, licensing requirements under the Medicines Act do not require that new preparations are tested against the best existing treatment. Many drugs are only tested against placebos and so it is unsure whether the new treatment will be better than existing treatments.

EQUIVALENCE, EFFICACY AND EFFECTIVENESS

Sometimes new drugs are tested against existing drugs not to demonstrate that one is better than another but to demonstrate that they are the same in order to gain a foothold in the market. Such trials are called equivalence trials and are open to many biases. A good critique of such trials is available by Jones et al (1996).

Most drug trials aim to test the efficacy or effectiveness of the therapeutic agent. Efficacy trials test whether the agent works in the best possible circumstances and in such cases only those who actually received a full course of the agent are compared with those who did not. Effectiveness trials test whether the agent works in ordinary practice and these are analysed on an intention to treat basis, whereby people who are randomised to receive the agent but do not for one reason or other, or who receive a smaller dose or shorter course, are included in the analysis as if they had received a full course of the agent.

DETECTING ADVERSE EFFECTS

Very few drug trials are sufficiently large or are run for a sufficiently long time to detect all adverse drug events.

The detection of many adverse drug events depends on post marketing surveillance and the reporting of adverse events thought to be linked to the drug once it has entered general use.

However, when a drug has been used on limited numbers of people it is still possible to estimate the risk of a serious adverse event using a statistical formula derived from 95% confidence intervals. A 95% confidence interval is a range in which we are 95% certain that the true population value lies and is derived from a study of a sample of the population.

Suppose 100 people have tried a new drug (or had a new operation) and there have been no adverse events. What is the risk to a person taking the drug of having an adverse event? With our knowledge of confidence intervals we can say that we are 95% certain that the risk of an adverse event is no more than $3/n$ where n = number of people who have had the drug. Here $n = 100$ and $3/n = 3\%$. We are 95% sure that the risk of an adverse event after taking the drug is no more than 3%. The rule of $3/n$ is very useful when people ask about serious adverse events of new therapies.

MEASURES OF EFFECTIVENESS

How effective a treatment is can be expressed in many ways.

Relative risk and odds ratios

This is the risk of an event in a group which receives treatment A versus the risk in a group receiving placebo treatment B. Suppose 80 of 100 people receiving A improve compared with 40 of 100 receiving B. The relative risk of improvement of A over B is $80/100 \div 40/100 = 2.0$, i.e. twice as many improve. Sometimes a slightly different measure, the odds ratio, is used instead of the relative risk.

The following standard 2 × 2 table shows the difference between relative risk and odds ratio.

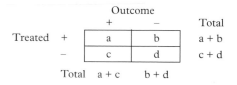

		Outcome		Total
		+	−	
Treated	+	a	b	a + b
	−	c	d	c + d
	Total	a + c	b + d	

a, b, c, d are numbers of people who are treated (+) or not (−) and have a dichotomous, good (+) or bad (−), outcome.

The relative risk of a favourable outcome given treatment is $a/(a + b)$ divided by $c/(c + d)$. The odds ratio of a favourable outcome given treatment is a/b divided by c/d or $\dfrac{a \times d}{b \times c}$.

Odds ratios are often used as they suit a greater variety of statistical tests, e.g. meta analysis.

The 95% confidence interval for the above relative risk is from 1.5 to 2.6 so that we can be 95% certain that the true effect of the drug is a 1.5 to 2.6 times improvement. 95% confidence intervals for relative risks and odds ratios which exclude 1.0 are statistically significant i.e. $p < 0.05$.

Improvement in survival or reduction in symptoms

Suppose 100 people receiving drug A survive on average 80 months and 100 receiving drug B survive on average 40 months. The net average survival effect of drug A is 40 months and the 95% confidence interval from a 37.2 months survival advantage to a 42.8 months survival advantage. 95% confidence intervals for improvements in survival or symptom reduction which exclude 0.0 are statistically significant i.e. $p < 0.05$.

Number needed to treat (NNT)

In evidence based practice the number of people needed to treat to produce (on average) one additional successful outcome is currently the most used measure of effectiveness. It is used instead of the relative risk because it gives more information by taking into account the baseline risk. In the above example $80/100$ people improved with drug A and $40/100$ with drug B. The absolute risk reduction (ARR) with drug A is $80/100 - 40/100 = 40/100$ or 0.4. The number needed to treat with drug A to produce an additional successful outcome is the inverse of the absolute risk reduction (NNT = $1/$ARR), here $1/0.4 = 2.5$. This means that on average it is necessary to treat 2.5 people with drug A to make one of them better. Suppose a successful outcome with drug A occurred in $80/1000$ and $40/1000$ with drug B. The relative risk of improvement would still be 2.0 but the NNT would now be 25. Clearly NNTs give a better feel for how effective a drug is. It is also possible to calculate 95% confidence intervals for NNTs.

Graphical representation

Meta analyses often demonstrate the effect size and confidence intervals of each of the individual studies and the pooled results in a graph are often referred to as a blobbogram by those teaching critical appraisal skills. Figure 4.1 is an example of a blobbogram.

The lines with dots in the centre represent four studies. The dots represent the odds ratios of the treatment relative to placebo in achieving a desired outcome. The length of the line represents the confidence interval around the odds ratio. The central vertical line represents an odds ratio of 1, that is, no treatment effect. Two of the studies do not cross the line of no effect and demonstrate statistically significant improvement in outcome with treatment. In the other two studies the confidence intervals cross the line of no effect and whilst on average are positive are also consistent with the treatment having a negative effect. The diamond represents the odds ratio of the combined estimate of effectiveness in the meta analysis.

Effective interventions for individuals

So much for the principles of evidence based practice. What happens when a clinician wishes to put EBP into practice with an individual patient? Trials tell us whether on average a group of people with a certain condition will be better or worse off with treatment but not whether it is in the best interest of any one individual to accept treatment.

To make a decision for an individual further information is required. It is necessary to know (a) how effective the treatment is (relative risks from meta analyses or RCTs), (b) the risk of the event which it is hoped to prevent happening to an individual patient of a particular age, sex, race, and with certain risk factors (should come from multi-variate risk equations derived from cohort studies) and (c) the risk of harm from treatment (data on frequency of adverse events). Only if the reduction in absolute risk with treatment exceeds the risk of

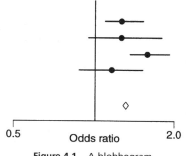

Figure 4.1 A blobbogram.

an adverse event is treatment worthwhile for the individual. It is often worthwhile treating individuals at high risk of illness but not often worth treating low risk individuals. An example of how to work out these risks in practice is explained by Glasziou and Irwig (1995).

Sources of evidence

Whilst there is an increasing number of systematic reviews available it will be a long time before reviews are ready for all but a sizeable minority of clinical problems. The following sources are particularly useful. Current internet addresses are provided on contact points (these may change).

International Cochrane Collaboration
This group facilitates the creation, review, and dissemination of reviews of the effectiveness of health care.

Internet address: http://hiru.mcmaster.ca:80/cochrane/default.htm

NHS Centre for Reviews and Dissemination
The centre produced two publicly available databases (a) Database of Abstract of Reviews of Effectiveness (DARE) and (b) NHS Economic Evaluation Database (NEED). The NHS CRD also produces Effective Healthcare (along with Nuffield Institute) and Effectiveness Matters. Both papers contain copies of reviews.

Internet address: http://www.york.ac.uk/inst/crd/list.htm

Bandolier
Paper copies of reviews and interpretations of statistical tests used in evidence based health care. Funded by NHS Management Executive and Anglia and Oxford Regional Health Authority.

Internet address: http://www.jr2.ox.ac.uk/bandolier/

Evidence Based Purchasing
This is produced by the R & D directorate of the South and West Regional Health Authority and the NHS Executive.

Internet address: http://www.epi.bris.ac.uk/rd/publicat/
ebpurch/index.htm

It is also possible to search databases (e.g. Medline, Embase)
for RCTs where reviews have not been carried out. To ensure
your search strategy is comprehensive and scientific please
consult a librarian for advice as amateur attempts generally
only acquire 15–20% of the appropriate literature.

If you are asked to carry out a systematic review yourself
help is available in the form of a report produced by the NHS
Centre for Reviews and Dissemination (1996). Carrying out a
systematic review is a daunting task not to be undertaken
lightly or by the untrained.

CRITICAL APPRAISAL

It is much more likely that you might be asked to carry out a
critical appraisal of existing literature. Critical appraisal is a
systematic method for assessing the scientific quality and relevance of the literature on a particular topic. Critical appraisal
of a systematic review involves assessing whether the following
steps listed in Box 4.1 have been carried out.

BOX 4.1 Steps in critical appraisal of systematic reviews

1. Is the review focused in terms of clearly describing
   — the population or types of patients studied
   — the intervention
   — the outcomes measured?

2. Were the right type of studies to answer the question
   included in the review?
   — randomised controlled trials to assess efficacy and
     effectiveness?
   — controlled trials, post-marketing surveillance, adverse
     event reporting for side-effects?

3. Were all the relevant studies included?
   — need a comprehensive search strategy to uncover
     published and unpublished studies and foreign
     language studies.

4. Were the decisions to include/exclude studies in/from the
   review reasonable?
   — specified inclusion/exclusion criteria described
     preferably before results of study seen?
   — do you agree with them?

---

5. If the overall results have been summarised in a meta
   analysis was it reasonable to do so?
   — A meta analysis is a statistical technique for combining
     the results of studies to form a group averaged result
     with narrower confidence intervals and so more
     precision.

   Meta analysis can be validly carried out when:
   — similar type studies are compared (similar
     interventions, outcome measures and populations)
   — the results of the different studies are clearly displayed
   — the reasons for differences in results are explicable.

6. Have the overall results been clearly displayed?
   — estimate of effect (odds ratio, mean etc.)?
   — confidence interval for above?
   — numbers needed to treat to produce one extra positive
     outcome?
   — cost of producing one extra positive outcome?

> You need to form a judgment as to whether the
> benefits are worth the harm and costs of the intervention.
>
> • Remember other important outcomes will not have been
>   measured. All interventions have multiple outcomes (e.g.
>   NHS, patient, carers, society, death, disability etc.) which are
>   time dependent. Only a few will have been measured.
> • Compare the cost of a positive outcome with other
>   interventions which are currently funded (health economics
>   literature) to see whether priorities should change.

> Training in critical appraisal skills is available from
> many sources. One of the best is the Critical Appraisal Skills
> Programme.
> Internet address: http://www.ihs.ox.ac.uk/casp/

GETTING RESEARCH INTO PRACTICE — IMPLEMENTING CLINICAL PRACTICE GUIDELINES

There is always a considerable delay in implementing the findings of research into routine clinical practice. There are many
reasons for this including clinicians' lack of awareness of
research, which is hardly surprising given the volume of literature on any one topic. Textbooks are nearly always written by

individuals without recourse to systematic reviews and often contain outdated or erroneous material. For example, while definitive evidence of the effectiveness of thrombolytic agents in acute myocardial infarction was available in the early 1970s, most textbooks written in the 1980s omitted the topic and the therapy was not widely introduced until the 1990s. One way to keep up with substantial changes in clinical practice is to subscribe to a journal which contains lists of reviews such as the ACP Journal Club which is available on the Internet.

Internet address: http://www.acponline.org

Clinical guidelines are increasingly used to implement evidence based practice. It is important that the guidelines are themselves evidence based. Some of the best evidence based guidelines have been developed by the Agency for Health Care Policy and Research (AHCPR) in the US. AHCPR guidelines on many clinical issues can be found on the Internet.

Internet address: http://text.nlm.nih.gov

The Canadian Medical Association also provides access to useful guidelines on the Internet.

Internet address: http://www.cma.ca/cpgs/index.htm

In 1994 the Effective Health Care Bulletin produced a report on implementing clinical guidelines. The reviewers found that guidelines could change clinical practice and affect patient outcome but that the method of development and implementation affected the likelihood of successfully improving outcomes. Guidelines were more likely to be effective if they took into account local circumstances, were disseminated by an active educational intervention, and were implemented by patient specific reminders relating directly to clinical activity. Those intending to introduce clinical practice guidelines should read the reviews before starting.

BOX 4.2 Pharmacy sources on the Internet

This section on evidence based practice has made much reference to what is available on the Internet. *Since the Internet is unregulated, addresses may change or new services may start or existing ones stop.* At the time of going to press the following sources can provide valuable information to the clinical pharmacist (n.b. remember to log on in the morning before America awakes as increased traffic slows the access and data exchange):

- http://www.cpb.uokhsc.edu from the University of Oklahoma College of Pharmacy contains a list of pharmacy resources on the Internet and is particularly useful as the first place to visit
- http://www.pharmweb.net is used to e-mail emergency information on drugs, such as product recalls, to prescribers registered with the service
- http://www.premec.org.nz – The New Zealand National Preferred Medlines Centre Inc. was founded by GPs for GPs and provides best practice and evidence based prescribing advice.

REFERENCES

CRD 1996 Undertaking systematic reviews of research on effectiveness. CRD guidelines for those carrying out or commissioning reviews. CRD Report No. 4. University of York and NHS Centre for Reviews and Dissemination, York
Egger M, Smith D 1995 Misleading meta analysis. British Medical Journal 310:752–754
Glasziou PP, Irwig LM 1995 An evidence based approach to individualising treatment. British Medical Journal 311:1356–1359
Jones B, Jarvis P, Lewis JA, Ebbutt AF 1996 Trials to assess equivalence: the importance of rigorous methods. British Medical Journal 313:36–39
Nuffield Institute for Health 1996 Effective health care: implementing clinical practice guidelines. University of Leeds, Leeds

CLINICAL TRIAL DESIGN

J Hyde, W Kingdom

5

Clinical trials are scientific experiments and, as such, require research and planning at the outset.

OBJECTIVES

The purpose of a clinical trial is to answer a question about a treatment or therapeutic intervention. The question is referred to as the *objective* of the trial and, like all objectives, it must be **SMART**.

Specific: Is Drug A effective at lowering diastolic blood pressure in hypertensive patients?

Measurable: Peak expiratory flow rate must increase from < 250 L/min to > 350 L/min.

Attainable: Not only must the defined therapeutic outcome be achievable, but the number of patients to be recruited must also be possible.

Reasonable: Can the number of episodes of chemotherapy induced vomiting be reduced to zero in all patients? Or is this so unlikely as to be unrealistic?

Timed: The treatment period will be 4 weeks. Any adverse events occurring more than 2 weeks after the last dose of study medication will not be reported. The study will start March 1999 and recruitment will continue until November 1999.

In addition, the objectives of a trial must be ethical. Whilst Ethics Committee approval is mandatory before a study may start, it is a waste of time to submit a protocol for a study which is unethical. As a guide, you must be willing to participate in the trial yourself.

SAMPLE SIZE, ERRORS AND POWER

A study must have sufficient *power* to achieve its objective. A study with insufficient power is wasteful since a meaningful result cannot be obtained, but also unethical since subjects will be treated with an unproven/unlicensed treatment or therapeutic intervention, with no possibility of the data being usable.

The objective of the trial is to determine whether the treatment or intervention has a beneficial effect. The null hypothesis, H_0, assumes that the treatment has no effect. The alternative hypothesis, H_1, assumes that the null hypothesis is false and that the treatment has an effect, which could be better or worse.

The chance of rejecting the null hypothesis when it is really true is known as an α or *Type I error*. A β or *Type II error* is the chance of accepting the null hypothesis when it is really false. The probability of making a Type I error is inferred from the significance level of the study, and the probability of making a Type II error is inferred from the power of the study. Both the power and the significance level have a direct effect on the sample size. Now, it is not very sensible to conduct a study and then to calculate its power. An acceptable level of power is defined, the significance level to be tested is set, then the number of patients necessary is calculated.

For a test of significance between two means:

$$n = \frac{2(Z_{\alpha/2} + Z_{1-\beta})^2 \cdot \sigma^2}{\delta^2}$$

where:

n is the sample size per group, $Z_{\alpha/2}$ is the value cutting off the $100(\alpha/2)\%$ of the upper tail of the Normal distribution, $Z_{1-\beta}$ is the value cutting off the $100(1-\beta)\%$ of the upper tail of the Normal distribution, σ is the standard deviation of the population (assumed equal within each group) and δ is the difference you wish to detect (assuming one exists).

From the equation, it can be seen that the values of $Z_{\alpha/2}$ and $Z_{1-\beta}$ have an effect on the sample size. By convention, statistical tests of significance are usually made at the 5% ($\alpha = 0.05$) or 1% ($\alpha = 0.01$) level. Also, a power of 90 or 95% ($\beta = 0.1$ or 0.05) is usual. The difference you wish to detect also has a large effect on sample size. If the difference you are looking for is small, the sample you will need to detect it will be large, and vice versa. However, the greatest influence on the sample size is the standard deviation.

Clearly, the standard deviation for the population is not known before the study is conducted. Frequently, an estimate may be obtained from published literature, but, occasionally, it might be necessary to conduct a pilot study (usually 10–20 subjects) to obtain the data from which the sample size can be calculated.

TYPES OF TRIAL DESIGN

Trial designs may be *crossover*, *parallel group*, *placebo controlled*, *active comparator*, or *not controlled*. The most appropriate design primarily depends on the indication for dosing.

Crossover trials

Crossover trials are where subjects act as their own control. Each subject receives each possible treatment in successive periods, the order of application being determined randomly. For example, in a two-way crossover trial, subjects receive one of two treatments for a specified period, then they cross over to the other treatment for the remainder of the study. For every treatment, baseline assessments must be made at the start of each treatment period, and a washout phase must normally be allowed in between periods to avoid the effect of one treatment being carried over to the next period. A crossover trial may have any number of periods, but the greater the duration of the study, the higher the risk of subjects failing to complete.

However, the main advantage of crossover trials is that they require fewer patients than parallel studies hence the variability of the data should be less.

Parallel group

Parallel group studies are necessary where (a) The treatment is a single dose or single treatment period e.g. trials for an anti-infective agent or early phase I volunteer studies, or (b) the disease process is progressive. For example, to test a new treatment in Parkinson's disease, the study would have to be parallel group. If the study were crossover, then the baseline assessments at the start of each period would be different, and there is a high risk that patients would respond differently depending on the stage of their disease at the time of starting treatment.

Placebo controlled

In a placebo controlled study, a dummy formulation of the test product is made, which is identical in appearance (and hopefully taste and smell) to the active product. Subjects frequently respond to treatment, even if there is no active ingredient. Therefore, without a comparator, a conclusion might be drawn that the active treatment is efficacious, when subjects might well have had the same response without any treatment at all. In a placebo controlled trial, the possibility of making this mistake is avoided.

Active comparator

As a rule, active comparator trials are performed for one of two reasons. Either the objective of the trial is to show that the test treatment is better than standard treatment, or withholding active treatment is unethical. It is possible that the active comparator may not be better than placebo, hence conclusions drawn from comparator trials should be restricted to statements about the relative efficacy of the treatments.

Not controlled

A study which is not controlled does not have a comparator to the test product. Pharmacokinetic studies are frequently not controlled since the objective of the study is to measure blood levels of the test substance, an outcome which is not susceptible to bias.

NUMBER OF CENTRES

Study designs can be *single* or *multicentre*. A single centre study is simple to administrate and is subject to minimal variability in test observations. However, the results obtained may be influenced by local medical practices which may differ at other centres. Also, if recruitment is poor, the study will have insufficient power to be meaningful and the data will be of little value.

Multicentre studies are complex to administrate and steps must be taken to standardise assessments. It has been known for consultant cardiologists to be sent on a course on how to take blood pressure, to ensure that every investigator in a study is following the same protocol. However, multicentre studies increase the pool of patients available for recruitment, and are less susceptible to local effects than single centre studies.

MINIMISING BIAS

We are all curious, not only the scientists conducting the study, but also the patients taking part. It is natural for us to question and, whether we mean to or not, we all try and decide which treatment is which. Study investigators and monitors may assume a subject has received a certain treatment based on the adverse event profile. Patients waiting to see the investigator may chat about the taste or odour of the product. The study could ultimately be deemed to be worthless because of *bias*.

Clearly, an objective measure of assessment is helpful, if it is possible. However, even objective measures are subject to bias. How long can a patient with angina carry on with a treadmill exercise test (a) with encouragement from the investigator, or (b) without encouragement? There are two key methods for minimising the bias: *randomisation* and *blinding*.

Randomisation

Randomisation is the process of assigning subjects to treatment, without prior knowledge of the treatment to be allocated. In addition, treatment phases in crossover trials are randomised in order to balance any carry-over effect from one treatment period into the next.

Blinding

Blinding is the process of concealing knowledge of the treatment so that any bias in observations is random. Blinding can be at several different levels.

Open — i.e. no blinding at all. Reasons for conducting an open study might include the following.

- The primary outcome is objective e.g. taking blood samples for pharmacokinetic analysis.
- The trial is a pilot for a larger study.
- The appearance/taste/odour of the treatment is unique so that it is impossible to match with a comparator.

Open studies are simple, but have little scientific value because they are liable to bias.

In a *single blind* study, one party (usually the patient) does not know which treatment has been administered. Single blind studies are used where the active treatment cannot be matched with a comparator (as above). They are useful where the assessment of efficacy is objective, but are subject to bias by the observer.

One possibility for minimising bias in a single blind study is *observer blind*. In this study design, the person who dispenses and/or administers the medication is not the same person who measures the results. The chief advantage is that bias by both the observer and the patient is eliminated, but it is more difficult to organise in that several people have to be available at the same time.

A *double blind* study is the ideal design for clinical trials because no-one involved in the collection of data knows which treatment is being assessed. However, it is important to protect the safety of the subjects participating in double blind studies and clear procedures for emergency code breaking must be in place before the study starts.

An alternative form of double blind study is the *double dummy* technique. Double dummy means that each treatment has a matched placebo, but that the two active treatments do not match each other. This form of trial is used when treatments cannot be matched and an open or single blind study is not appropriate. However, patient compliance is challenged by the necessity for taking a large number of treatments. Also, obtaining placebo to match comparator products is expensive and may be refused by the manufacturer. Nonetheless, the advantages of the study being double blind may outweigh the practical problems.

Finally, the person performing the analysis of a double blind study may not know the treatment identities until after conclusions have been reached. This is sometimes referred to as *triple blind*.

SOME PRACTICAL POINTS

When designing a study it is important to consider that the greater the demands on the subjects, the more difficult it will be to recruit, and studies tend to lose momentum when they drag on. Also, the longer the study, the higher the risk of subjects dropping out due to adverse events, or withdrawing their consent, perhaps due to boredom.

Consider the target population. People who work or have young children will not be available for numerous clinic visits. Elderly patients usually require transport. A study which takes the needs of the patients into account has a greater chance of success than one which makes unrealistic demands.

Clinical trial design is multifaceted. Studies must have sufficient power to achieve the objectives, take account of the underlying disease process (if any) both in terms of study design and availability of patient population, be unbiased, and practical.

DRUG LICENSING

6

D Scholey

The registration of medicinal products in Europe and the USA is regulated by a wide variety of national legislation. In order for a medicinal product to obtain a product licence in a country it must have been shown to be safe and efficacious in its intended population and therapeutic area.

An integral part of the marketing authorisation in Europe is the Summary of Product Characteristics (SmPC) which sets out the position of the product, its licensed indication, patient populations, expected adverse events, contraindications, posology, etc. All the information provided in the SmPC must be supported by relevant clinical or pharmaceutical data. It is the definitive statement between the competent authority and the company and provides a common basis of communication between regulatory authorities in all member states.

The process of drug development from molecule to product licence can take 10–12 years, although the pharmaceutical industry has in recent years undergone dramatic changes to focus on reducing the time to market for new products by improving efficiencies in processes and conducting studies in parallel. Specific aspects of the drug development process are described below, including some aspects of post-marketing.

PRE-CLINICAL DEVELOPMENT

The purpose of pre-clinical testing is to evaluate pharmaco-dynamics, pharmacokinetic and toxicological properties of the product when administered to animals both within and above the intended therapeutic range. The extent of pre-clinical testing will depend on the intended human use of the product. There are a number of EU guidelines which provide insight into the type of pre-clinical testing necessary for different products, e.g. anti-cancer medicinal products, materials derived from biotechnology processes, etc. In Europe, if a product is to be used for up to 30 days, repeat dose toxicity studies must be of equal duration and if the product is only intended for single dose use 2 weeks repeat dose studies are necessary. The guidelines are intended to prevent unnecessary testing prior to the clinical development phase and may include *in vitro* testing as well as animal models in some limited kinetics parameters, e.g. AUC, peak plasma levels, at doses around the maximum tolerated doses. Further studies are conducted during the human phase. The aims of toxicity studies are to establish a maximal tolerated dose prior to commencing Phase I trials and to identify target organ toxicity.

CLINICAL DEVELOPMENT

The purpose of the clinical programme is to demonstrate safety and efficacy of the product in the intended population. There are four phases of clinical studies. Phase I, the first human study, is typically a single dose study in healthy volunteers. In some cases, such as anti-cancer drugs, it is more appropriate to use patients for these early trials. The Phase II studies in patients are designed to demonstrate the dose response characteristics and to define a suitable dose for larger scale Phase III trials. The Phase III pivotal efficacy trials form the basis of the clinical data and may, depending on the indication, be long-term studies intended to evaluate long-term efficacy over several months or years. These trials would generally involve several hundred patients in a double blind design with either placebo or active comparators and be conducted in a multicentre, multinational environment. Further details can be found in the section on Clinical Trial Design. Again there is a plethora of EU guidelines designed to provide guidance on the types of study designs that are required to support a licensed indication in particular therapeutic areas, including specific guidelines in therapeutic areas such as epilepsy, hypertension, depression, Alzheimer's disease, etc.

PRODUCT LICENCE APPLICATION

The product licence application (PLA) in Europe or New Drug Application (NDA) in the USA is a compilation document including manufacturing processes and quality validation, pre-clinical safety evaluation and clinical and pharmacological data. The presentation format of a PLA has been standardised across Europe but remains different to the USA format for an NDA. The US Food and Drug Administration (FDA) requires more extensive raw data thus allowing further analysis whereas in Europe the data is presented in a summary format supported by Expert Reports.

A product licence is only granted for use in the population that has been adequately studied in the clinical programme. A company is unlikely to be granted use in an indication that has not been fully studied in the clinical trial programme. Additional studies in a broader or different indication can be used to vary the original product licence at a later stage. If a product is used 'off label', i.e. outside the licensed indication, the doctor takes responsibility for its use, not the pharmaceutical company. Generally 'off label' use is not recommended although in the USA it occurs particularly if it is supported by publications.

European product licence approval procedures

Within Europe new registration procedures have been in operation since 1995 which streamline the approval of new products across Europe. There is now a European Medicines Evaluation Agency whose role is to coordinate central applications, thus allowing a single product licence application to be approved across Europe. A second system, known as the mutual recognition system, allows the approval from one country to be recognised by other country regulatory authorities, thereby preventing multiple reviews of the same documentation.

Orphan drug status

A typical clinical development programme for a new chemical entity may include 1500 patients. Such an extensive programme cannot be justified if the intended disease is relatively rare. In cases where the disease has an incidence of $\leq 200\,000$ cases per annum it is possible in the USA to apply for 'orphan drug status'. In this case a reduced clinical programme is acceptable on the basis that the risk to the human population is much less than larger disease areas. It is also impractical to conduct large scale studies in rare diseases. Within the European regulatory arena draft proposals are in circulation to define similar orphan regulations to the USA, although no such system exists at the present time.

The advantage of this system is a rapid approval for new products with limited indications to treat rare diseases. Since the registration package will only have limited long-term safety data, a prerequisite for an orphan drug status is for the conduct of post marketing surveillance studies to monitor drug safety.

PHARMACOVIGILANCE

Following the granting of a product licence within the EU, pharmaceutical companies are required to monitor drug safety and to provide, according to EU regulations, periodic safety reports describing the reported adverse events of the product during its early post-marketing phase. This information is gathered from a number of sources; routine reporting to regulatory agencies, publications and ongoing risk/assessment studies. It must be provided to the European agencies every 6 months for the first 2 years, annually for the next 3 years and thereafter every 5 years when the product licence has to be renewed. If during this process there are major safety concerns the European Committee for Pharmaceutical Medicinal Products will review the data and may recommend changes to the labelling or if appropriate recommend product withdrawal. Product licence withdrawal is essentially only made on the basis of safety concerns where it is apparent that there are concerns to public health.

This article provides only a brief overview of the drug licensing process, highlighting the major components of the product licence application and the importance of the SmPC as the basis of the product licence. It summarises some of the procedural aspects, such as orphan drug status and the requirements to monitor safety of products during the post-licensing phase.

PHARMACOECONOMICS

R Elliott

7

WHAT ARE HEALTH ECONOMICS AND PHARMACOECONOMICS?

- *Health economics* applies economics to health and health care and considers the choices concerned with allocating scarce resources.
- *Pharmacoeconomics* is the branch of health economics that is specifically concerned with pharmaceutical products and services.

THE ROLE OF HEALTH ECONOMICS AND PHARMACOECONOMICS

Containing the rate of increase in health care spending is a principal concern in health policy. 'Cost-effectiveness' is now an important criterion for selection of therapies by providers and purchasers of health care.

Health economics and pharmacoeconomics analyse the relationship between the costs and consequences of health care. This analysis of new and existing therapies is needed to inform decisions about allocating scarce resources. The method used to analyse this relationship is *economic evaluation*.

Pharmacists need to critically assess these economic evaluations as they are increasingly integrated into the decision-making process by purchasers and formulary committees.

ECONOMIC EVALUATION

What is economic evaluation?

> Economic evaluation is the comparative analysis of the costs and consequences of two or more courses of action.

In Europe and the USA, economic evaluations of drugs are undertaken voluntarily by pharmaceutical companies to provide information for purchasers. In Australia and some Provinces in Canada, these companies have to include economic evaluation of their products in any application for reimbursement.

Components of economic evaluation

Principal components are costs and consequences (outcomes).

Costs

The inputs in an intervention are the resources used. The value attached to this resource use is the *cost*. Costs can be divided into:

1. *Direct costs*: occur within the health sector, e.g. drugs, laboratory tests and staff time. Direct non-medical costs are incurred by other parts of the public sector or by patients and families, e.g. travel costs.

2. *Indirect costs*: relate to lost productivity of patients and families due to treatment, illness or death, e.g. time off work and premature mortality. Inclusion of indirect costs, e.g. cost of illness, in economic evaluation usually has a significant effect on conclusions.

3. *Intangible costs*: cannot easily be measured, e.g. pain and suffering experienced by patients. Due to measurement problems they are often left out of an analysis.

Costs are also divided into:

4. *Fixed costs*: incurred whether patients are treated or not. *Capital costs* occur when major capital assets are purchased, e.g. building a counselling room. *Overhead* costs include services such as lighting, heating and security.

5. *Semi-fixed costs*: remain unchanged over a range of activity. Given sufficient changes in activity, they increase or decrease, e.g. staff costs.

6. *Variable costs*: incurred from a patient's treatment, e.g. drugs, blood products and laboratory investigations.

Outcome measures

1. *Effectiveness*: single measures of outcome, such as impact on survival (life years gained). Clinical indicators are also used (intermediate outcome measures), e.g. reduction in blood pressure.

2. *Health related quality of life (QoL)*: a complex concept with many functional, social, psychological, cognitive and subjective components. QoL measures can be divided into:

- *Disease specific*: These measures have been developed for specific diseases, e.g. Arthritis Impact Measurement Scale (AIMS) in rheumatoid arthritis.
- *Generic*: These measures are useful when looking at groups of patients who may have different illnesses and can be used to compare health gains in different patient groups, e.g. the Nottingham Health Profile and the EuroQol.
- *Utility*: This is a measure of the relative preference for a specific level of health status. It can be directly measured or derived from generic QoL measures. It is expressed as quality-adjusted life-years (QALYs) or healthy years equivalent (HYEs).

> e.g. 1 year in 'perfect health' = 1 QALY
> 2 years in a health state valued as 50% 'perfect health' = 1 QALY.

3. *Expressing benefits as monetary values*: simple for some measures, such as loss of earnings, cost to the health service or social services for treatment and care. It is more difficult to attach monetary values to disability, distress, uncertainty or threat to life. One method, 'willingness to pay', seeks to elicit how much an individual would be willing to pay to avoid an illness or obtain the benefits of a treatment.

Types of economic evaluation

There are four types:

- Cost-effectiveness analysis (CEA)
- Cost minimisation analysis (CMA)
- Cost utility analysis (CUA)
- Cost benefit analysis (CBA).

They measure inputs (costs) in the same way, but differ in the type of outcome measure used (see Table 7.1).

WHAT TO LOOK FOR IN AN ECONOMIC EVALUATION

Apply the following questions to identify strengths and weaknesses in published economic evaluations.

1. Was a well-defined question posed in answerable form?
The study should include justification of the economic analysis technique chosen. Assess whether the study compared both costs and consequences of alternatives. Make sure the viewpoint has been stated, e.g. 'From the viewpoint of this community trust, is it more cost-effective to initiate therapy of major depressive disorder in the community with an SSRI or a TCA antidepressant?' (Not 'Is treating depression worth it?').

Table 7.1 Measurements of inputs and outcomes in different forms of economic evaluations

Form of analysis	Measurement of input	Measurement of outcome	Use of results
Cost-effectiveness analysis	Costs	Natural units (cases successfully treated, life-years gained, disease-free time)	Comparison of interventions with the same unit of benefit but a different magnitude: cost per unit of effect
Cost minimisation analysis	Costs (often only direct)	No measurement within study	Cost comparison (lowest cost to achieve an identical result): cost per case
Cost utility analysis	Costs	Quality-adjusted life-years (QALYs), healthy years equivalents (HYEs)	Summary of multiple dimensions into one scale; comparison of treatments with initial different outcome measures: cost per QALY
Cost benefit analysis	Costs	Monetary benefit	Cost minus benefit: net benefit

(Source: Kobelt 1996)

The viewpoint, or *perspective*, of the study determines which costs need to be included, e.g. the cost to a hospital of initiating lipid-lowering treatment will be less than the cost to the whole NHS, which will also include primary care costs.

Ideally, the viewpoint should be societal. In practice, the viewpoint is usually that of the funder of the service, e.g. a trust, a community trust or the NHS.

2. Was a comprehensive description of the competing alternatives given?

Can you tell *who* did *what* to *whom*, *where* and *how often*? Assess whether any important alternatives have been left out (e.g. 'do-nothing' or current practice). To assess the cost effectiveness of a pharmacist-run anticoagulant clinic, comparison with an existing clinician-led clinic could be valid.

The treatment paths of the alternatives should be described. *Decision analytic* techniques are often used.

3. Was there evidence that the programme's effectiveness had been established?

This is preferably done via randomised controlled trials. Sources of evidence need to be identified and justified.

> Is the evidence relevant to the economic evaluation (i.e. setting, patient group, treatment pathways, outcome measures used)?
>
> Are the trial treatment protocols relevant to everyday clinical practice?

e.g. An economic evaluation of antibiotic treatment of community-acquired pneumonia (CAP) requires evidence of the efficacy of antibiotics used for CAP in patients likely to acquire CAP.

Assumptions of equal effectiveness of alternatives in CMAs should be stated.

4. Have all relevant costs been identified, measured and valued?

All resource use needs to be identified and measured, e.g. drugs, staff time. Methods used to measure resource use need to be described in detail, e.g. computerised dispensing records.

Costs should then be attached to resources used. The sources and methods of valuation of costs must be clearly stated. For example, market prices may be used for resource use such as drugs. Methods used to allocate resource use such as overheads must be reported. Make sure that costs have not been inadvertently counted twice, i.e. *double-counting*. This can happen when overheads are allocated.

'Top-down' costs, 'bottom-up' costs or charges?   Studies often use costs provided by accounting departments in the form of *average costs*, e.g. cost per day in hospital. These are 'top-down' costs which divide total running costs for a department by total number of patient-days. Average costs often over or underestimate actual costs.

Studies may use *charges* instead of costs. These are less accurate than costs because they usually include cross-subsidisation, which makes up for losses on one service by making a profit on another.

'Bottom-up' costs represent the actual resource use associated with an individual patient's treatment. They are the most relevant in an economic evaluation because they are the most sensitive to treatment differences.

Some studies report only additional costs of the alternative under investigation. This is valid as long as all changes in resource use have been identified.

5. Have all relevant outcomes been identified, measured and valued?

Outcome measures should be identified and their selection justified. Those used are dictated by the study objective. For example, looking at the impact of lipid-lowering agents on survival means that long-term mortality is the outcome measure.

Intermediate outcome measures, such as infection rates, can be used as long as the study makes explicit the link to a final health outcome, e.g. survival or QoL.

Studies may report more than one outcome measure such as reduction in blood pressure, myocardial infarction rates and QoL.

In CUA, proven generic QoL measures should be used.

In CBA, accepted methods for attaching monetary values to benefits should be used, e.g. willingness-to-pay, contingent valuation.

6. Have costs and consequences been discounted?

Discounting is a technique that allows comparison between costs and consequences that occur at different times. In health care, costs often occur immediately, while benefits occur later. Discounting is not a correction for inflation. It reflects that we prefer to receive benefits now and postpone costs. It also reflects the returns that could have been gained if the resources were invested elsewhere, e.g. based on a discount rate of 5%, a cost of £1000 occurring in one year's time is considered to be worth only about 95% at present value, i.e. £950.

Discounting is done on an annual basis, so studies shorter than one year do not need to use it.

OHE Recommendations for Discounting (Kobelt 1996). Two methods should be used:
1. All costs and outcomes discounted at the prevailing rate recommended by the treasury.
2. All costs and monetary outcomes discounted at the Treasury rate (currently 6% per annum) but non-monetary outcomes not discounted.

---

7. Was an incremental analysis of costs and consequences of alternatives performed?

Incremental analysis is the preferred method of comparing the costs and consequences of a health care intervention.

If one alternative is more effective and less costly, it is the *dominant* therapy. When one alternative is more effective, but requires more resources, the cost required to achieve each extra unit of outcome is calculated. This is the incremental cost/outcome ratio.

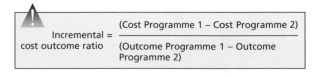

$$\text{Incremental cost outcome ratio} = \frac{(\text{Cost Programme 1} - \text{Cost Programme 2})}{(\text{Outcome Programme 1} - \text{Outcome Programme 2})}$$

8. Was sensitivity analysis performed?

This examines the effect on the results of changes in key assumptions or parameters. For example, what effect does it have if the effectiveness of a treatment is doubled or halved, the incidence of side effects lowered or increased? It identifies which parameters or assumptions have the most significant effect on the outcome and stability of the results.

Make sure that the study has justified the choice and range of parameters to vary.

9. Did the discussion of the study results include all issues of concern to users?

Assess whether the study has sufficiently dealt with related issues such as ethical concerns and equity, generalisability and implementation.

Comparison with other studies should take into account differences in methods (e.g. which costs are included) and setting (e.g. patient groups). Published league tables of economic evaluations, such as cost per QALY league tables, should be interpreted and used with caution due to these differences.

A final note

The appraisal above assesses whether the results of an economic evaluation are valid. It is then necessary to ask:

If the results are valid, would they apply to my setting?

GLOSSARY

Cost-effectiveness   Efficient use of scarce resources

Decision analysis   Explicit quantitative approach to decision-making under uncertainty

Direct medical costs   Fixed and variable costs directly associated with a health care intervention

Effectiveness   Therapeutic consequence of a treatment in real world conditions

Efficacy   Consequence of a treatment under controlled clinical conditions

Incremental cost-effectiveness ratio   Additional cost of producing an extra unit of outcome by one therapy compared with another

Indirect costs   Cost of reduced productivity resulting from illness or treatment

Intangible costs   The cost of pain and suffering resulting from illness or treatment

Marginal costs   The extra cost of one extra unit of product or service delivered

Sensitivity analysis   Assessment of the robustness of study results through systematic variation of key variables

Utility   A measure of the relative preference for, or desirability of, a specific level of health status or a specific health outcome

REFERENCES

Department of Health 1994 Guidance on good practice in the conduct of economic evaluations of medicines. National Health Service and Association of the British Pharmaceutical Industry

Drummond MF, Stoddart GL, Torrance GW 1987 Methods for the economic evaluation of health care programmes. Oxford University Press, Oxford

Kobelt G 1996 Health economics: an introduction to economic evaluation. Office of Health Economics, London

Choice

OVER-THE-COUNTER PRESCRIBING AND ADVICE

8

C Mackie

On average, there is one pharmacy for approximately 5000 people, although this distribution is uneven. There are reported to be six million visits made to pharmacies in Britain every day. The public thus has far more opportunities for contact with the pharmacist than with any other health care professional. This is important when we consider that at any time 33% of the population are self-medicating, and a further 33% are taking prescribed medication. In 1994 sales of over-the-counter drugs accounted for 23% of total medicine sales (EPMMA 1995). Self-medication is a cost-effective component of all health care systems. It is an area the Government is actively encouraging, which is not surprising when one considers that public expectations of health care are continuing to rise and will be unable to be met out of current resource allocations.

DEVELOPMENT OF THE PHARMACIST'S ADVISORY ROLE

The Nuffield Enquiry Report (1986) proposed that the pharmacist should concentrate on providing an advisory service on all aspects of medicines, including health promotion and response to symptoms:

> The pharmacist's place is not in the dispensary counting, pouring or labelling, but in virtually constant contact with those who will benefit most from direct involvement with the pharmacist.

This shift in emphasis from dispensing to an extended role was enthusiastically supported by the White Papers 'Promoting Better Health' (HMSO 1988) and 'Working For Patients' (HMSO 1989) which proposed that more emphasis should be placed on the advisory role of the community pharmacist:

> People want to understand more about their treatment and side-effects and to accept greater responsibility for their own health care.

The Joint Working Party Report Pharmaceutical Care: The Future for Community Pharmacy (RPS 1992) made 30 recommendations including extending the patient medication record scheme and the provision of confidential areas for advice and counselling.

More recently, Pharmacy in a New Age (RPS 1996) and Choice and Opportunity (HMSO 1996) have identified community pharmacists as the first port of call for common ailments. There is much talk of pharmacists acting as gatekeepers to the NHS, because they are often the first point of contact; however the reality is that the service of response to symptoms is outwith the NHS. Although advice is freely given, if a medicine is required its supply will depend on the patient's ability to pay.

PROTOCOLS AND STAFF TRAINING

Since 1 January 1995, community pharmacies are required to have a written protocol covering medicine sales and from 1 July 1996, all staff whose work regularly includes the sale of medicines must have completed a recognised training course or be undertaking such a course. However, there is no standard protocol for medicine sales; resulting in a large variation in the quality of this service in practice.

RESPONDING TO SYMPTOMS

Ideally the pharmacist should respond to all patient requests for advice, however due to time constraints this is often impractical. It is therefore necessary in practice for pharmacy staff to operate a system of triage to help identify those patients who could potentially benefit from direct involvement with the pharmacist. In an attempt to structure questioning, a number of mnemonics have been developed. Two of the most frequently used—WWHAM and AS METHOD—are given in Box 8.1. Whilst these mnemonics may be a useful tool for training and triage purposes, in practice great care must be taken to avoid the patient feeling as if they are being interrogated.

BOX 8.1 Mnemonics to assist in responding to symptoms (Blenkinsopp & Paxton 1989)

W Who is the patient	A Age and appearance
W What are the symptoms	S Self or someone else
H How long have symptoms been present	M Medication taken regularly
A Action taken, medicines tried	E Extra medicines taken for current symptoms
M Medicines taken for other conditions	T Time persisting
	H History
	O Other symptoms
	D Danger symptoms

Maintenance of good comprehensive patient medication records is an asset when responding to symptoms. Knowledge of the patient's current medical conditions may help identify symptoms due to poor disease control or iatrogenic disease. Detailed records of both prescribed and purchased medicines will reduce the potential for drug interactions.

When responding to symptoms, pharmacists have a number of options; they may:

- provide reassurance and advice on management
- supply an OTC medicine
- refer the patient.

In practice one may choose a combination of all three. Referral may be direct or conditional, based on symptoms persisting or worsening over a specific period.

These options were examined in a study of 716 tape recorded consultations occurring in a random sample of 64 community pharmacies in London (Smith 1993). If we consider the outcome of the consultations, 75% were given advice on management and supplied with an OTC medicine and 25% were given advice only. Overall 15% were referred to another health care professional. It is interesting to compare the cases presented in this study with those in the study of GP consultations for minor conditions. The top five conditions for both are given in Table 8.1.

Table 8.1 Comparison of case mix for GPs and pharmacists		
Symptom	**GP consultations for minor conditions (Fry 1993) (%)**	**Pharmacist consultations (Smith 1993) (%)**
Upper respiratory	30	30
Skin	15	15
Pain	12	5% pain/5% dental
Minor trauma	10	–
Gastrointestinal	8	11

The case mixes for common ailments presented to both pharmacists and GPs are remarkably similar. It is possible that in the future pharmacists may help to reduce GPs' workloads by managing common ailments. However for this to work, a change to the current remuneration structure would be required so that common ailments can be managed within the NHS, allowing community pharmacists to develop their role as the first port of call for common ailments and gatekeepers to the NHS. Pharmacists currently consult an average of 10–17 patients per day, and this is likely to increase in the future due to growth in demand, and the availability of more potent drugs OTC because of reclassification of medicines from Prescription Only Medicine (POM) to Pharmacy (P) status.

POM to P switches

Traditionally, community pharmacists have advised patients on the management of common self-limiting conditions and referred other conditions to the GP to manage. However this has changed recently due to the reclassification of medicines from POM to P; pharmacists can now counter prescribe for recurrent and/or persistent conditions that can be managed following an initial doctor diagnosis. Recurrent conditions include vaginal thrush and labial herpes and persistent conditions include eczema and psoriasis. For a medicine to be reclassified from POM to P it must meet the data requirements in Box 8.2. However, it should be noted that OTC doses are often lower and that the licence may be restricted in terms of both indication and duration of therapy. Table 8.2 lists drugs by BNF chapter, which have been switched from POM to P status in the last 15 years and includes both dosage and licensed indications. Restrictions are intended to reduce the risks of OTC prescribing, namely drug interactions, adverse effects and delays in diagnosis of more serious conditions. However, pharmacists should be alert that once purchased, patients may use these products outside their licence. Therefore counselling is important, particularly regarding duration of therapy.

BOX 8.2 Data requirements for POM to P switch (Lawson 1995)

Safety
- Epidemiological evidence showing safety in use over time.
- Reference to the adverse drug reaction profile of the dose and form proposed for non-prescription sale, which should be minor in nature.

- Information relating to the possibility of risk to potential customers of wrong or delayed diagnosis arising from the availability of non-prescription medicine.

Efficacy
- Evidence for both the indications and dosage being suitable for self-medication.
- Appropriateness of the indications being recognised by consumers and not confused with potentially serious, treatable diseases.

Information
- Product information leading to safe use, including warnings and advice on duration of treatment and when medical attention should be sought.

In the past 15 years, over 50 medicines have been reclassified from POM to P. This wider availability of a range of potent drugs will allow the community pharmacist to deliver his OTC advisory role more effectively. Indeed this may lead to other health care professionals referring patients to the pharmacist.

Table 8.2 Medicines reclassified from POM to P 1982–97 (Adapted from RPS 1997) md= maximum dose; mdd= maximum daily dose; ms= maximum strength. All products are licensed for adults and children over 12 years of age unless otherwise stated.

BNF ref.	Drug	Indication(s)	Restrictions on OTC sale	Licensed products
1.2 Antispasmodics	Mebeverine hydrochloride	Symptomatic relief of irritable bowel syndrome	md 135 mg mdd 405 mg (> 10 years)	Colofac IBS 100 mg tablets
	Hyoscine butylbromide	Relief of spasm of the gastrointestinal or genitourinary tracts, dysmenorrhoea, irritable bowel syndrome	md 20 mg mdd 80 mg max pack 240 mg children 6–12 years: 10 mg tid	Buscopan 10 mg tablets
1.3.1 Ulcerhealing drugs	Cimetidine	Short-term symptomatic relief of heartburn dyspepsia and hyperacidity, prophylaxis of meal induced and nocturnal heartburn	md 200 mg mdd 800 mg maximum 14 days (> 16 years)	Tagamet 100 tablets and dual action liquid
	Famotidine	As for cimetidine	md 10 mg mdd 20 mg maximum 14 days (> 16 years)	Pepcid AC 10 mg tablets
	Ranitidine	Short-term symptomatic relief of heartburn dyspepsia and hyperacidity	md 75 mg mdd 300 mg maximum 14 days (> 16 years)	Zantac 75 tablets

(contd)

Table 8.2 Medicines reclassified from POM to P 1982–97 (Adapted from RPS 1997) md= maximum dose; mdd= maximum daily dose; ms= maximum strength. All products are licensed for adults and children over 12 years of age unless otherwise stated. (contd)

BNF ref.	Drug	Indication (s)	Restrictions on OTC sale	Licensed products
	Nizatidine	Prevention of symptoms of food related heartburn	md 75 mg maximum of 4 doses in any 14 days (> 16 years)	None available at the present time
1.4.2 Anti-diarrhoeal drugs	Loperamide	Symptomatic relief of acute diarrhoea	md 4 mg mdd 16 mg max pack 12 capsules	Imodium 2 mg capsules and liquid, Arret, Diocalm ultra and a number of other brands
1.7.2 Haemor-rhoids	Hydro-cortisone rectal	Symptomatic relief of uncomplicated internal and external haemorrhoids	Maximum use 7 days (> 18 years)	Anusol plus HC supposi-tories and ointment
	Hydro-cortisone rectal	Symptomatic relief of uncomplicated internal and external haemorrhoids and pruritis ani	maximum 4 times daily for 7 days (> 18 years)	Proctofoam HC cream
	Hydro-cortisone/ lignocaine spray	Symptomatic relief of uncomplicated internal and external haemorrhoids	maximum use 7 days (> 18 years)	None available at the present time
2.6.1 Nitrates	Isosorbide dinitrate	Prophylaxis of angina	20 mg three times daily	Cedocard 20

(contd)

BNF ref.	Drug	Indication (s)	Restrictions on OTC sale	Licensed products
3.4.1	Astemizole	Symptomatic relief of hayfever only	mdd 10 mg max pack 100 mg	Hismanal, Pollen-eze
	Loratadine	Symptomatic relief of hayfever and perennial rhinitis	mdd 10 mg max pack 100 mg	Clarityn 10 mg tablets
	Acrivastine	Symptomatic relief of hayfever	mdd 24 mg max pack 240 mg	None available at the present time
	Cetirizine	Symptomatic relief of hayfever, allergic rhinitis and allergic skin conditions	mdd 10 mg max pack 100 mg	Zirtek
	Hydroxyzine hydro-chloride	Pruritus associated with acute or chronic urticaria or atopic dermatitis in adults and children > 6 years	md 25 mg mdd 75 mg* max pack 240 mg *mdd 50 mg for child aged 6–12 years	None available at the present time
3.9.1 Cough prepar-ations	Dextro-methorphan controlled release	Symptomatic relief of dry unproductive cough	md 30 mg mdd 75 mg	None available at the present time
3.10 Systemic nasal decong-estants	Pseudo-ephedrine controlled release	Symptomatic relief of nasal congestion	md 120 mg mdd 240 mg	None available at the present time

(contd)

Table 8.2 Medicines reclassified from POM to P 1982–97 (Adapted from RPS 1997) md= maximum dose; mdd= maximum daily dose; ms= maximum strength. All products are licensed for adults and children over 12 years of age unless otherwise stated. (contd)

BNF ref.	Drug	Indication (s)	Restrictions on OTC sale	Licensed products
	Pseudo-ephedrine hydro-chloride	Symptomatic relief of nasal congestion	md 60 mg mdd 240 mg	Sudafed and Galpseud
4.7.2 Analgesics	Paracetamol/dihydro-codeine	Relief of mild to moderate pain and/or fever	Maximum 8 in 24 hours	Paramol tablets
4.10 Substance depen-dence	Nicotine gum 2 mg and 4 mg	Treatment of nicotine dependence and relief of symptoms of nicotine withdrawal	Maximum 15 in 24 hours	Nicorette 2 mg, Nicorette plus 4 mg, Nicotinell 2 mg
	Nicotine patches	Treatment of nicotine dependence and relief of symptoms of nicotine withdrawal	One patch daily (> 18 years)	Nicotinell TTS, Nicorette, Nicabate
5.2 Antifungal drugs	Fluconazole	Oral treatment of vaginal candidiasis in patients not less than 16 years and not over 60 years	md 150 mg maximum pack 150 mg (> 16 yrs, < 60 yrs)	Diflucan one capsule
5.5.1 Anthel-mintics	Meben-dazole	Oral treatment of enterobiasis (threadworm) in adults and children > 2 years	md 100 mg max pack 400 mg (> 2 years)	Ovex 1, Ovex 4 pack and Pripsen meben-dazole tablets

(contd)

Table 8.2 Medicines reclassified from POM to P 1982–97 (Adapted from RPS 1997) md= maximum dose; mdd= maximum daily dose; ms= maximum strength. All products are licensed for adults and children over 12 years of age unless otherwise stated. (contd)

BNF ref.	Drug	Indication (s)	Restrictions on OTC sale	Licensed products
	Pyrantel embonate	Oral treatment of enterobiasis in adults and children > 2 years	Max pack 400 mg (> 2 years)	None available at the present time
7.2.2 Vaginal and vulval conditions	Clotrimazole pessaries	Vaginal candidiasis	For external use in adults only	Canesten 100 mg, 200 mg and 500 mg pessaries
	Econazole pessaries	Vaginal candidiasis	For external use in adults only	Ecostatin 150 mg pessaries and Gyno-Pevaryl 150 mg pessaries
	Isoconazole pessaries	Vaginal candidiasis	For external use in adults only	Travogyn 300 mg pessaries
	Miconazole pessaries	Vaginal candidiasis	For external use in adults only	Femeron 1200 mg soft pessary, Gyno-daktarin 1200 mg pessary
10.1.1 Rheumatic disease	Ibuprofen oral	Rheumatic and muscular pain, backache, neuralgia, migraine, headache, dysmenorrhoea	md 400 mg mdd 1200 mg Max pack 12 doses of 200 mg for GSL status	Cuprofen, Nurofen, Proflex and a number of other brands

(contd)

Table 8.2 Medicines reclassified from POM to P 1982–97 (Adapted from RPS 1997) md= maximum dose; mdd= maximum daily dose; ms= maximum strength. All products are licensed for adults and children over 12 years of age unless otherwise stated. (contd)

BNF ref.	Drug	Indication (s)	Restrictions on OTC sale	Licensed products
	Ibuprofen sr oral	Sustained relief of mild to moderate pain, symptomatic relief of sprains, rheumatic pain, lumbago, muscular aches and pains	md 600 mg mdd 1200 mg	Proflex 300 mg sustained release capsules
	Ibuprofen suspension	Reduction of fever and relief of mild to moderate pain	100 mg/ 5 ml dose depends on age, max 4 doses in 24 hours (child > 1 year)	Junifen suspension
10.3.2 Soft-tissue inflamma-tion	Ibuprofen topical	Rheumatic pain, muscular aches and pains or swellings	ms 5.0% P status md 125 mg mdd 500 mg max pack 2.5 g for GSL status	Ibuleve gel, Ibuleve spray, Proflex pain relief cream
	Ketoprofen topical	Rheumatic and muscular pain	ms 2.5% max pack 30 g for max 7 days	Oruvail gel, Solpaflex gel
	Diclofenac topical	Pain and inflammation in trauma of tendons, ligaments, muscles, joints and soft tissues	ms 1.16% max pack 30 g	None available at the present time

(contd)

Table 8.2 Medicines reclassified from POM to P 1982–97 (Adapted from RPS 1997) md= maximum dose; mdd= maximum daily dose; ms= maximum strength. All products are licensed for adults and children over 12 years of age unless otherwise stated. (contd)

BNF ref.	Drug	Indication (s)	Restrictions on OTC sale	Licensed products
	Felbinac topical	Soft tissue injury	ms 3.17% max pack 30 g	Traxam pain relief gel
	Piroxicam topical	Rheumatic pain, muscular aches, pains and swellings	ms 0.5% 30 g	Feldene P gel
11.4.2 Anti-inflammatory preparations for the eye	Sodium cromo-glycate 2% drops and ointment	Acute seasonal allergic conjunctivitis	Eye drops ms 2% max pack 10 ml eye ointment 4% max pack 5 g	Opticrom allergy, Brolene, Optrex hayfever
12.2.1 Drugs acting on the nose	Beclo-methasone dipropionate	Seasonal allergic rhinitis and allergic rhinitis	md 100 mcg mdd 200 mcg per nostril max pack 200 doses	Beconase hayfever nasal spray
	Flunisolide nasal	Seasonal allergic rhinitis	md 50 mcg mdd 100 mcg* per nostril max pack 240 doses *md 25 mcg mdd 75 mcg for child 12–16 years	Syntaris Hayfever nasal spray
	Budesonide nasal	Seasonal allergic rhinitis	md 200 mcg mdd 200 mcg per nostril max pack 50 doses	None available at the present time

(contd)

Table 8.2 Medicines reclassified from POM to P 1982–97 (Adapted from RPS 1997) md= maximum dose; mdd= maximum daily strength. All products are licensed for adults and children over 12 years of age unless otherwise stated. (contd)

BNF ref.	Drug	Indication (s)	Restrictions on OTC sale	Licensed products
	Azelastine nasal	Seasonal allergic rhinitis	md 140 mcg mdd 280 mcg per nostril max pack 36 doses	None available at the present time
12.3.1 Drugs acting on the orophar-ynx	Carbe-noxolone granules	Mouth ulcers	md 20 mg mdd 80 mg max pack 560 mg	Bioplex granules
	Hydro-cortisone pellets	Mouth ulcers	Exemption from POM control applies to named products only	Corlan pellets
	Triam-cinolone dental paste	Mouth ulcers	Maximum 5 days	Adcortyl in orabase for mouth-ulcers
13.4 Topical cortico-steroids	Hydro-cortisone topical 1%	Irritant contact dermatitis, allergic contact dermatitis, insect bite reactions and mild to moderate eczema	exemption from POM control applies to named products only	HC45, Lanacort, Dermacort and a number of other brands

(contd)

Table 8.2 Medicines reclassified from POM to P 1982–97 (Adapted from RPS 1997) md= maximum dose; mdd= maximum daily dose; ms= maximum strength. All products are licensed for adults and children over 12 years of age unless otherwise stated. (contd)

BNF ref.	Drug	Indication (s)	Restrictions on OTC sale	Licensed products
	Hydro-cortisone/crotamiton	Irritant contact dermatitis, allergic contact dermatitis, insect bite reactions and mild to moderate eczema	Exemption from POM control applies to named products only	Eurax HC cream
13.7 Preparations for warts	Podo-phyllum resin	Plantar warts	ms 20%	Posalfilin
13.9 Scalp preparations	Minoxidil	Male pattern baldness	ms 2% for external use only	Regaine
13.10.2 Anti-infective skin preparations	Ketocona-zole shampoo	Dandruff and seborrhoeic dermatitis of the scalp for adults and children	ms 2% max pack 120 ml max frequency once every 3 days	Nizoral shampoo
	Tioconazole 2%	Dermal skin infections	ms 2%	Trosyl cream 1%
13.10.3	Aciclovir 5% cream	Herpes simplex virus infections of the lips and face	Named product only	Zovirax cold sore cream, Herpetad, Soothelip, Zaclivir
13.12 Anti-perspirants	Aluminium chloride	Hyperhidrosis affecting axillae, hands or feet	No restrictions	Anhydrol forte, Driclor

(contd)

Table 8.2 Medicines reclassified from POM to P 1982–97 (Adapted from RPS 1997) md= maximum dose; mdd= maximum daily dose; ms= maximum strength. All products are licensed for adults and children over 12 years of age unless otherwise stated. (contd)

BNF ref.	Drug	Indication (s)	Restrictions on OTC sale	Licensed products
13.13.8 Wound management	Dextra-nomer topical	Exudative and infected wounds and leg ulcers	No restrictions	Debrisan
	Cadexomer iodine	Venous leg ulcers and pressure sores	No restrictions	Iodosorb ointment

REFERENCES

Blenkinsopp A, Paxton P 1989 Symptoms in the pharmacy. Blackwell Scientific Publications, London

European Proprietary Medicines Manufacturers' Association 1995 Economic and legal framework for non-prescription medicines in Europe. EPMMA, London

Fry J 1993 General Practice: The facts. Radcliffe Medical Press, Oxford

HMSO 1988 Promoting better health: CM 249. HMSO, London

HMSO 1989 Working for patients: CM555. HMSO, London

HMSO 1996 Choice and opportunity. Primary care: the future HMSO, London

Lawson D 1995 Treatments for common ailments. In: OTC directory 1995/96. Proprietary Association of Great Britain, London

Nuffield Foundation 1986 Pharmacy: A report to the Nuffield Foundation. Nuffield Foundation, London

Royal Pharmaceutical Society 1992 Pharmaceutical care: The future role of the community pharmaceutical services. RPS, London

Royal Pharmaceutical Society 1996 Pharmacy in a new age: The new horizon. RPS, London

Royal Pharmaceutical Society 1997 Bibliography: Prescription only medicines reclassified to pharmacy only medicines. RPS, London

Smith FJ 1993 Referral of clients by community pharmacists in primary care consultations. International Journal of Pharmacy Practice 2:86–89

PAIN

9

B Hughes

Pain is a perception arising from a sensory stimulus, usually to reveal an underlying problem which requires attention. It is a physiological *alarm* and demands a response. It is only the patient who can judge its nature and severity, and his perception must be respected.

- Unless the cause is obvious, such as surgical trauma, attempt to discern the origin and treat accordingly (e.g. nitrates for angina) before considering analgesia.
- Note the distinction between pain (nociception) and decreased pain threshold (hypersensitivity). Bradykinin is a primary mediator of pain whereas prostaglandins increase afferent receptor sensitivity and lower the pain threshold. The distinction is important in treatment since NSAIDs, which suppress prostaglandin formation, may raise the pain threshold independently of any possible intrinsic analgesic action (*see* Arthritis, p. 64). Their effects may not be evident for 12 to 72 hours but may facilitate a reduction in the dose of primary analgesic.

Since the central nervous system (CNS) can modulate pain perception by amplification or attenuation, the general principle is to rapidly achieve relief from pain then to maintain adequate control by regular treatment, even in the acute situation, rather than to treat pro re nata (p.r.n.) in response to breakthrough of pain.

ACUTE PAIN

Do not treat with analgesics until the cause has been ascertained as this may mask diagnosis, impede correct treatment and thus worsen the prognosis. Following diagnosis, use the analgesic ladder (Box 9.1) to determine appropriate treatment for pain control. Where possible, facilitate a multidisciplinary acute pain service within the hospital as this greatly improves care.

Dental pain

- *Sublingual buprenorphine* is particularly effective in severe dental pain.

Dysmenorrhoea (period pain)

- *Ibuprofen* or *aspirin* is the treatment of choice with
  mefenamic acid or other NSAIDs as second line treatment.
- *Oestrogen* treatment should be considered for regular severe
  dysmenorrhoea.

Wound pain

If the wound becomes inflamed, use appropriate systemic antimicrobial or antifungal agents.

- A short-acting analgesic such as dextromoramide or
  pethidine can be given 30 minutes before removing the
  tube from a painful drainage site.
- *Entonox*® is particularly effective when changing dressings
  on painful wounds.
- Consider infiltration with local anaesthetic.

BOX 9.1 The Analgesic Ladder

STRONG			
Opioids (*see* section)	**MODERATE**		
Opioids + NSAIDs	Buprenorphine		
Tramadol	Dihydrocodeine		
	Aspav®		
	Co-dydramol		
	Co-codamol		
	Co-proxamol	**MILD**	
	NSAIDs	Aspirin	
	Tramadol*	Ibuprofen	
		Paracetamol	

*Opioids, *see* p. 67; Tramadol, *see* p. 64
Hepatic or renal impairment
Opioid analgesics can precipitate hepatic encephalopathy and
in renal impairment excretion of opioid metabolites is slower. In
either situation, where opioids are indicated, monitor the
effects of dosage carefully and reduce the frequency of dosage
where necessary (e.g. morphine 6–8 hourly). NSAIDs, aspirin
and corticosteroids will exacerbate fluid retention in hepatic
failure and should best be avoided unless absolutely necessary.
In renal impairment NSAIDs and aspirin may cause deterioration
of renal function: BNF classifies this as a mild interaction.
(Tiaprofenic acid is contraindicated in renal impairment).

POSTOPERATIVE PAIN

Although there is a marked variation in the degree of pain experienced or at least expressed by different individuals undergoing the same operative procedure, the expected norm for most procedures can be anticipated. Where the expected level of pain is sufficient to impede movement and the beginning of rehabilitation, thereby impairing gas exchange and increasing the risk of emboli and deep vein thrombosis, a parenteral narcotic analgesic (unless contraindicated) should be commenced shortly before full consciousness is regained.

Parenteral analgesics

To minimise respiratory depression post-extubation, continuous i.v. or epidural analgesic following a bolus dose of say i.v. morphine injection 5 mg is preferable to intermittent i.m. or oral drug for the initial period, though monitoring is essential. The duration of analgesia should be appropriate to the assessed need but could be up to 48 hours or even longer. Patient controlled analgesia enables the dose to be titrated by the patient and confers distinct advantages in management.

Typical dosage schedules are shown in Table 9.1

Table 9.1 Typical dosage schedules for parenteral analgesics		
Method	**Solution**	**Rate**
Continuous i.v.	Morphine salt 1 mg/ml	2–10 mg/h
PCA — i.v. (Patient controlled analgesia)	Morphine salt 2 mg/ml	Maximum 10 mg/h (6 min lock out)
Epidural	Diamorphine HCl 0.5 mg/ml (not morphine injection because it contains preservative)	2–5 mg/h

• *Opioid* analgesics cause constipation normally by day 3 postoperatively. Where appropriate a laxative should be given in anticipation. Senna is the drug of choice, but note that if lactulose is used it takes 2 days to be effective, therefore initiate on Day 1. Laxatives should be given on a regular basis.

• *Pethidine* has no advantage over morphine and is equally effective though less potent and shorter acting. It will require supplementary analgesia within 2 hours of cessation of continuous i.v. compared to 4 hours after cessation of morphine.

• *Droperidol* 1–3 mg per hour may be added to the morphine injection to control nausea and vomiting: 200 micrograms/ml added to the solution is the maximum concentration for stability of the solution.

• *Bupivacaine* may be added to the epidural diamorphine solution to potentiate activity: thus typically the solution would contain 0.1% bupivacaine.

• *Tramadol* is a recently introduced drug and is recommended by the CSM (October 1996) only for short-term/intermittent use in moderate and severe pain.

Oral analgesics

For procedures with low trauma or for follow-up after i.v./epidural opioids use moderate or mild analgesics as in the analgesic ladder.

• *Buprenorphine* sublingually up to 400 micrograms 8-hourly is useful, particularly for dental pain. Higher doses rarely increase the degree of analgesia as this drug is a partial agonist. Another opioid should be used if greater analgesia is required but reassess dosage during 4–12 hours as the receptor blocking effect of buprenorphine is reversed.
• *Pentazocine* offers no advantages over other drugs and is erratically absorbed orally. It has a high incidence of dysphoria.
• *NSAIDs* are useful adjuncts if not contraindicated, as inflammation often accompanies surgery, particularly orthopaedic surgery.

CHRONIC PAIN

Arthritis

Pain is an integral part of both osteo- and rheumatoid arthritis. It is a measure of the state of the condition and as such cannot be treated in isolation. The full management of arthritis cannot be adequately considered in this monograph.

In rheumatoid arthritis relief is principally through reduction of the inflammatory process by non-steroidal anti-inflammatory drugs (NSAIDs). Since their action is primarily through inhibition of prostaglandin formation, and in particular of the COX-2 enzyme, onset of relief may take hours and the full effect not be noted for 2 to 3 days. Morning stiffness is a particular problem and therefore pre-treatment is essential.

- Where *aspirin* or *ibuprofen* is used ensure that full anti-inflammatory dosage is given and not the lower analgesic dosage.
- Ensure that measures are taken to minimise gastrointestinal effects (irritancy and ulceration).

Osteoarthritis is relieved by surgery or by means of minimising the burden on the relevant joints. Use drugs as indicated in the analgesic ladder to give relief until appropriate surgery is available.

Musculoskeletal pain

After consideration of the causes of the pain and initiating appropriate treatment where possible, pain should be relieved in accordance with the analgesic ladder.

> ⚠ As the degree of musculoskeletal pain will be modified according to the circumstances (physical, temporal and emotional) it is ***essential to review regularly***.

- Spasm may be relieved by *diazepam* 5–10 mg daily or *baclofen* 5–10 mg tds.
- Localised pain may be beneficially treated by nerve block or transcutaneous electrical nerve stimulation (TENS).

Neuralgia and causalgia

Some anti-convulsants and anti-depressants are useful treatments and, to avoid undue anxiety, it may be advisable to inform the patient that these are not being used for their normal indications. They should usually begin with a small dose, increasing gradually until relief is achieved or side-effects become evident.

- *Amitriptyline*   25–150 mg at night for constant burning pain.
- *Carbamazepine* 50–400 mg bd for intermittent shooting/stabbing pain. (See BNF 4.7.3 for dosing schedule).

For trigeminal neuralgia, both drugs together may be more effective. The drugs may take at least one week to be fully effective and if successful, an attempt should be made to reduce the dose by one decrement after a further 1 to 2 weeks.

- *TENS* may occasionally be beneficial.
See also Malignant neuropathy (p.67)

MALIGNANCY AND PALLIATIVE CARE

Many cancers are not painful whilst others arouse considerable pain. Both experience and the fear of pain can impair the quality of life. Often, however, exacerbations of pain are due to secondary causes and these should be ascertained and treated or relieved before considering further analgesics. For many patients referred to hospital for pain control, relief of constipation due to opioid analgesics or to low mobility is a more satisfactory solution than increasing the opioid!

• Carefully consider possible secondary causes of pain (e.g. constipation, dyspepsia, locus of infection in necrotic tissue, cranial pressure).
— Treat accordingly.

• Identify locus of pain.
— Consider whether an adjuvant would be more appropriate than an analgesic (*see* p.67).
— Select control from analgesic ladder.
— Add a NSAID, as many cancers including lung cancers, bony metastases and breast cancers release prostaglandins which lower the pain threshold.

• Assure the patient that the aim is to bring down the level of pain to a minimum and to retain such relief by *regular* analgesia.
— If relief is not achieved fairly rapidly progress to opioids without undue delay.

• Consider the necessity to relieve nausea and vomiting and the possible onset of constipation. For nausea and vomiting due to malignancy or narcotic analgesics the following are normally effective:
— *Haloperidol* 0.5 mg orally bd or 1.5 mg at night
— *Prochlorperazine* 12.5 mg i.m. then 5 mg po 4- to 8-hourly (suppositories 25 mg tds). Chlorpromazine is a more sedative alternative to prochlorperazine.
— *Cyclizine* 50 mg orally tds: useful for iatrogenic N & V if patient is normally prone to travel sickness.

• Ensure that doses are evenly spread over 24 hours and if necessary use all three drugs additively rather than increasing the dose of one class of drug.
— *Metoclopromide* is normally too short acting unless given by continuous infusion.

• For constipation *senna preparations* are the drugs of choice for maintenance but they should not be used if the faeces is already impacted.

REVIEW REGULARLY

Analgesic adjuvants

Bone metastases

- *NSAIDs* will enable reduction of the opioid dosage after about 2 days of treatment (n.b. suppositories available).
- *Corticosteroids*
- Focal radiotherapy
- Radioactive isotopes of strontium (Metastron®)

Headache from cerebral secondaries

- *Dexamethasone* 16 mg orally daily for 4–5 days reducing to 4–6 mg daily if possible.

Neuropathy

Antidepressants and anticonvulsants are first-line treatment. *See* Chronic pain — neuralgia and causalgia (p.65)

Persistent neuropathy may benefit from membrane stabilising agents but note that such use is outside the current product licences.

- *Flecainide* 100–150 mg orally bd or
- *Mexiletine* m/r 360 mg orally bd (if renal function poor).

They may take 7–10 days to be effective. An ECG should be performed before initiating the drug.

Nerve compression may be relieved by

- *Dexamethasone* 8 mg daily.

Localised pain

Consider nerve block, TENS, focal radiotherapy and acupuncture.

Opioids

Concerns for dependence and respiratory depression have been overstressed with regard to the use of opioids as analgesics. Except for the immediate postoperative period, when care in titration is needed because of the opioid/anaesthetic interaction, respiratory depression is not normally a problem. Dependence does not generally occur even with high doses of opioid provided that the dosage is regularly reviewed and adjusted to maintain an acceptable level of relief from pain.

Morphine is the most useful opioid analgesic. For regular parenteral administration diamorphine, because of its greater solubility, has an advantage in that low volume injections can be used, with particular benefit in small portable syringe drivers: see BNF 'Guidance on prescribing in palliative care' for details.

> *Legal note* — diamorphine is an illegal drug in most countries other than the UK and Belgium. Do not commence use in patients returning abroad.

Transdermal patches of fentanyl are effective for long-term maintenance where other routes of administration are less appropriate. There are also opioid suppositories available.

- *Morphine salts.* By mouth start at 5–10 mg 4-hourly to replace a mild to moderate analgesic and 10–20 mg a stronger one. Increase by dose increments of $1^1/_2$ to 2 fold to provide adequate relief and, as recommended in the BNF, 'there should be no hesitation in increasing the dose to 30–60 mg or occasionally to 90–150 mg or higher if necessary.'

- Once relief is established, try reducing the dose by small increments (15–20%) to optimise the benefits whilst minimising the side-effects.

- Drowsiness is common for 2–3 days after increasing the dose but will usually subside thereafter to a more tolerable level.

Useful oral morphine preparations (Check BNF for latest preparations)

To establish control use 4-hourly regular dosage of standard preparations.

- *Sevredol*® *tablets* scored 10 mg, 20 mg, 50 mg
- *Oramorph*® *oral solution* 10 mg/5 ml, 100 mg/5 ml
- *Oramorph*® *UDV* 10 mg, 30 mg, 100 mg vials

For continuation transfer to sustained release preparations.

— 12-hourly dosage:

- *MST Continus*® *tablets* 5 mg, 10 mg, 15 mg, 30 mg, 60 mg, 100 mg, 200 mg
- *Oramorph*® *SR tablets* 10 mg, 30 mg, 60 mg, 100 mg
- *MST Continus*® *suspension* 20 mg, 30 mg, 60 mg, 100 mg, 200 mg

— 24-hourly dosage:

- *MXL*® *capsules* 30 mg, 60 mg, 90 mg, 120 mg, 150 mg, 200 mg

When using these modified release preparations use the non-sustained release preparations (e.g. Sevredol or Oramorph) for breakthrough pain and whilst reaching 'steady state', then adjust the 12 h or 24 h MR dosage accordingly.

Newer opioids

With the long established opioids there is little difference between the drugs in dose ratio of side-effects to analgesia; that is, their efficacy is similar despite vast differences in potency. Although with more recent drugs there has been some selectivity in action, none has minimised the untoward effects whilst maintaining the full analgesic profile of morphine. Any contender should have thoroughly proven benefit before being substituted for the established analgesics.

EQUIVALENT DOSES

These drugs vary in the potency of their active metabolites and in their duration of action. Dose equivalents are given as a starting guide (Box 9.2).

BOX 9.2 Equivalent doses and conversions

EQUIVALENT DOSES — Intramuscular (single dose)

Morphine salts	**10 mg**
Papaveretum	12 mg
Diamorphine HCl	4 mg
Pethidine HCl	80 mg

thus	**Morphine sulphate 10 mg/ml**	**1.0 ml**
	Papaveretum 14.4 mg/ml	0.75 ml
	Diamorphine HCl 5 mg/ml	0.8 ml
	Pethidine HCl 100 mg/ml	0.8 ml

EQUIVALENT DOSES — Oral (single dose)

Morphine salts	**30 mg**
Buprenorphine (*sublingual*)	0.4 mg
Codeine phosphate	200 mg*
Dextromoramide	20 mg
Diamorphine HCl	20 mg
Dihydrocodeine tartrate	300 mg*
Methadone HCl	10 mg
Papaveretum	35 mg
Pethidine HCl	150 mg
Phenazocine HBr	10 mg

(contd)

CONVERSIONS (continuous dosing)
  i.m. Morphine salts : oral Morphine salts   = 1 : 2
  i.m. Diamorphine HCl : oral Morphine salts   = 1 : 3
  transdermal Fentanyl–Durogesic® '25' ≡ oral Morphine
  salts 90 mg/24 h

*Higher doses are not normally used due to the increased ratio of constipation and side-effects to pain relief. Some studies indicate a greater potency for dihydrocodeine.

10

ANTI-INFECTIVES

A Boyter, S Hudson

Anti-infective agents account for on average one third of drug costs and 10% of a general hospital's material running costs. They are widely used and they exert major effects on morbidity, mortality and duration of hospitalisation. The consequences of misuse are wide in terms of drug-related toxicity, emergence of resistance and economic considerations. The prevention and control of infection is based on multi-disciplinary cooperation to implement infection control procedures and to apply voluntary controls through guidelines. Local policies aim to manage the environment by making most use of established agents and prolonging the effectiveness of the newer ones.

Pharmacists can provide continuous educational support towards the implementation of agreed policies. Guidelines for the use of anti-infective agents wherever possible should be supported by evidence from controlled trials. However data from such trials are not always available and therefore guidelines should be seen as providing a general framework rather than a prescriptive policy for the selection and use of agents in individual patients.

SELECTION AND USE

In individual patient care the selection and use of anti-infective agents depends upon the following factors.

Clinical

1. Diagnosis and likely source of infection
2. Localisation/dissemination of the infection
3. Clinical severity including potential severity
4. Patient's underlying condition and vulnerability.

Bacteriological (Figure 10.1)

5. Presumed pathogen(s), initially by inference, subject to laboratory confirmation
6. Sensitivity of the organism to particular anti-infective agents including local variations.

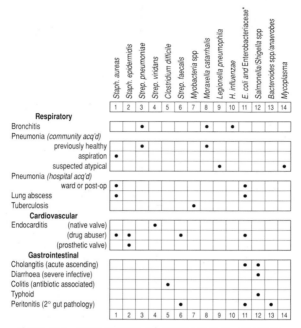

Figure 10.1 Some common infections and likely organisms.

Pharmaceutical

7. Evidence of clinical efficacy
8. Suitability of route of administration
9. Potential toxicity and drug interactions of possible anti-infective agents
10. Cost of treatment.

Clinical assessment

Sources of infection may be exogenous (transfer via host or from the environment) or endogenous (migration of flora from normal body site of residence). Portal of entry or primary locus of infection (skin and soft tissues, lungs, gastrointestinal and urinary tracts) is sought from history and examination.

	Anaerobic cocci	Staph. aureus	Staph. epidermidis	Strep. pyogenes and Group B strep.	Strep. pneumoniae	Strep. faecalis	Clostridium spp	Neisseria meningitidis	Neisseria gonorrhoeae	H. influenzae	E. coli & Enterobacteriaceae*	Bacteroides spp/anaerobes	Spyrochaetes	Chlamydia spp
	1	2	3	4	5	6	7	8	9	10	11	12	13	14
Skin/soft tissue/bone														
Cellulitis/erysipelas		•		•										
Lyme disease													•	
Toxic shock syndrome		•												
Bite (animal)	•	•				•						•		
Bite (human)	•	•		•								•		
Acute osteomyelitis/septic arthritis		•												
Central nervous system														
Bacterial meningitis elderly					•									
infant < 2mo				•				•						
child 2 mo – 12 yr								•		•				
young adult								•						
Brain abscess		•		•										
Ear, nose, throat														
Otitis media, acute			•		•					•				
Sinusitis			•		•					•				
Tonsilitis			•											
Quinsy			•											
Genitourinary														
UTI (lower)/cystitis		•	•								•	•		
Pyelonephritis (acute)		•	•								•	•		
Prostatitis (acute)			•								•			
Epididymo-orchitis		•	•											
Gonorrhoea									•					
Non-specific urethritis														•
Pelvic inflammatory (acute)									•					
	1	2	3	4	5	6	7	8	9	10	11	12	13	14

Figure 10.1   Some common infections and likely organisms. (continued)

BOX 10.1 Clinical assessment: Signs and symptoms of infection

- Temperature >38°C or <36°C (*perhaps afebrile in uncomplicated/localised infections*)
- Tachycardia: heart rate >90 bpm
- Tachypnoea: respiratory rate >20 per min, pCO_2 <4.3 kpa
- White blood cells >12.0 or <4.0 × 10^{-9}/L *polymorphocytosis in bacterial infection/ lymphocytosis in viral infection*
- Local signs of inflammation/purulence
- Hypotension
- Hyperglycaemia
- ↑Erythrocyte sedimentation rate/plasma viscosity
- ↑Serum complement
- ↑C-reactive protein

BOX 10.2 Patients with CNS infections (lumbar puncture)

↓ CSF glucose
↓ white blood cells
↓ CSF protein

⚠️ **Confounding factors:**
Corticosteroid use may mask signs of infection. Drugs (especially anti-infectives) may cause febrile reactions.

Patients at risk

Hospital acquired (nosocomial) infections characteristically arise in:

- Immune compromised patients
- Patients in intensive care
- Patients who are malnourished
- Patients with cancer
- Patients with diabetes
- Elderly and infirm patients
- Infants and neonates.

Nosocomial infections often involve environmental or commensal organisms, normally possessing low virulence but increasing antibiotic resistance. In debilitated patients there is increased risk of dissemination and its consequences:

- Disseminated intravascular coagulation (DIC)
- Acute respiratory distress syndrome (ARDS)
- Septicaemic (endotoxic) shock.

Bacteriological assessment

Endogenous infection involves the contamination of normally sterile tissues by organisms known to colonise body spaces above the diaphragm (typically Gram-positive bacteria) or below the diaphragm (typically Gram-negative bacteria).

- Clinical diagnosis leads to best guess source of infection and likely pathogen(s) (Fig. 10.1)
- Before treatment, samples taken depending on site of infection (blood, sputum, mid-stream urine, pus/wound swabs)
- After sampling, empirical treatment started on basis of best guess pathogen(s) (taking into account local sensitivities)
- Culture and in vitro sensitivity results guide continuation or modification of regimen.

Urgent microscopy gives morphology and Gram stain characteristics which may help (e.g. in bacterial meningitis). Full bacteriological diagnosis requires 18–24 h for culture and in vitro sensitivity testing (disk diffusion). Tuberculosis organism sensitivities require up to 6 weeks because of slow organism growth. MIC estimates which may be used in specific infections, such as bacterial endocarditis, require broth dilution techniques.

A positive culture may not always signify infection but may represent colonization of the organism or contamination of the sample. Hospital acquired infections characteristically involve a greater diversity of microbes than community acquired infections.

Pharmaceutical assessment

Choice of agent (Figure 10.2)

Rational use of anti-infective agents requires confidence in the clinical efficacy of preferred agents, based on published clinical trial evidence in the particular indications for which they are to be selected for inclusion in the formulary. Although effective dosing with a single agent is the preferred strategy, a combination of agents is sometimes used for:

- Broad spectrum coverage of potential pathogens (e.g. prophylaxis in abdominal surgery)
- Synergy between two agents (e.g. aminoglycoside + β lactam antibiotic)
- Prevention of resistance emerging during treatment (e.g. antitubercular chemotherapy)
- Serious infections presenting physiological barriers (e.g. bacterial meningitis)
- Avoidance of high doses to reduce risk of toxicity (e.g. systemic antifungal therapy)

There are theoretical objections to the non-rational combinations of bacteriostatic with bactericidal agents which have not been borne out by clinical evidence.

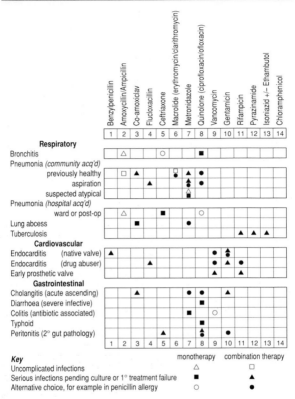

Figure 10.2 Infections and first choice agents.
(Based on proposed first choice agents of Infection and
Immunodeficiency Service, Dundee Teaching Hospitals)

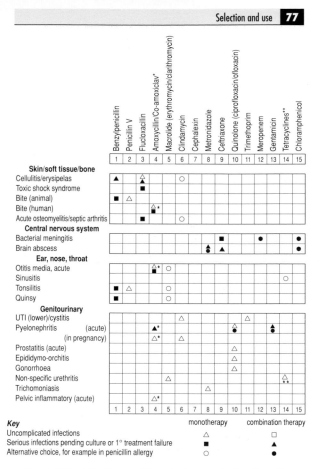

Figure 10.2 Infections and first choice agents. (continued)

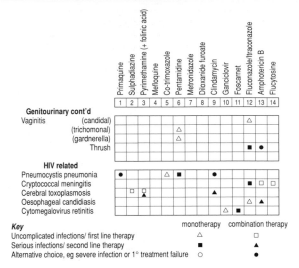

	Primaquine	Sulphadiazine	Pyrimethamine (+ folinic acid)	Mefloquine	Co-trimoxazole	Pentamidine	Metronidazole	Diloxanide furoate	Clindamycin	Ganciclovir	Foscarnet	Fluconazole/Itraconazole	Amphotericin B	Flucytosine
	1	2	3	4	5	6	7	8	9	10	11	12	13	14
Genitourinary cont'd														
Vaginitis (candidal)												△		
(trichomonal)							△							
(gardnerella)							△							
Thrush												■	●	
HIV related														
Pneumocystis pneumonia	●				△	■			●					
Cryptococcal meningitis												■	□	□
Cerebral toxoplasmosis		□	□ ▲						▲					
Oesophageal candidiasis												△	▲	
Cytomegalovirus retinitis										△	■			

Key

	monotherapy	combination therapy
Uncomplicated infections/ first line therapy	△	□
Serious infections/ second line therapy	■	▲
Alternative choice, eg severe infection or 1° treatment failure	○	●

Figure 10.2 Infections and first choice agents. (continued)

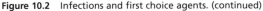

- Check medical and drug history for possible contraindications/interactions.
- Check for previous allergic reactions and look for current signs. Allergies are common.
- Confirm true allergies, where possible, and ensure they are clearly documented.
- Drug interactions are common and preventable, check the patient's current medication.
- Check present renal and hepatic status for contraindications or dosing precautions.

Choice of route

Oral administration with adequate doses is preferred where possible.

BOX 10.3 Parenteral use of anti-infectives

- Intravenous administration is necessary for serious/life threatening infections.
- Comparative safety by i.v. route is an important consideration in choice of agent.
- I.V. administration should be continued until there is clinical control of the infection.
- Comparative efficiency of oral absorption is an important practical consideration (*Switch early from parenteral to oral administration if agent is well absorbed*).
- Intramuscular route is often less reliable than i.v.; avoid where possible.

BOX 10.4 Topical use of anti-infectives

- Avoid topical therapy with agents used systemically
- Topical care (debridement, drainage, lavage) needed with localised infections and consider additional systemic treatment to achieve control of infection/dissemination.
- Aerosolised anti-infective agents may supplement parenteral use in intractable/recurrent pulmonary infections.

Oral absorption of many anti-infective agents is limited by acid/pepsin degradation in the stomach or inefficient absorption in the small intestine. Confidence in the efficacy of an anti-infective agent requires achievement of effective concentrations at the site of infection and so requires the support of pharmacokinetic studies and clinical trials.

Comparative spectra of some anti-infective agents are shown in Figure 10.3.

Choice of dose regimen

Use of inadequate doses of anti-infectives: *subtherapeutic dosing is a common cause of treatment failure.*

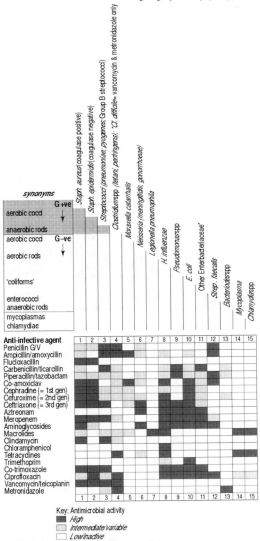

Figure 10.3 Comparative spectra of some anti-infective agents.

BOX 10.5 Dose regimen for anti-infectives

- Ensure adequately high doses.
- Check doses are being *given* at the correct dose interval.
- Consider any dose-related toxicity (such as renal, hepatic, haematological or CNS effects).
- Assess renal function and where necessary adjust doses accordingly.
- Unnecessary switching to second-line agents will prolong an infective episode.
- Mode and duration of parenteral therapy greatly affect outcome and cost of treatment.

The best use of an appropriately chosen anti-infective agent therefore relies on adjustments to the dose, the route and the duration of administration to suit the individual patient. These additional decisions contribute considerably to the overall effectiveness and cost of a treatment episode. Economic considerations are especially important in the choice of anti-infectives in non life-threatening infections and for routine chemoprophylaxis. Local protocols with automatic stop orders enable pharmacists to control the duration of routine courses of anti-infectives.

EVALUATION AND MONITORING

Clear signs of effectiveness should be sought within the first 3–5 days by attention to clinical and laboratory parameters. Monitoring should include screening for signs of toxicity.

BOX 10.6 Clinical monitoring

- Temperature
- Pulse
- Blood pressure
- Respiratory rate
- Physical examination signs
  — (e.g. chest sounds, local redness, swelling, induration, suppuration, peripheral stigmata such as skin rashes, splinter haemorrhages)
- WBC count
- X-ray findings
- Symptomatic improvement
  — (e.g. weakness, dyspnoea, anorexia, malaise, headache, delerium, pain, fever and chills).

> **BOX 10.7 Laboratory monitoring**
>
> • Plasma drug concentrations
>   — to optimise efficacy, minimise toxicity (aminoglycosides, parenteral vancomycin, flucytosine)
> • Biochemical and haematological signs of toxicity
> • Cultures (may take days or weeks for culture negativity)
> • Serum bactericidal titres during use of anti-infectives (target peaks ≥1:8 dilution or ≥1:16 dilution)
>   — used for specific infections (e.g. in neutropenia, endocarditis, acute osteomyelitis in children)

SPECIAL CONSIDERATIONS

Microbial resistance

The increasing availability and use of anti-infective agents has been accompanied by resistance and local patterns of resistance vary widely. Emergence of resistance has affected a range of different organisms with the following presenting particular clinical problems: *S. aureus* (commonly β-lactamase producers and occasionally methicillin resistant *S. aureus* — MRSA); *S. epidermidis* (also methicillin resistant *S. epidermidis* — MRSE); *H. influenzae* and *E. coli* (β-lactamase producers); enterobacteriaceae and pseudomonads (aminoglycoside resistance); and more recently *S. pneumoniae* (penicillin resistance) and *S. faecalis* (aminoglycoside resistance, while vancomycin resistance has been reported in the USA).

Antimicrobial prophylaxis

Medical indications
Control of spread of infection in particular epidemics (tuberculosis, bacterial meningitis, whooping cough) may require use of prophylaxis for treating contacts.

Surgical indications
Prophylaxis requires effective doses administered immediately preoperatively and/or perioperatively to ensure tissue concentrations at the point of incision. Antibacterial use beyond 24 hours constitutes *treatment* and should be discouraged in the absence of infection. Surgical prophylaxis usually requires parenteral administration. These simple points of effective use require continuous pharmaceutical vigilance to ensure adherence to guidelines for optimum effectiveness, cost control and the prevention of emergence of resistance.

BOX 10.8 Antimicrobial prophylaxis: acceptable indications

- Where postoperative infection is a common complication (e.g. after surgery to colon/rectum, female genital tract, head/neck and gastroduodenum — especially in patients receiving gastric acid suppression treatment; and contaminated wounds due to surgery on already infected tissues such as infected biliary and urinary tracts).

  In this category there is surgical entry into an area of the body which has its own resident bacterial flora. In colorectal surgery, the gross contamination during surgery also requires prior preparation of the bowel with lavage/purging/additional oral non-absorbed anti-infectives.
- Where infection may destroy the viability of a graft/prosthesis/repair in cardiac, vascular and orthopaedic surgery.
- Prevention of endocarditis in patients with valvular heart disease immediately prior to procedures associated with bacteraemia (e.g. dental surgery, urological investigations).

Treatment of acute sepsis

Pyrexia of unknown origin and other bacteriologically undiagnosed episodes of acute sepsis require the use of a combination of agents to provide broad spectrum cover against G+ve and G−ve aerobes (β-lactam + aminoglycoside or a fluoroquinolone) with additional metronidazole (for anaerobes). Corticosteroids are not effective in septic shock and may be counterproductive.

Immune compromised patients

Patients with haematological malignancies, on cytotoxic chemotherapy or steroids and following organ or bone marrow transplantation are at special risk of infection from a wide range of organisms. Patients with HIV infection are at particular risk of bacterial, fungal and protozoal infections (see Figure 10.2). Profound immune suppression severely affects the patient's capacity to eradicate an infection and often necessitates vigorous prolonged treatment courses with multiple anti-infective agents. Antibacterial coverage requires combinations of two or more of the following: aminoglycosides, extended spectrum β-lactams, or vancomycin (if MRSA is a local problem). Combination treatment is also required to minimise the emergence of resistance during treatment. Serum bactericidal titres are useful for optimising treatment (peak ≥1:16 dilution are associated with increased clinical success). Continuous administration as an option for the use of β-lactam antibiotics remains controversial.

INSULINS

11

K. Taxis

Name of preparations	Species	pH	Physical state	Absorption and effect (hours)		
				Onset	Peak	Duration
Humalog	H	7.0–7.8	Solution	0.25	0.5–1.5	2–5
Humalog Mix25	H	7.0–7.8	Insulin lispro 25%, insulin lispro protamine suspension 75%	0.25	0.5–2	22
Human Actrapid	H	7.0	Solution	0.5	2.5–5.5	8
Human Insulatard	H	7.0	Isophane insulin	2	4–12	24
Human Mixtard 10	H	7.2–7.4	Soluble 10%, isophane 90%	0.5	2–12	24
Human Mixtard 20	H	7.2–7.4	Soluble 20%, isophane 80%	0.5	2–12	24
Human Mixtard 30	H	7.2–7.4	Soluble 30%, isophane 70%	0.5	2–12	24
Human Mixtard 40	H	7.2–7.4	Soluble 40%, isophane 60%	0.5	2–12	24
Human Mixtard 50	H	7.2–7.4	Soluble 50%, isophane 50%	0.5	2–12	24
Human Monotard	H	7.0	Insulin zinc suspension (amorphous 30%, crystalline 70%)	3	7–15	24
Human Ultratard	H	7.0	Crystalline insulin zinc suspension	4–8	8–24	24–28
Human Velosulin	H	7.0	Solution	0.5	1–3	8
Humulin I	H	6.9–7.5	Crystalline isophane insulin	0.5	2–8	22
Humulin Lente	H	7.0–7.8	Insulin zinc suspension (amorphous 30%, crystalline 70%)	1	3–9	23
Humulin M1	H	6.9–7.5	Soluble 10%, isophane 90%	0.5	1–12	22
Humulin M2	H	6.9–7.5	Soluble 20%, isophane 80%	0.5	1–12	22
Humulin M3	H	6.9–7.5	Soluble 30%, isophane 70%	0.5	1–12	22

Table 11.1 Insulin preparations currently marketed in the UK

(contd)

Table 11.1	Insulin preparations currently marketed in the UK (contd)					

Name of preparations	Species	pH	Physical state	Absorption and effect (hours)		
				Onset	Peak	Duration
Humulin M4	H	6.9–7.5	Soluble 40%, isophane 60%	0.5	1–12	23
Humulin M5	H	6.9–7.5	Soluble 50%, isophane 50%	0.5	1–12	22
Humulin S	H	7.0–7.8	Solution	0.5	1–6	12
Humulin Zn	H	7.0–7.8	Crystalline insulin zinc suspension	2	4–20	25
Hypurin Bovine Isophane	B	7.2	Isophane insulin	0.5–2	6–12	18–24
Hypurin Bovine Lente	B	7.3	Insulin zinc suspension (amorphous 30%, crystalline 70%)	2	8–12	30
Hypurin Bovine Neutral	B	7.0	Solution	0.5–1	2–5	6–8
Hypurin Bovine PZI	B	7.2	Protamine zinc sulfate suspension	4–6	10–20	24–36
Hypurin Porcine Biphasic Isophane	P	6.9–7.8	Soluble 30%, isophane 70%	0.5–1	4–12	18–24
Hypurin Porcine Isophane	P	6.9–7.8	Isophane insulin	0.5–2	6–12	18–24
Hypurin Porcine Neutral	P	7.0	Solution	0.5–1	2–5	6–8
Lentard MC	P,B	7.0	Insulin zinc suspension (amorphous porcine MC insulin 30%, crystalline bovine MC insulin 70%)	3	7–16	24
Pork Actrapid	P	7.0	Solution	0.5	1–3	8
Pork Insulatard	P	7.3	Isophane insulin	2	4–12	24
Pork Mixtard 30	P	7.0	Soluble 30%, microcystalline isophane insulin 70%	0.5	4–8	22

H = Human, B = Bovine, P = Porcine
Time for absorption and effect may be prolonged in patients with high titres of anti-insulin antibodies.

PARENTERAL NUTRITION IN ADULTS 12

A. Scott, M. Lee

The decision to provide nutritional support should be made on the basis of an informed assessment of the patient's condition. Parenteral nutrition (PN) should be reserved for conditions when the gut is not available or requires rest and certain catabolic states where the nitrogen/energy requirements cannot be met by the enteral route. It must be remembered that parenteral nutrition requires considerable expertise and calls for heavy commitment in back-up services compared with those needed for enteral nutrition. Enteral feeding should be used wherever possible either by mouth, nasogastric or percutaneous endoscopic gastrostomy (PEG) tube.

A team approach to nutritional support is the recommended way to coordinate the management of patient feeding within a hospital. The team should include a doctor, specialist nurse, dietician, biochemist and pharmacist.

COMPONENTS OF A PARENTERAL NUTRITION SOLUTION

Parenteral nutrition regimens should be designed to provide all substances present in the normal diet, in similar amounts and proportions to those absorbed from the gastrointestinal tract. Parenteral nutrition should aim to supply fluid, nitrogen (as amino acids), energy (as carbohydrate and lipid), electrolytes, trace elements and vitamins.

1. Fluid

Requirements are approximately 2–2.5 litres water per day and in addition any abnormal losses e.g. fistula. This will vary for renal patients or patients with congestive heart failure who may require less.

2. Nitrogen

Patients require approximately 0.15–0.3 g/kg/day of nitrogen (1–2 g of amino acids/kg/day) Generally the average patient will receive between 9–14 g of nitrogen per day. Burns patients are extremely stressed and may require up to 2.5 g amino acids/kg/day. Hepatically compromised patients may require as little as 0.5–1 g amino acids/kg/day. Monitoring parameters include urea nitrogen concentrations in plasma and urine.

Different commercial sources of nitrogen are available in terms as grams of nitrogen per litre. They should contain both essential and non-essential amino acids. Commercial amino acid solutions are available which include electrolytes, minimising or eliminating the need for aseptic addition of electrolytes, or without electrolytes to give greater flexibility. The BNF contains information listing the contents of the different parenteral nutrition products available.

3. Energy

To avoid metabolic complications, the calculation of a patient's energy requirements should be based on assessment of a number of factors, in particular:

- age of patient — with younger patients requiring more calories than older patients
- disease state — requirements higher for first few days after surgery. Catabolic patients require extra calories
- level of activity — ambulant patients require more than bed-bound patients.

As a guide, 25–50 kcal/kg/day should be provided, with 30–40 kcal/kg/day the normal optimum range. A balanced combination of carbohydrate and fat provides the best source of energy with 30–50% of the daily energy requirements provided as lipid depending on the patient's clinical condition.

Carbohydrate as energy source

Glucose is the carbohydrate of choice for parenteral nutrition, available either in a range of concentrations of 5 to 70% w/v. A normal maximum of 5g/kg/24h should be used. The energy value of glucose is 4 kcal per gram. The approximate energy content of the various strengths of glucose available is shown in Table 12.1.

Table 12.1   Approximate energy content of various strengths of glucose

Glucose conc. w/v	Approx. energy content per litre (kcal)
5%	200
10%	400
15%	600
20%	800
40%	1600
50%	2000
70%	2800

BOX 12.1 Advantages and disadvantages of carbohydrate as an energy source

Advantages:
- cheap and readily available
- effectively metabolised in presence of insulin and phosphate
- stimulates insulin release therefore encouraging nitrogen retention in muscles.

Disadvantages:
- concentrated solutions are hypertonic which limits peripheral infusion depending on tonicity
- major complications — hyperglycaemia and glycosurea.
- fatty acid deficiency can occur if used alone as energy source.

Lipid as energy source

Available usually as soya bean oil in an oil in water emulsion (consisting of fractionated soya oil, phospholipids and glycerol) in 10, 20 and 30% w/v concentrations. The calorific value is 9 kcal per gram. Infusions containing long chain triglycerides (LCT) and combinations of long and medium chain triglycerides (LCT/MCT) are available. There is evidence that medium chain triglycerides are more beneficial in critically ill patients. The approximate energy content of the various strengths of lipid emulsion available is shown in Table 12.2.

BOX 12.2 Advantages and disadvantages of lipid as an energy source

Advantages:
- high energy content per unit volume
- isotonic allowing peripheral infusion
- source of essential fatty acids and vitamin E.

Disadvantages:
- expensive compared to glucose
- lipid droplets may interfere with routine blood tests
- some patients may have reduced ability to clear fat from bloodstream.

If the patient has increased prothrombin times or abnormal liver function tests, their capacity to handle lipid may be impaired.

Table 12.2 Approximate energy content of various strengths of emulsion		
Lipid conc. w/v	Volume (ml)	Approx. energy content (kcal)
10%	500	550
20%	500	1000
30%	333	1000

4. Electrolytes

Fluid and electrolyte abnormalities should be corrected whenever possible before starting parenteral nutrition. Electrolyte contents in parenteral nutrition tend to be empirical depending on urine and blood monitoring results (Table 12.3).

Table 12.3 Electrolytes in parenteral nutrition			
Electrolyte	Average daily requirement (mmol)	Recommended blood monitoring frequency	Normal serum range (mmol/l)
Sodium	80–120	Daily	135–145
Potassium	80–120	Daily	3.5–5.0
Calcium*	5–10	Twice weekly	2.15–2.55
Magnesium	5–14	Twice weekly	0.7–1.0
Phosphate	10–30	Twice weekly	0.6–1.25
Chloride	Varies, decrease if acidotic	Daily	95–105
Bicarbonate	Varies — acetate more stable	Daily	23–30

*Calcium is extensively bound to albumin. Only 'corrected' calcium results which take into account albumin levels should be used.

5. Trace elements

Trace elements are essential components of enzymes and co-enzymes in many biochemical processes within the body (e.g. synthesis of nucleic acids, membrane transport and prevention of free radical damage by active oxygen species).

Small amounts of trace elements, e.g. zinc, copper, manganese, iron and selenium are considered essential for health. The usual adult basal requirements can be met by the administration of 10 ml of Additrace daily. This will supply Fe 20 micromol, Zn 100 micromol, Mn 5 micromol, Cu 20 micromol, Cr 0.2 micromol, Se 0.4 micromol, Mo 0.2 micromol, F 50 micromol, I 1 micromol.

6. Vitamins

Deficiencies can occur rapidly in malnourished patients. Water and fat soluble vitamin preparations are available.

- *Multibionta*: water soluble vitamins and fat soluble vitamins A and E
- *Solivito N*: nine water soluble vitamins
- *Vitlipid N Adult*: fat soluble vitamins A, D_2, E and K_1 as an oil in water emulsion
- *Cernevit*: combination of both water soluble and fat soluble vitamins (but not vitamin K).

The high vitamin A content of Multibionta is undesirable in patients with liver disease in whom B and C complex injection (Pabrinex i.v.) with the higher thiamine content, alternated with Solivito N, may be an advantage.

> ⚠ Loading doses of vitamin B_{12}, folic acid and Vitamin K_1 are advised when deficiency is likely, e.g. malabsorption syndrome.

Table 12.4 gives the typical requirements of three types of patient and a suggested regimen suitable for peripheral administration.

Table 12.4 Typical Regimens	Postoperative	ICU trauma	Renal	Peripheral administration
Volume	2500 ml	2500 ml	1500 ml	3000 ml
Nitrogen	12 g	15 g	9 g	9 g
Total energy (kcal)	2000	2400	1550	1800
Lipid (kcal)	1000	1000	550	1100
Sodium (mmol)	100	100	70	70
Potassium (mmol)	80	120	30	80
Calcium (mmol)	5	7.5	5	7.5
Magnesium (mmol)	5	5	2	5
Phosphate* (mmol)	18	30	10	20

Does not include any phosphate present in lipid component.

METABOLIC COMPLICATIONS OF PN FEEDING

- *Dehydration and overhydration* — caused by fluid and electrolyte imbalances usually due to miscalculation and failure to account for fluid loss or intake.

Complications with carbohydrate

- *Hyperglycaemia* — if excessive glucose is administered, is too rapidly infused or when glucose tolerance is impaired, e.g. in stressed or septic patients. May lead to osmotic diuresis and dehydration.
- *Hypoglycaemia* — can occur if PN regimens containing highly concentrated glucose solution are stopped abruptly.
- *Hyperosmolar coma* — may develop following untreated hyperglycaemia and may be fatal.
- *Respiratory distress* — the infusion of excessive glucose can precipitate CO_2 accumulation in patients with impaired ventilatory capacity.

Complications with lipid

- *Over infusion* — caused by over infusion at excessive rates.
- *Acute reactions* — uncommon and transient, e.g. fever, shivering.
- *Impaired utilisation* — particularly in severely ill patients and those with renal or hepatic insufficiency and uncompensated diabetes.
- *Impaired pulmonary function* — especially if plasma hyperlipaemic.

> It is therefore important to check the clearance of infused lipid emulsions to avoid hyperlipidaemia.

Complications with amino acid infusions

- *Elevation of blood urea* — slightly elevated but not above normal if renal function adequate. Continued rise may be caused by dehydration or renal impairment.
- *Hyperammonaemia* — may occur in patients with liver disease.
- *Acid-base disturbances* — mainly hyperchloraemic metabolic acidosis especially in patients with renal impairment.
- *Hepatic toxicity* — elevation of AST, ALT, alkaline phosphatase and bilirubin levels reaching a peak after 1–4 weeks but usually returning to normal upon discontinuation. Sepsis may contribute to hepatic disturbance.

Other complications

- *Essential fatty acid deficiency* — when carbohydrate infused as sole energy source, avoided by infusion of lipid emulsion.
- *Mineral and trace element deficiency* — sodium and potassium imbalances, hypophosphataemia, hypomagnesaemia and hypocalcaemia can occur. Zinc, copper and other trace element deficiencies may become apparent with long-term PN.
- *Vitamin deficiency* — especially vitamin B1, biotin, folate and vitamin C. Acute folate deficiency has been reported with the precipitation of pancytopaenia.

FORMULATION COMPATIBILITY AND STABILITY

The degradation of amino acids and vitamins in compounded PN formulations is affected by temperature, daylight and oxygen content. Compounded mixtures should be stored in a refrigerator until shortly before administration. PN mixtures should be protected from exposure to daylight during administration especially if the formulation does not include lipid.

The oxygen content of compounded PN bags is affected by the filling technique used. The greater the oxygen content, the higher the rate of ascorbic acid degradation. The use of multi-layer bags will reduce oxygen permeability and they are preferable to EVA bags.

Precipitation of calcium phosphate in particular can occur in PN mixtures. The causes of the reaction are relatively complex.

- *pH of the solution* — precipitation unlikely to occur in solutions at or below pH 5.4 but more likely as the solution rises towards neutrality (pH 7). The main determinants of pH in PN mixtures are the commercial source of the amino acid, concentration of amino acids in final mixture and inorganic phosphate source. As calcium and phosphate ions form soluble complexes with amino acids, larger quantities of each ion can be added to PN solutions as the amino acid concentration increases before precipitation occurs.
- *Presence of other divalent cations* — especially magnesium.
- *Type of phosphate solution* — organic phosphate injection does not contain free phosphate ions so precipitation of calcium phosphate is not seen in mixtures containing organic phosphates.
- *Calcium salt used* — in general, proportionately more calcium can be added as the gluconate than the chloride.

• *Temperature* — Calcium gluconate is largely unionised, however, ionisation increases with temperature therefore precipitations is more likely after removal from cold storage. Rising temperature causes a greater dissociation of the calcium salt and increases the likelihood of precipitation. Calcium phosphate precipitation may take up to 24 hours to occur in borderline combinations.

• *Order of addition* — the addition of the phosphate injection to the mixture before the calcium salt can reduce the possibility of precipitation.

Thus the solubility of calcium phosphate is affected by many factors and requires the assessment for precipitation in any particular mixture.

Emulsion stability is influenced by the cation content of a PN bag. As a guide, this can be calculated using the following scoring system:
• Monovalent cations (Na^+, K^+ etc.) — contribution 1 'point' per mmol
• Divalent cations (Ca^{2+}, Mg^{2+} etc.) — contribution 64 'points' per mmol
• Trivalent cations (Fe^{3+} etc.) — contribution 729 'points' per mmol
• No. of points per litre = {($1 \times$ total M^+) + ($64 \times$ total M^{2+}) + ($729 \times M^{3+}$)}/bag volume in litres.

In practice, this means that changes in sodium and potassium content will not significantly affect the stability but calcium and magnesium being divalent ions will have a considerable effect on the emulsion stability. Trivalent ions are present in such small quantities that although their 'point' contribution is high the effect on stability is low.

Emulsion stability is also affected by:

• low pH, especially below pH 5
• low and high glucose concentrations
• low lipid concentrations
• commercial source of amino acid solution and concentration of amino acids.

Bicarbonate is often used to correct metabolic acidosis, however, it is too unstable for prolonged storage in PN bags — although short-term stability is acceptable. Acetate is a metabolic precursor of bicarbonate and is more stable in solution. The conversion of acetate is not impaired in those patients with severe hepatic disease. Many amino acid solutions now contain acetate as well as chloride to prevent patients becoming acidotic. Sodium acetate 30% is available commercially as a 'special' within the UK.

Stability data are available by request from companies such as Geistlich, Pharmacia & Upjohn and Baxter Clintec.

Additions to PN bags

All additions must be made under strict aseptic conditions and no additions should be made to bags on the ward. Drugs must never be added to compounded bags unless adequate compatibility and stability data exists. Insulin is adsorbed onto the plastic of PN bags and giving sets, giving rise to unpredictable delivery to the patient.

ADMINISTRATION OF PN

Peripheral

This route is usually recommended for short-term use only. As it usually involves administration into a small blood vessel with low blood flow, the infusion of irritant (hypertonic and low pH) solutions usually causes pain and carries a risk of thrombophlebitis at the vein site. Solutions should ideally be isotonic, however, in practice this is difficult to achieve. As a guide, osmolarity of the final mixture should be not more than 700–800 mOsm/kg.

A small gauge silastic or polyurethane catheter should be used, e.g. 23 gauge. Teflon coated cannulae should not be used. Blood flow to the area can be improved by the use of a 5 mg GTN patch applied daily, distal to the cannula. Hydrocortisone 1% cream should be applied twice daily distal to the cannula site. The site should be changed on evidence of phlebitis.

Central

Carbohydrate based, low pH parenteral nutrition regimens are usually hypertonic and therefore require infusion through a central venous catheter into the superior vena cava. A dedicated lumen must be used for intravenous feeding and this should not be used for the administration of drugs or blood, routine sampling or measurement of central venous pressure.

Flushing

The line should be flushed with sodium chloride 0.9% w/v injection (5–10 ml) before and after administration of PN. Heparinised saline injection (10 units per ml) should then be used to keep the line patent if administration is interrupted.

Blockage

Catheter obstruction may be caused by thrombus formation, precipitation of minerals or by the deposit of waxy substances from lipid containing feeds and endogenous lipids. Should a blockage occur it may be possible to remove the obstruction by gentle irrigation with heparinised saline. Do not exert excessive pressure. If irrigation does not work, consider the use of urokinase (5000 units in 2 ml of sodium chloride 0.9% injection) to lyse any fibrin clots. Urokinase is not effective against mineral or lipid deposits.

Ethanol 70% injection can be used to dissolve waxy lipid deposits and aseptically prepared 0.1 M hydrochloric acid has been used to clear mineral deposits.

Suspected infection of central line

If infection of the line is suspected, discontinue the PN immediately and discard the remainder of the bag. Inject heparinised saline into the catheter. A sample of blood for culture should be taken. A peripheral venous blood culture should also be performed. Establish a peripheral intravenous infusion to administer electrolytes and fluid. The catheter entry site should be inspected using aseptic technique. If the entry site is red, inflamed or discharging a swab for culture should be taken. Obtain a specimen of urine and swabs from other wound sites and look for other sources of infection.

If the patient is stable but febrile the catheter may be left in position but not used. If no organisms are identified from the blood culture within 48 hours the catheter may be used again for infusion.

The catheter should be removed if the patient is severely ill and no other source of infection can be found. The tip of the catheter should be sent for microbiological culture.

For susceptible gram positive bacteria, consider the use of Teicoplanin injection. It is recommended that all the lumen of multi-lumen catheters be treated.

Filters.   Bacteria and endotoxin retaining particulate filters are available with a pore size of 0.2 micron that allows the infusion of non-lipid containing PN solutions. For feeds with a lipid component, a 1.2 micron filter is available that removes the particulates and precipitates that can contaminate nutrient admixtures.

Infusion pumps.   Parenteral nutrition is usually infused over a 12–24 hour period on hospital wards using a volumetric infusion pump. If glucose has not be given prior to the start of the feed, the first PN bag may be administered at a reduced infusion rate for the first six hours then the infusion rate increased gradually to full rate to reduce the risk of hyperglycaemia.

Home PN patients may infuse over 10–16 hours with 'step-up' and 'step-down' administration, although this may not always be necessary.

Should the nutrition bag be damaged, e.g. spiked during insertion of the administration sets, and no other bag be available, administer a glucose infusion of a strength as close as possible to the concentration contained in the compounded bag at the same rate.

PATIENT MONITORING

Successful monitoring prevents most of the complications associated with parenteral nutritional support. Table 12.5 shows suggested monitoring parameters and frequency.

Table 12.5 Suggested monitoring parameters	
Clinical	**Frequency**
Patient examination	Daily
TPR and BP	4 hourly
Fluid balance	Daily
Ward urine analysis	4–6 hourly
Body weight	Daily if possible
Biochemistry	
Urea, electrolytes, creatinine	Daily
Glucose*	4 hourly BM sticks initially for 2 days then daily or as indicated
Calcium, magnesium, phosphate	Twice weekly
Liver function test	Twice weekly
Trace elements	Monthly if possible
Acid-base balance	Daily
Haematology	
Full blood count	Daily
Prothrombin time	Twice weekly
Albumin	Twice weekly

Hyperglycaemia can be corrected by administering, via a syringe pump, a short acting insulin e.g. Actrapid insulin, according to a sliding scale. Never add insulin to PN bags.

HOME PARENTERAL NUTRITION

With the issue in 1995 of the Department of Health's Executive Letter (95)5 'Purchasing high-tech healthcare for patients at home', which changed the method by which the NHS in England funds parenteral nutrition at home, the contract for the provision of nutrient solutions, equipment and all other needs has now to be between a Health Authority, acting as purchaser, and a supplier. Pharmacists are increasingly being required to be involved in decisions regarding the specifications of contracts for these patients. For these patients to have a good quality of life, they require not only management of the disease state, but also a clinical support programme, training in techniques of PN and an organised system for the provision of solutions and equipment.

There should be a discharge plan specific to home parenteral nutrition and a protocol for teaching patients/carers prior to discharge.

Pharmacists should be involved in:

- formulation of the nutrient solution to meet the needs of the patient
- the specification of the quality of nutrient solutions in regard to stability and safety with the aim being to reduce manipulation of the feed to a minimum
- how to store and check nutrient solutions, flushing solutions and other drugs
- how the solutions will be packed and delivered
- how the 'cold chain' will be maintained during transportation to the home
- selection of the infusion pump, repair and servicing arrangements.

Quality criteria for clinical services and the supply of nutrient fluids and equipment are contained in 'Home Parenteral Nutrition' published by the British Association for Parenteral and Enteral Nutrition.

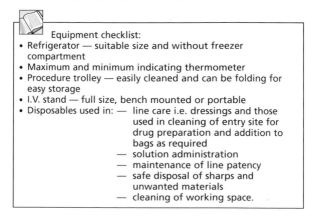

Equipment checklist:
- Refrigerator — suitable size and without freezer compartment
- Maximum and minimum indicating thermometer
- Procedure trolley — easily cleaned and can be folding for easy storage
- I.V. stand — full size, bench mounted or portable
- Disposables used in: — line care i.e. dressings and those used in cleaning of entry site for drug preparation and addition to bags as required
  — solution administration
  — maintenance of line patency
  — safe disposal of sharps and unwanted materials
  — cleaning of working space.

REFERENCES

Department of Health 1995 Purchasing high-tech healthcare for patients at home. Department of Health Executive letter (95) 5. HMSO, London

FURTHER READING

Barnet M, Cosslett A 1995 Parenteral nutritional formulation. In: Payne-James J, Grimble G, Silk D (eds) Artificial nutrition in clinical practice. Edward Arnold, London

Baumgartner TG (ed) 1991 Clinical guide to parenteral micronutrition, 2nd edn. Fujisawa, USA

Hammersmith Hospitals NHS Trust 1995 Drug and blood products policies. Hammersmith Hospitals NHS Trust, London

Trissel LA 1988 Handbook of injectable drugs, 9th edn. AHSP, Bethesda, USA

Wood S (ed) 1994 Home parenteral nutrition. The British Association for Parenteral and Enteral Nutrition, Maidenhead

Monitoring

PRESCRIPTION MONITORING

13

R Batty, K Brackley

SCREENS FOR MONITORING PRESCRIPTIONS

Ideally, pharmacists would be in a position to review all patient data and play a major role in tailoring individual drug therapy, but there is simply not enough time to do so. It is therefore imperative that they develop skills of problem detection using readily available data, i.e. the prescription, the appearance of the patient and other circumstantial evidence of drug related problems. Talking to the patient may help corroborate the circumstantial information and also provide extra information.

Most prescriptions are seen on the hospital ward, or in the community pharmacist's shop. The types of accessible patient data in these locations differ, thus the prescription monitoring screens will differ. This chapter summarises structured approaches for prescription monitoring for each location. They are intended as a stimulus for discussion rather than authoritative documents.

Prescription monitoring on the hospital ward

During their regular visits to the wards, pharmacists need to provide a fast, efficient service that is of benefit to patients. Observing the patient, reviewing the prescription chart and talking to him/her allows the pharmacist to identify drug related problems. This may lead the pharmacist to check specific information in the patient's notes or elsewhere. Using these data from the prescription and elsewhere, along with their own clinical knowledge, leads to the problem orientated approach to patient monitoring. Full details of the approach can be found elsewhere (Wood 1993, Hart et al 1988). The following describes the approach to prescription review.

Information sources

It is assumed that the prescription sheets and observations such as temperature and blood pressure are kept at the end of the patients' beds. The pharmacist visits each bed in turn, observing the patient, talking to him/her and reviewing the charts at the end of the bed. The pharmacist would not scrutinise the case notes or the nursing Kardex routinely; only if the initial screen indicated a need to do so. It is assumed that the pharmacist understands local prescribing procedures.

The screen. The approach can be summarised in the LANOT checklist (Batty & Barber 1991) (Table 13.1). There follows some further explanation of the questions asked in the LANOT. This explanation is not exhaustive and there are many other examples of each point in the checklist.

Table 13.1 LANOT prescription monitoring checklist for ward pharmacists (Look Around, New drugs, Old drugs, TTAs) (Batty & Barber 1991)

'LANOT' prescription monitoring checklist for ward pharmacists

---

Look around
Before you look at the prescribed drugs, ask yourself the following questions.

1. Has the patient more than one prescription sheet? (e.g. separate i.v., cytotoxic, TPN, variable dose).
2. Ward name/consultant/junior doctor — do they give clues as to the disease the patient may be suffering from?
3. Age and weight of patient — have they any implications for dose?
4. Diet — does it indicate renal failure, obesity, liver failure, patient unable to swallow solids (i.e. diet), etc?
5. What is the patient's appearance (jaundiced, oedematous, cyanosed, breathless or unconscious)? What is their race?

You will not have time to look in every patient's notes, so look for pointers of certain diseases and refer to case notes to confirm your suspicions of the diagnoses. Pointers may include (i) appearance of patient (ii) diet (iii) other drugs (for example Titralac in renal patients; vitamins B and C strong i.v. injection in liver patients; frusemide in congestive cardiac failure (CCF)).

New drugs
For each drug prescribed, ask yourself the following questions.

1. Is this the most effective drug for the disease — is there a less expensive, but equally effective drug available?
2. Is the dose and/or frequency appropriate, particularly with regard to renal and hepatic function, cardiac status (CCF), age and weight of the patient?
3. Is the form or route the most appropriate (e.g. consider SR tablets with nasogastric tube, oral/IM/i.v./rectal bioavailability etc)?
4. Does the patient have a documented allergy to the drug or to a drug with a similar structure?
5. Will the drug interact with other drugs the patient is receiving, either to antagonise or duplicate a pharmacological action?
6. Does the patient have another disease that would contraindicate or caution the use of the drug?

7. For a drug to be given by the i.v. route — is it compatible with the infusion fluid? Is the duration of infusion appropriate. Is it compatible with other drugs it might mix with in the drug tubing or cannula?

8. Has the drug been added to treat a symptom caused by another drug (e.g. the addition of an anti-emetic may be because the patient is nauseated by theophylline, potassium chloride, digoxin etc)?

9. Is there anything in diet which will affect drug therapy or vice versa?

10. Do we stock it? Is it in the formulary?
   Yes — is it ward stock or does it need to be dispensed?
   No — has the patient their own supply? What alternatives with a similar effect do we stock?

Old drugs
For drugs already in the patient's regimen, the following questions should be asked.

1. Did the dispensary supply it and did the dispenser check all points in the section above?

2. Is the drug still needed (especially antibiotic agent)?

3. Is the drug working?

4. Does the dose need modifying (e.g. chlormethiazole in alcoholics)?

5. Is the patient receiving the drug (check for 'X' in administration record section)?

6. Is there a relationship between the drugs the patient is taking and events noted at the end of the bed?

TTAs
For TTA drugs, the following questions should be asked.

1. Are inpatient details the same as TTAs? If no, are the differences reasonable?

2. Does the patient still need the items?

3. Has steady state been achieved?

4. Are items from all prescription sheets included?

Pharmaceutical Journal 1991; **247**:242–244

Look around. The patient's environment should be considered. This can give important clues about the patient, the types of disease(s) they may be suffering from, drug handling and/or administration problems.

• *Has the patient more than one prescription sheet?*
A drug on one sheet may interact with a drug on another sheet. Sometimes duplication of therapy can occur, e.g. an antibiotic prescribed intravenously on one sheet and orally on another.

- *Ward name/consultant/junior doctor*

A patient on a liver ward may have abnormal handling of drug eliminated by hepatic metabolism. It may also be advisable to avoid hepatotoxic drugs in such a patient. Similarly a patient under the care of a doctor specialising in renal medicine may have impaired renal function, necessitating dosage adjustment of some drugs.

- *Age and weight of the patient*

Neonates often have poor hepatic and renal clearance and absorption via the gastrointestinal tract may be variable.

The elderly often have declining end organ function and altered target organ sensitivity.

- *Diet — does it indicate a patient problem?*

Special dietary requirements are sometimes listed among the end of bed information and altered protein, sodium and/or potassium may indicate liver or renal disease. Patients who are fluid restricted may have poor renal or cardiac function.

- *What is the patient's appearance?*

A patient who has 'nil by mouth' signs, or is vomiting may need drugs to be administered by a non-oral route, while a patient with a nasogastric tube may need oral drugs administered as liquids. Certain races may have altered drug handling, e.g. some black hypertensives do not respond well to ACE inhibitors.

New drugs.

- *Is this the most effective drug for the disease?*

The drug should be the most effective for the disease, considering other concurrent disease, other prescribed drugs, age, known drug allergies, hepatic and renal function, convenience and cost.

- *Is the dose and/or frequency appropriate?*

The dosage regimen should be appropriate for the patient's age, weight, hepatic, renal and cardiac function. Concomitant drugs may affect dose.

- *Is the form and/or route the most appropriate?*

The form and route should be appropriate for the patients. A patient with a nasogastric tube will require liquid forms of oral medicines or non-oral routes. Patients with a history of non-compliance may benefit from modified release preparations which can be given less frequently.

- *Does the patient have a documented allergy to the drug?*

The choice of drug may be influenced by an allergy to the drug or one of a similar structure.

- *Will the drug interact with other drugs?*
Some drugs antagonise the effects of others while some duplicate and enhance the effects of others. Any such drug interactions should be managed so that the dose of each drug is appropriate. Alternatively, the pharmacist can recommend changing one of the drugs to another which is also indicated for the disease and is from a different drug class.

- *Has a drug been added to treat a symptom caused by another drug?*
The adverse drug effect should be assessed and a decision taken as to whether it is better to change to another therapy rather than introduce a drug to treat the adverse effect.

- *Is there anything in the diet which will affect drug therapy or vice versa?*
Where food can affect the absorption of a drug, the drug should be given at an appropriate time in relation to meals. Where the diet restricts the intake of a particular nutrient, e.g. sodium, a drug formulated to have non or low levels of that nutrient may need to be chosen.

- *Do we stock it?*
Once the above questions have been answered, a supply of the drug should be initiated according to local policies.

Old drugs.

- *Did the dispensary staff supply it and did the dispenser complete the new drugs check?*
Dispensary staff do not have access to the information around the patient and so cannot fully assess if the prescribed drugs are appropriate. This can be checked at the next ward visit by a pharmacist.

- *Is the drug still needed?*
Some drug therapies should be continued for life, while others need be given for a short period, often as a course. Sometimes a patient is continued on therapy long after the 'course' has finished.

- *Is the drug working?*
The response to the drug should be assessed to ensure it is adequate and appropriate. If it is inadequate or causing unacceptable side-effects, the dose and/or the drug should be changed.

- *Does the dose need modifying?*
Sometimes the dose of a drug needs adjusting as therapy continues. This may be a dose increase because the drug induces its own metabolism (e.g. carbamazepine) or a tailing down of the dose before stopping the drug, e.g. prednisolone for some acute asthma attacks.

• *Is the patient receiving the drug?*
The administration record section of the prescription sheet may indicate the patient is not receiving the drug. Failure to follow the prescribed regimen may be a reason for an inadequate response. The reasons for non-administration should be followed up. If appropriate, alternative ways of ensuring the drug is given should be offered.

• *Is there a relationship between the drugs the patient is taking and the events at the end of the bed?*
The end of bed information can give indication of some common side-effects of drugs such as altered bowel habits, nausea and vomiting. Such effects should be assessed and managed appropriately.

Prescription monitoring in the community

Like prescription monitoring in hospital, monitoring in the community should be patient focused. The patient's condition and therapy should be considered as a whole. Items presented singly for dispensing should not be viewed out of context of the patient's entire regimen, including over-the-counter (OTC) medicines and alternative therapies.

This presents several challenges in the community as, unlike colleagues in hospital, community pharmacists do not have ready access to patients' medical records, and the pharmacist may only see the patient's representative.

Information sources
Although access to GP held records may be limited, the community pharmacist has three valuable information sources available.

Patient medication record (PMR). In addition to the record of dispensed medicines, information about the indication for each medicine should be elicited from the patient or prescriber. This, and additional information, can be built on successive occasions if necessary.

OTC medicines purchased for the patient should be recorded wherever possible as these can provide valuable information about the effectiveness or side-effects of prescribed therapy, e.g. a patient buying regular laxatives who is taking co-dydramol may require a review of their analgesic therapy.

In order to maximise the PMR, information should be recorded in an easily used format. It should include a profile of:

• patient's current therapy
• indications for the use of each medicine
• past medication history

- allergies
- any personal information such as age and weight, special diets
- any other relevant medical information such as hepatic and renal function
- pharmaceutical care issues such as preferences for plain lids, use of compliance aids.

The patient.   Talking to the patient is an essential step in determining what medicines they are currently taking. This may vary from the regimen recorded on both GP and pharmacy records.

Talking to the patient and *probing* can determine:

- *what* medicines (prescribed and purchased) they are taking
- *how* they are taking them
- *why* there are variations from the expected regimen
- *what* medicine related problems they are experiencing (including any side-effects)
- *what* measures they have taken themselves (if any) to overcome any medicine-related problems.

Personal knowledge.   A community pharmacist will build up considerable knowledge of the patient and local prescribing preferences which will assist in the review process.

When access to GP held records is possible, these may supplement pharmacists' knowledge of the patient. Discussion with the GP may yield the same information. If the prescriber is not willing to release this information a signed consent from the patient may be necessary. Ideally the GP and pharmacist can work together as part of the health care team to optimise therapy. To achieve this face-to-face meetings on a regular basis may be beneficial.

Prioritising

Ideally a community pharmacist would review the therapy of each patient. However, time constraints make this difficult, therefore prioritising of patients is important. Patient groups such as the elderly, house bound and those on multiple medication should be targeted.

Once the available patient information is collected, therapy should be reviewed. The following adaptation of LANOT (Batty & Barber 1991) could be used as a guide for both new and existing drugs.

- *Is the patient still taking the drug?* The regular prescribing and dispensing of a drug does not ensure it is being taken or taken as intended. Likely adherence can be determined by talking to the patient.

• *Is therapy still required for an indication?* Some drug therapies should be continued for life, while others need to be given for a short period, often as a course. Sometimes a patient is continued on therapy long after the 'course' has finished, e.g. a patient still taking a NSAID intended for short-term use after a back injury 6 months ago.

• *Is the drug still working?* The response to the drug should be assessed to ensure it is adequate and appropriate. If inadequate or causing side-effects, the dose and/or drug should be changed.

• *Is this the most effective drug for this indication?* The drug should be the most effective for the disease, considering other concurrent disease, other prescribed drugs, age, known drug allergies, hepatic and renal function, convenience, patient preference and cost.

— Does current evidence show that there is a less expensive, but equally effective alternative available?

— Does current evidence show medication should be added to the regimen? e.g. a steroid inhaler needs adding to a bronchodilator inhaler only therapy when the patient requires the bronchodilator more than once a day.

• *Is the dose and frequency appropriate?* The dosage regimen should be appropriate, particularly with regard to renal and hepatic function, cardiac status, age and weight of the patient. Concomitant drugs may affect dose.

• *Is the timing of doses appropriate?* The timing of some drugs is critical for maximum effectiveness, e.g. the timing of taking long acting nitrates to allow for nitrate-free periods.

• *Is the dosage form the most appropriate?* The dosage form should be appropriate for the patient, drug and condition treated, e.g. modified release nifedipine — is the frequency correct for specific preparation? Has a modified release NSAID formulation been prescribed for occasional analgesic use?

• *Does the patient have a documented allergy?* Does the patient have a documented allergy to the drug or to a drug with a similar structure?

• *Will the drug interact with other drugs?* Will the drug interact with other drugs the patient is receiving (prescribed and purchased), either to antagonise or duplicate a pharmacological action? If your computer highlights an interaction how significant is it for *this* patient? e.g. a patient prescribed warfarin and aspirin — is the patient taking regular low dose aspirin or using larger doses intermittently for analgesia?

• *Any contraindications?* Does the patient have another disease that would contraindicate or caution the use of the drug? e.g. use of a beta-blocker in an asthmatic patient.

• *Has the drug been added to treat a symptom caused by another drug?* The adverse drug effect should be assessed and a decision taken as to whether it is better to change to another therapy rather than introduce a drug to treat the adverse effect, e.g. ranitidine prescribed to treat NSAID induced dyspepsia.

• *Is there anything in the diet which will affect drug therapy or vice versa?* If the patient is on a special diet, will anything in it affect drug therapy or vice versa? e.g. effect of a low fat diet on griseofulvin absorption.

REFERENCES

Batty R, Barber N 1991 Prescription monitoring for ward pharmacists. Pharmaceutical Journal 247:242–244

Hart LL, Gourley DR, Herfindal ET 1988 Workbook for clinical pharmacy and therapeutics. Williams and Wilkins, Baltimore

Wood J 1993 Clinical skills for the hospital pharmacist: case analysis. Hospital Pharmacy Practice 3:305–309

MEDICATION ADHERENCE

R Walker

14

The term compliance was formerly used when referring to medication-taking behaviour. It is, however, now considered to reflect an authoritarian attitude and has been replaced by the term adherence. As such, adherence to a prescribed medication regimen can be defined as:

> the extent to which a patient's behaviour coincides with the intention of the health advice given.

The success of a medication regimen and the associated level of adherence is multifactorial and influenced by the dynamics of the relationship between the patient and their health care adviser (doctor, nurse, pharmacist etc.), the nature and format of any advice given, and the patient's cognitive and socio-demographic characteristics. One must also be careful not to focus solely on medicine-taking behaviour in isolation. Non-adherence with behavioural recommendations such as diet, exercise, weight loss or smoking cessation, are equally well known and are issues that must also be understood and addressed to ensure the patient has every chance of achieving optimum health gain from any disease management strategy.

Health care advisers are often too enthusiastic and blindly pursue a desire to ensure an individual takes their medication as prescribed. This approach overlooks the autonomy of the individual and the fact that the patient's analysis and actions may be correct, or more appropriate than those of the health care adviser.

No longer is it acceptable that the patient unquestioningly follows the orders of the health professional. The concept of an alliance between the patient and the health professional has emerged and the term 'concordance' introduced to reflect this therapeutic alliance between two parties of equal importance (RPSGB 1997).

MEDICATION NON-ADHERENCE

There are many categories (Box 14.1) and causes of non-adherence (Box 14.2). It is evident that the health care team have a poor understanding of the patient when one realises that between 10% and 20% of prescriptions are not even presented for dispensing (Beardon et al 1993).

BOX 14.1   Categories of non-adherence

- Not having prescription dispensed
- Not taking dose prescribed
- Not taking medicine at prescribed time
- Not taking medication
- Not taking medication for required duration
- Taking additional, non-prescribed medication.

BOX 14.2 Examples of factors that may contribute to poor adherence with a prescribed medication regimen

- Breakdown in communication with health team
- Lack of faith in doctors or medicine
- Dissatisfaction with consultation
- Little perception of seriousness of condition to be treated
- Inadequate understanding of medication regimen
- Absence of long-term support monitoring or follow-up from health care workers
- Occurrence of side-effects
- Packaging/presentation of medication.

Whilst many attempts have been made to classify individuals as adherent or non-adherent, in reality, most people fall between the two extremes. Moreover, the extent of an individual's adherence probably varies on a day to day basis with individuals adherent in one situation, or on one day, not being so on another. A number of methodologies have been developed to monitor non-adherence (Table 14.1) none of which are 100% foolproof.

Table 14.1   Methods to detect medication non-adherence

Method	Comment
Patient interview	Ask patient if they adhere to prescribed regimen. Method of questionable reliability.
Tablet count	Count tablets remaining in container. Tablets absent do not necessarily equate to tablets taken.
Clinic attendance	Opportunity to counsel and/or interview patient. Clinic non-attenders have greater likelihood of being non-adherers.
Measure blood levels of drug	Generally gives indication of short-term adherence unless drug has long half-life.

Table 14.1 Methods to detect medication non-adherence (contd)	
Measure blood levels of marker	Add marker to medicine and measure levels in body. Ethical issues on the safety of a given marker are always a concern.
Electronic medication containers	Opening and closure times of container recorded on a micro-processor in lid of container. Opening of container does not equate to tablets taken. The lids/ containers are expensive. Increased likelihood of Hawthorn effect.

WHEN IS ADHERENCE IMPORTANT?

Adherence with a prescribed medication regimen is particularly important when the level of the drug in blood has to be maintained to control a particular disorder, e.g. anticonvulsant; when a pharmacological effect has to be sustained, e.g. antihypertensive; or when replacement therapy is required, e.g. thyroxine. Some drugs reduce mortality, e.g. angiotensin converting enzyme inhibitors in heart failure; or postpone a morbid event, e.g. use of antihypertensives to avoid stroke, but the majority are given in the hope that they will make people feel better. Unfortunately, whilst physiological measurements may improve, or the treatment brings about the desired effect in terms of reduced mortality or morbidity, the medicine may not make the individual feel better with a consequent adverse influence on adherence.

STRATEGIES TO IMPROVE ADHERENCE

To promote better adherence with prescribed regimens the approach of health care professionals must change. More effort must be made to involve the patients and their carers in the decision-making process. Whilst there is a clear preference for the elderly, or those with a serious acute illness to have greater faith in the treatment proposed by their physician, this must not be assumed and is always worthy of assessment.

In general terms, adherence is more likely to be favourable if the patient is involved in the decision-making process. A well-informed patient, actively participating in his or her own health care with the support of the health care team, is likely to take more responsibility to manage their own health and adhere to the treatment plan. In order to produce this well-informed and motivated patient, it is essential for all members of the team to work together and be aware of each other's input. Good communication by all parties is perhaps one of the critical factors that influences adherence and yet has been overlooked by many. Whilst convention dictates that the pharmacist and physician are key individuals in giving advice and support to the patient, the influence and impact of advice from other sources of health care such as a nurse, or home support from a relative, carer or friend should not be overlooked (Figure 14.1). If the chain of communication breaks down at any point, there is every likelihood that the patient may deviate from optimum adherence.

Pharmacists often provide verbal education and written, individualised information for the patient although the benefits of these strategies alone is unclear. It has been demonstrated that knowledge and satisfaction can be enhanced by using patient information leaflets. Similarly, adherence may be improved by counselling and education, whilst written information has been shown to be most beneficial when used in conjunction with verbal reinforcement. However, few studies have shown benefits to adherence and outcomes, the two most important end-points of any successful strategy (Haynes et al 1996).

What is clear is that patients want more information about the medicines that are prescribed for them. The order of

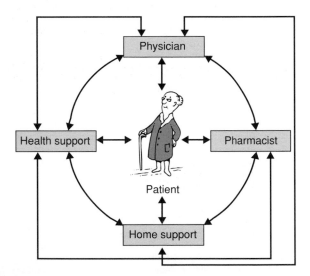

Figure 14.1 Adherence with prescribed medication is influenced by the quality of the communication cycle.

priority that patients place on the various bits of information that may be presented to them is shown in Table 14.2. Provision of this information alone is unlikely to have a significant impact on adherence but is the starting point for the counsel of excellence.

Overall there is little evidence to suggest that low adherence to the taking of medication is disease-specific or regimen-specific except, perhaps, with the exception of psychiatric disorders. Poor adherence is common, even with life threatening conditions (Wright 1993). A systematic review of randomised trials of interventions to assist patients' adherence to their prescribed medication regimen (Haynes et al 1996) revealed a small number of successful strategies to improve adherence with long-term medication (Box 14.3). Although associated with successful outcomes, many of the strategies listed are complex and labour intensive and consequently their relevance to the practice setting must be questioned. What is clear is that there is no simple solution to poor adherence although a list of the more pragmatic approaches for the pharmacist to adopt is presented in Box 14.4.

In addition to the strategies listed in Box 14.4 some workers would also advocate the use of multicompartment containers, such as the Medidos and Dosett, to improve adherence. These devices can hold up to 7 days of medication arranged in day compartments. However, they are not suitable for many patients because they do not provide appropriate storage conditions for

Table 14.2 Patient priority ranking of information given by pharmacist (Lyons et al 1996)

Information	Importance to patient
Dosing frequency	1
Side-effects noted	2
Reason prescribed	3
Pharmacological effect	4
Side-effects explained	5
Name of medication	6
Duration of therapy	7
Missed dose effects	8
Refill needed	9
Take with food	10
Missed dose resolution	11
Special directions	12
Take on empty stomach	13
Storage conditions	14
Need to revisit doctor	15
Drug interaction	16

their medicines or they require a level of dexterity that exceeds the patient's capabilities. These devices should not be considered a general aid to promote adherence although their judicious use in selected individuals may prove beneficial.

BOX 14.3 Strategies that have been shown to improve adherence when applied in various combinations

- Combinations of more convenient care e.g. worksite care
- Information
- Counselling
- Reminders
- Self-monitoring
- Reinforcement
- Family therapy
- Additional supervision or attention.

BOX 14.4 Strategies to improve adherence

- Be aware of patient's wishes
- Involve patient in treatment decisions
- Provide information required by patient
- Promote informed prescribing
- Simplify prescribed regimen
- Undertake medication review
- Improve home support
- Monitor beneficial effects
- Monitor side-effects
- Ensure good communications between health care team and carers
- Provide long-term support to patient.

REFERENCES

Beardon PHG, McGilchrist MM, McKendrick AD, McDevitt DG, MacDonald TM 1993 Primary non-compliance with prescribed medication in primary care. British Medical Journal 307:846–848

Haynes RB, McKibbon KA, Kanani R 1996 Systematic review of randomised trials of interventions to assist patients to follow prescriptions for medications. Lancet 348:383–386

Lyons RF, Rumore MM, Merola MR 1996 An analysis of drug information desired by the patient. Journal of Clinical Pharmacy and Therapeutics 21:221–228

Royal Pharmaceutical Society of Great Britain (RPSGB) 1997 From compliance to concordance: achieving shared goals in medicine taking. RPSGB, London

Wright EC 1993 Non-compliance — or how many aunts has Matilda? Lancet 342:909–913

SUBSTANCE MISUSE

J Sheridan

15

This chapter will focus briefly on certain aspects of drug misuse; the management of drug misuse as it pertains to pharmacy practice in the UK, other related services which pharmacists may find themselves involved in, and dealing with any dependent patients in a hospital context. Readers are also directed to other reference sources for more detailed information.

Substance misuse is not a new phenomenon. However, the context in which we view substance misuse today is shaped by the legal status of the drugs, the effects of drug misuse on health and social well-being, Government and medical policy on drug misuse and by the effect of substance misuse on the rest of society. The number of drug misusers continues to grow each year, especially those dependent on opioids. From a pharmacy perspective, it is these individuals with whom most pharmacists will come into contact, either through dispensing their prescriptions or through selling or exchanging clean injecting equipment.

HARM REDUCTION

Much of the service provision for drug misusers is based on the philosophy of harm reduction — i.e. enabling drug takers who cannot or will not abstain, to take drugs in a way which causes least harm to them (and to society).

> Personal harm, in the context of harm reduction includes:
> - blood-borne diseases such as hepatitis B and C, HIV
> - problems surrounding injecting — abscesses, gangrene, ulcers, septicaemia
> - overdose
> - poor health status (including oral health)
> - deep vein thrombosis.

For many drug misusers, abstinence is not possible (at least not in the short-term) and harm reduction embraces the concept of intermediate goals such as not sharing injecting equipment, reducing the frequency of injecting, reducing the amount of drug injecting, switching from injecting drugs to taking them orally (or in other ways less harmful than injecting, such as smoking, inhaling etc).

The following sections deal briefly with just a few of the many aspects of service provision for drug misusers.

CONTROLLED DRUGS

Misuse of drugs act and regulations

Under the Misuse of Drugs Act of 1971, drugs are categorised into classes. This classification system is used to determine penalties for criminal acts. However, for the purposes of pharmacy practice it is the classification under the Misuse of Drugs Regulations (1985) which is of relevance. These regulations permit the use of certain controlled drugs and regulate, amongst other things, their supply, storage and manufacture. There are five schedules, details of which may be found in 'Medicines, Ethics and Practice: a Guide for Pharmacists' (MEPG). Emergency supplies of controlled drugs (CDs) in Schedules 1, 2 and 3 are not allowed (with the exception of phenobarbitone or phenobarbitone sodium — see MEPG for full details). A table of the main types of controlled drugs by schedule and class may be obtained in a leaflet from Release.

Expired controlled drugs
Destruction of date-expired controlled drugs must be supervised 'by a person authorised by the Secretary of State either personally or as a member of a class', usually a member of the RPSGB inspectorate or a police officer. Details of this procedure are given in the MEPG.

Dispensed controlled drugs returned to the pharmacy

Where a patient's controlled drugs are returned to the pharmacy, they should be destroyed immediately. Although a witness is not required, it is advisable to get a member of staff to witness, and to make an entry in the back of the prescription register. Otherwise, the controlled drugs could be rendered unrecoverable by making up a slurry, e.g. using washing up liquid or cat litter (the resultant mixture then becomes POM). It can then be destroyed along with other clinical waste. Special destruction kits (DOOP kits) may also be obtained (see list of useful phone numbers at the end of the chapter). Always contact the RPSGB Professional Standards Directorate for advice.

Requests to identify a suspected controlled drug
Confidentiality should not be breached, for example where a parent finds a substance which they think belongs to their child.

Further guidance on this difficult matter may be obtained from the RPSGB Professional Standards Directorate. Hospital pharmacists may find useful information on this in the MEPG (Schedule 1 drugs) with reference to substances removed from patients on admission. Fact sheets are available from the RPSGB Professional Standards Directorate.

COMMUNICATING WITH OTHER MEMBERS OF THE HEALTH CARE TEAM

Dealing with phone calls from prescribers

If a prescriber/member of clinic staff calls to give information or to advise you of the arrival of a script, call them back, using the telephone number YOU have obtained from directory enquiries. Prescriptions for CDs in Schedules 2 and 3 given over the telephone are not valid (with the exception of those for phenobarbitone for the treatment of epilepsy, provided it does not contain any other Schedule 2 or 3 drugs). Faxed prescriptions for controlled drugs in Schedules 2 and 3 are never valid.

Confidentiality

Clients often have concerns about confidentiality, and are anxious about others knowing about their drug misuse, often because drug users are held in low esteem and have worries about children being taken into care. They may not have told their own GP. It is important to be clear with clients about who you have a professional responsibility to communicate with, for example the drug clinic/prescriber.

Confidentiality issues may be a problem for pharmacists when a client uses two or more services, e.g. dispensing methadone and utilising the needle exchange. Information should not normally be shared between the two services.

METHADONE AND OTHER OPIOIDS

The most commonly prescribed drug for the treatment of opioid dependence is methadone. Other opioids such as diamorphine and dihydrocodeine are less frequently prescribed.

Methadone

This section will look at the important points to remember when working with methadone.

Pharmacokinetics and metabolism
Methadone is soluble in lipids and is metabolised mainly in the liver. Mean half-life of first oral dose is 15 hours (range 12–18) and after repeated doses a mean of 25 hours (range 13–47) (Dollery 1991). However, it may be much longer than this. It is therefore usually prescribed as a single daily dose. The fact that methadone induces its own metabolism is a further confounding factor.

Drug interactions
Any drugs which affect the cytochrome p450 pathways will interact with methadone, e.g. rifampicin increases the metabolism of methadone and higher doses of methadone are often needed. Drugs which cause CNS depression will cause increased sedation (e.g. alcohol, hypnotics, tricyclics and anxiolytics) and possibly increased respiratory depression. See The Methadone Briefing for more information. A number of drugs used in the management of HIV/AIDS interact with methadone, e.g. AZT. Protease inhibitors also have the potential for significant interactions as they affect microsomal enzymes.

Dosage forms
Methadone is available as mixture 1 mg/ml (most commonly prescribed, other strengths are available), linctus 2mg/5ml (licensed for cough), ampoules in various strengths and 5mg tablets. The prescribing of tablets is not recommended as drug misusers may crush and inject them, which can result in damage at the site of injection, possibly leading to abscesses and gangrene.

Tolerance and overdose
Tolerance develops within 2 weeks after repeated doses, so the same dose has less effect. Tolerance may be lost as quickly as it develops, so that taking the same dose after several days without opioids may result in overdose. It is therefore advisable to discuss with prescribers, the procedure for dealing with patients who have missed several (usually three or more) consecutive days of medication, as their tolerance may have fallen. Patients should be informed of such procedures. Death by overdose is mainly caused by respiratory depression. Naloxone (a short acting opioid antagonist) is used to reverse opioid overdose. Repeated doses may be required as its effect wears off and the patient slips back into overdose. Methadone should not be dispensed to clients intoxicated with alcohol and/or drugs, as this increases the risk of overdose. Consult the prescriber before dispensing.

> ⚠️ Signs of overdose include:
> nausea and vomiting, pin-point pupils, drowsiness, cold,
> clammy bluish skin, reduced heart rate, breathlessness,
> cyanosis, pulmonary oedema.

Withdrawal syndrome

This syndrome is a result of rebound activity at opiate receptors
causing a release of large amounts of noradrenaline (noradrenaline 'storm'). Symptoms may be heightened by anxiety about
withdrawal.

> ⚠️ Symptoms of withdrawal include:
> weakness, yawning, sneezing, sweating, goose bumps, tremors,
> insomnia, muscle spasms, diarrhoea.

Patients who gain a lot of weight may also find their dose
does not 'hold them' leading to symptoms of withdrawal.

> 📝 Advice to new clients:
> • Don't take the first dose of prescribed methadone while
>   alone — have someone with you for the first 2–4 hours.
> • Don't mix methadone with other drugs or alcohol.
> • Beware of using other opioids (e.g. street heroin) as well as
>   methadone.

For regular patients, discuss with prescribers what information they would like to be fed back to them, for example missed
doses, chaotic behaviour, etc. You should normally let the
patient know that you are liaising with the prescriber.

Dispensing methadone

Methadone is in Schedule 2 of the Misuse of Drugs Regulations.
Prescription writing requirements, handwriting requirements,
record keeping and safe storage requirements all apply (see
MEPG for details). Prescribers may have a handwriting exemp-
tion from the Home Office (this can be verified with the Home
Office).

The details of instalment prescriptions may not be varied,
e.g. if a patient should receive two days supply on a Monday,
and does not collect on this day, they may not obtain their
Tuesday supply on Tuesday. A new prescription will be required
for that supply, although not invalidating the remaining instal-

ments if collected on the correct days. The RPSGB law department may be contacted with queries relating to controlled drug prescription requirements.

Where a client wishes a representative to collect their supply, a note signed by the client should be obtained for each separate supply (for more details see Pharmaceutical Journal (May 18) 1996, vol. 256: 677).

Supervised consumption of methadone in the community pharmacy

You may be asked by a local prescriber to supervise the consumption of methadone for an individual patient, or there may be a locally set up scheme in conjunction with a clinic or GP. Sometimes the request may be made by the patient, to help with compliance, or possibly because they are being threatened by other drug misusers to hand over their medication. Guidelines may be obtained from the RPSGB. Additional information may be obtained from your local Pharmaceutical Adviser, local Drug Action Team and Drug Reference Group, and the RPSGB library.

Supervision may be requested for a number of reasons:
- as an aid to compliance
- to give clients some stability
- to prevent diversion on to the illicit market
- to reduce risks of accidental overdose by having less methadone in the community (particularly a risk with small children).

To ensure methadone has been swallowed:
- talk to clients — it's difficult to talk with a mouthful of methadone
- offer them a drink of water — this also helps to reduce tooth decay and offers another opportunity for some health education.

Things to remember:
- ensure all locums understand the procedure and are willing to supervise
- ensure that clients can be identified by locums
- check your insurance covers you
- consider hepatitis B vaccinations for you (and key staff)
- methadone should be dispensed in bottles with child proof closures and labelled in accordance with the Medicines Act
- remove labels from used containers before disposal to maintain client confidentiality
- procedures for missed doses (see under Tolerance)
- do not administer to intoxicated clients – consult prescriber first.

Diamorphine

A prescriber must have a licence from the Home Office to prescribe diamorphine *for the treatment of addiction*, and such prescribers will normally be hospital specialists prescribing on pink FP10HP (ad) forms. You may check that a prescriber has a licence by calling the Home Office.

Diamorphine has a shorter half-life than methadone and requires divided daily doses.

Prescriptions for reefers (heroin cigarettes)

The RPSGB has published guidelines for the manufacture of diamorphine reefers. You may also receive prescriptions for methadone reefers. Contact the RPSGB for more information before dispensing.

Buprenorphine

Buprenorphine is a partial agonist and is prescribed for the management of opioid dependence. It has recently been licensed for this in the UK as Subutex®

LOFEXIDINE

Lofexidine is an α_2 adrenergic agonist similar to clonidine. It is used in the management of opioid withdrawal as it suppresses noradrenergic neuronal hyperactivity. Side-effects of lofexidine include drowsiness and dry mouth, and it can cause hypotension. Patients will have their blood pressure monitored while on lofexidine, although for most patients the hypotensive effect is not clinically significant.

OTHER DRUGS

You may come into contact with clients being prescribed benzodiazepines and amphetamines for the treatment of substance misuse. It is outside the scope of this chapter to deal with each of these groups individually. However, useful information on treatment may be obtained from your local drug misuse clinic and/ or the Institute for the Study of Drug Dependency (ISDD) library.

Over the counter medicines

Care should be exerted over requests for antihistamines (e.g. cyclizine and diphenhydramine), and products containing opioid analgesics, as they may be misused. Where a methadone patient requests something for pain, paracetamol, aspirin and non-steroidal anti-inflammatory drugs may be recommended.

Watch out for excessive requests for cimetidine (in theory a drug interaction between cimetidine and cytochrome p450 pathway could reduce the metabolism of methadone).

The RPSGB does not condone the sales of citric acid or ascorbic acid when used to facilitate the dissolving of street heroin. (Selling could constitute an offence under the Misuse of Drugs Act section 9a and the Drugs Trafficking Offences Act — injecting paraphernalia). Watch out for sales of powdered substances which may be used to dilute the injected substance, e.g. glucose.

NEEDLE EXCHANGE SCHEMES

Health Authorities arrange for adequate needle exchange facilities to meet local demand. Some of this will be from stand alone needle exchanges, others from drug agencies, and others through pharmacy schemes. Each health authority will have a needle exchange coordinator responsible for pharmacy needle exchange. If you feel you want to be involved in the local scheme, contact the health authority.

Issues surrounding confidentiality with regard to clients need to be clear. Information on clients using the needle exchange should not be given to others, such as their prescriber.

Things to consider before becoming involved in needle exchange.
- Is there any local demand (do you already get requests for sales of injecting equipment)?
- Are there other exchange facilities near by?
- How do your staff feel about this (they are often the first point of contact for clients and negative attitudes could ruin the scheme)?
- Do you have the necessary space, time and staff?
- Talk to someone else already providing this service — you will be able to allay most of your fears by seeing how the service functions in practice — usually without any problems at all.

HOSPITAL PHARMACY

A number of scenarios may occur with respect to substance misusers in the hospital context. These will be dealt with briefly. Your hospital or local Health Authority may have their own guidelines.

Opiate misusers admitted who need prescribed controlled drugs for the treatment of dependence

• You may need to supply drugs such as methadone to prevent the patient going into withdrawal.

• Where the patient states they are in receipt of a prescription for methadone (or another drug) you should contact the patient's prescriber to confirm this (n.b. confidentiality issues). Remember patients may not always be taking all the dose prescribed for them.

• You should contact the community pharmacist who dispensed the methadone to inform them of the situation and confirm when the last dose was dispensed. Is consumption of the drug supervised? How much is the client actually taking? Did they actually consume this last dose? What other drugs could they be taking?

• Where a patient is in withdrawal and there is no evidence of a prescription, the dose should be carefully titrated from a low dose, in accordance with local guidelines.

• If high doses are being prescribed or demanded by patients they should be titrated up from a low dose, in divided doses and the patient monitored for signs of overdose/withdrawal, in line with local guidelines.

Inform the patient's prescriber and the community pharmacist of:
• discharge date
• whether the patient received methadone on the day of discharge and how much
• details of any take-home doses given
• any other drugs being prescribed on discharge.

Discharge of such patients who are currently receiving prescriptions in the community for the treatment of their drug misuse

Arrange for a community prescription to be resumed or arrange for a new prescription to be written. It should be noted that clients referred for treatment are unlikely to be able to get a prescription immediately until a full assessment has been made. There may also be waiting lists for treatment. Check procedures with local drug services/GPs.

REFERENCES AND FURTHER READING

Beard JC 1995 Illicit drug use: acute and chronic pharmacological
  intervention. Quay Books, London
British National Formulary (latest edition). Pharmaceutical Press,
  London
Department of Health et al 1999 Drug misuse and dependence.
  Guidelines on clinical management. The Stationery Office, London
Dollery C 1991 Therapeutic drugs. Churchill Livingstone, Edinburgh
Martindale The extra pharmacopoeia. Pharmaceutical Press, London
Preston A 1993 The methadone handbook. CADAS, Dorchester
  (available from ISDD)
Preston A 1996 The methadone briefing ISDD, London
Preston A, Hunt N, Derricot J 1999 Safer injecting briefing. HIT,
  Liverpool
Preston A, Malinowski A 1994 The detox handbook a user's guide to
  getting off opiates. ISDD, London
Release 1996 The Misuse of Drugs Act explained. Release, London
RPSBG Medicines, ethics and practice – a guide for pharmacists
  (latest edition). RPSGB, London
Wills S 1997 Drugs of abuse. Pharmaceutical Press, London

USEFUL PHONE NUMBERS

DOOP 01491 612267
HIT 0151 227 4012
The Home Office 0171 273 3000
Institute for the Study of Drug Dependence (ISDD) 0171 928 1211
Release 0171 729 9904
Royal Pharmaceutical Society of Great Britain (RPSGB), Professional
  Standards Department and Library/Information 0171 735 9141
Standing Conference on Drug Abuse (SCODA) 0171 928 9500

ADVERSE REACTIONS TO DRUGS

SafeScript

16

Adverse reactions to drugs are common, so when a patient presents with a problem it is important to remember it may be caused by a drug. When a patient is on many drugs it can be time consuming to search through the ADR profile of all of them, so this chapter is constructed in reverse — the condition is listed (by Read code) and is followed by the pharmacological group of drugs that have been reported to cause that condition. Note that not all the drugs in a pharmacological group may cause the ADR. This list has been abstracted from a database package from SafeScript which, amongst other functions, holds the ADR profile for around 30 000 drug products and is updated monthly.

Hospital pharmacists can now fill in yellow cards and send them to the Committee on Safety of Medicines. It is essential that they do this for *all* suspected ADRs to black triangle drugs in the BNF and all serious suspected reactions to established drugs, even if the ADR is already well documented. If you are in doubt the BNF gives examples of what constitutes a serious reaction. Community pharmacists should alert the prescriber or the patient's GP if the reaction is to an over the counter drug.

ADR	Pharmacological Group
Abdomen feels bloated	Gastrointestinal agents
	Laxatives
	Somatotrophic hormones
Abdominal cramps	Anthelmintics
	Anthraquinone glycosides
	Anticholinesterase parasympathomimetics
	Antidiuretic hormones
	Antivirals
	Diagnostic agents
	Docusate
	Gastrointestinal agents
	Laxatives
	Monobactams
	Oestrogen antagonist antineoplastics
	Organic iodinated contrast media
	Parasympathomimetics
	Picosulphate
	Pilocarpine

Posterior pituitary hormones
Sweetening agents
Typhoid vaccines
Vasopressins

Abdominal discomfort

Anthelmintics
Antifungals
Antivirals
Bile acid binding resins
Calcium antagonist vasodilators
Diagnostic agents
Ergot compounds
Laxatives
Lincomycins
Lipid regulating agents
Macrolides
Medicinal enzymes
Sex hormones
Sweetening agents
Triazole antifungals

Abdominal distension

Bulk laxatives
Chloral sedatives
Hypoglycaemics

Abdominal pain

4 Methanolquinoline antimalarials
4 Quinolones
8 Aminoquinoline antimalarials
ACE inhibitors
Amino acids
Analgesics and anti-inflammatory drugs
Anthelmintics
Antiandrogens
Antianginal vasodilators
Anticholinesterase parasympathomimetics
Antidepressants
Antidiuretic hormones
Antidotes
Antiemetics
Antimalarials
Antimuscarinics
Antineoplastics
Antituberculous agents
Antiulcer agents
Antivirals
Aspartic acid
Benzimidazole anthelmintics
Bisphosphonates
Borates
Carbapenems
Cardiac glycosides
Catechol O-methyl transferase inhibitors
Central stimulants

Cephalosporins
Chelating agents
Cinchona antimalarials
Clofibrate and analogues
Colchicum alkaloids
Colony stimulating factors
Contrast media
Digitalis
Dopaminergic antiparkinsonian agents
E series prostaglandins
Ergolines
Ergot alkaloids
Ergot compounds
Essential amino acids
Gastrointestinal agents
Glycol and glycerol esters
Gonad regulating hormones
HMG CoA reductase inhibitors
Hydroxyquinoline antiprotozoals
Imidazole antifungals
Interleukins
Leukotriene inhibitors
Lipid regulating agents
Medicinal enzymes
Neuroleptics
Nutritional carbohydrates
Oestrogen antagonist antineoplastics
Opioid antagonists
Oral hypoglycaemics
Oxazolidinedione antiepileptics
Pilocarpine
Prophylactic antiasthmatics
Selective serotonin reuptake inhibiting
    antidepressants
Somatotrophic hormones
Triazole antifungals
Vasodilator antihypertensives
Vitamin E substances
Vitamins

Abnormal granulation tissue	Chlorine releasing substances
Abnormal uterine bleeding	Anabolics Beta sympathomimetic vasodilators Beta2 selective stimulants E series prostaglandins Oestrogen antagonist antineoplastics Sex hormones
Abnormal weight gain	Aliphatic phenothiazine neuroleptics Alpha blocking antihypertensives Anabolics Antiandrogens

Antidepressants
Antiepileptics
Antiulcer agents
Butyrophenone neuroleptics
Calcium antagonist vasodilators
Diphenylbutylpiperidine neuroleptics
Ergot compounds
Flupenthixols
Fluphenazine
GABA related antiepileptics
Gonad regulating hormones
H1 antagonist antihistamines
Haloperidols
Hydrazine monoamine oxidase inhibiting
    antidepressants
Immunosuppressants
Lithium
Monoamine oxidase inhibiting
    antidepressants
Neuroleptics
Norgestrels
Oestrogens
Phenothiazine neuroleptics
Piperazine phenothiazine neuroleptics
Piperidine phenothiazine neuroleptics
Progestogens
Prophylactic antiasthmatics
Sex hormones
Skeletal muscle relaxants
Tetracyclic antidepressants
Thioxanthene neuroleptics
Tricyclic antidepressants
Vasodilator antihypertensives
Zuclopenthixols

Abnormal weight loss

ACE inhibitors
Anabolics
Antiandrogens
Anticholinesterase parasympathomimetics
Antidepressants
Antiepileptics
Antifolate antineoplastics
Butyrophenone neuroleptics
Fat soluble vitamins
Gonad regulating hormones
Haloperidols
Norgestrels
Oestrogens
Oxazolidinedione antiepileptics
Progestogens
Selective serotonin reuptake inhibiting
    antidepressants
Sex hormones
Skeletal muscle relaxants

	Tetracyclic antidepressants
	Thyroid agents
	Tricyclic antidepressants
	Vitamin D substances
	Vitamins

| **Abnormalities of the hair** | Antiandrogens |

| **ACE inhibitor symptom complex – collagen vascular** | ACE inhibitors |

| **Acidosis** | Glycol and glycerol esters |

Acne	Anabolics
	Gonad regulating hormones
	Hydantoin antiepileptics
	Norgestrels
	Phenytoin
	Progestogens
	Sex hormones

| **Acne-like eruption** | Tars |

Acquired hypothyroidism	Antithyroid agents
	Antituberculous agents
	Class III antiarrhythmics
	Iodides
	Iodine compounds
	Iodophores
	Lithium

| **Acquired pyloric obstruction** | E series prostaglandins |

| **Acute alcoholic intoxication** | Glycols |

| **Acute bronchitis/bronchiolitis** | Antiulcer agents |

| **Acute chemical pulmon.oedema** | Aromatics |

| **Acute closed-angle glaucoma** | Skeletal muscle relaxants |

| **Acute confusional state** | Opioid analgesics |

Acute conjunctivitis	Anthelmintics
	Antifolate antineoplastics
	Antivirals
	Beta2 selective stimulants
	Carbonic anhydrase inhibitors
	Organic iodinated contrast media
	Retinoic acid dermatological agents
	Sedatives

Acute coronary insufficiency	Antidiuretic hormones
	Posterior pituitary hormones
	Vasopressins

Acute cystitis	Nitrogen mustards

Acute hepatic failure	Antiepileptics
	Antituberculous agents
	Imidazole antifungals
	Xanthine oxidase inhibitors

Acute hepatitis	4 Aminoquinoline antimalarials
	ACE inhibitors
	Aliphatic phenothiazine neuroleptics
	Analgesics and anti-inflammatory drugs
	Antiandrogens
	Antibacterial agents
	Antibiotic antituberculous agents
	Antifungals
	Antiprotozoals
	Antituberculous agents
	Beta lactamase inhibitors
	Calcium antagonist vasodilators
	Carbazepine antiepileptics
	Chelating agents
	Class I antiarrhythmics
	Gastrointestinal agents
	Gold salts
	Histamine H2 antagonists
	HMG CoA reductase inhibitors
	Hydantoin antiepileptics
	Hydrazine monoamine oxidase inhibiting antidepressants
	Imidazole antifungals
	Immunosuppressants
	Indanedione anticoagulants
	Inhalation anaesthetics
	Isoxazolyl penicillins
	Macrolides
	Methadone and analogues
	Monoamine oxidase inhibiting antidepressants
	Monoamine oxidase inhibiting antihypertensives
	Neuroleptics
	Nitrofuran antimicrobials
	Nitrofuran antiprotozoals
	Oestrogen antagonist antineoplastics
	Oral hypoglycaemics
	Oxazolidinedione antiepileptics
	Phenytoin
	Retinoic acid dermatological agents
	Sex hormones

Skeletal muscle relaxants
Sulphone antileprotics
Sulphonylurea hypoglycaemics
Thiouracil antithyroid agents
Thiourea antithyroid agents
Tricyclic antidepressants
Trimethoprim sulphonamide
  combinations
Uricosuric agents
Vitamin B substances

Acute laryngitis	Medicinal enzymes
Acute myocardial infarction	ACE inhibitors Alpha blocking vasodilators Ergot alkaloids Ergot compounds Erythropoietin Nitrogen mustards Serotonin and analogues
Acute myocarditis	Gastrointestinal agents Neuroleptics Salicylate analgesics
Acute nasopharyngitis	Analgesics and anti-inflammatory drugs
Acute necrosis of liver	Analgesics and anti-inflammatory drugs Antiepileptics Beta blockers Centrally acting antihypertensives Ester type anaesthetics Hydrazide antituberculous agents Inhalation anaesthetics Nitrogen mustards Salicylate analgesics Skeletal muscle relaxants Xanthine oxidase inhibitors
Acute pancreatitis	ACE inhibitors Analgesics and anti-inflammatory drugs Antiepileptics Antivirals Coumarin anticoagulants Diamidine antiprotozoals Gastrointestinal agents Histamine H2 antagonists HMG CoA reductase inhibitors Immunosuppressants Indanedione anticoagulants Loop diuretics Nitrofuran antimicrobials Oxytetracyclines

	Salicylate analgesics
	Selective serotonin reuptake inhibiting antidepressants
	Sulphonamides
	Tetracyclines
	Thiazide diuretics
	Trimethoprim sulphonamide combinations

Acute pericarditis	Colony stimulating factors
	Neuroleptics
	Skeletal muscle relaxants

Acute pharyngitis	Antiulcer agents
	GABA related antiepileptics
	H1 antagonist antihistamines
	Medicinal enzymes

Acute renal failure	Antibacterial agents
	Antibiotic antituberculous agents
	Antineoplastics
	Antivirals
	Borates
	Carbazepine antiepileptics
	Cinchona antimalarials
	Diamidine antiprotozoals
	Immunosuppressants
	Inhalation anaesthetics
	Leech products
	Organic iodinated contrast media
	Polyene antibiotics
	Uricosuric agents

Acute renal tubular necrosis	4 Quinolones
	Aminoglycosides
	Antibiotic antituberculous agents
	Antifolate antineoplastics
	Antineoplastics
	Edetates
	Immunosuppressants
	Polyene antibiotics

Acute respiratory infections	Anticholinesterase parasympathomimetics
	Lipid regulating agents

Acute sinusitis	Antiulcer agents
	H1 antagonist antihistamines

Acute/subacute liver necrosis	4 Quinolones
	Antiandrogens
	Antidepressants
	Hydrazine monoamine oxidase inhibiting antidepressants

Monoamine oxidase inhibiting
   antidepressants
Sulphonamides
Trimethoprim sulphonamide
   combinations
Uricosuric agents

Adult respiratory distress syndrome	Blood products

Aggression	Antiepileptics
	Benzodiazepine sedatives
	Carbamate sedatives
	Carbazepine antiepileptics
	Central stimulants
	GABA related antiepileptics
	Neuroleptics
	Sedatives
	Skeletal muscle relaxants

Agitation	4 Quinolones
	Aliphatic phenothiazine neuroleptics
	Anabolics
	Antianginal vasodilators
	Anticholinesterase parasympathomimetics
	Antidepressants
	Antiepileptics
	Antiulcer agents
	Antivirals
	Barbiturate sedatives
	Benzodiazepine antagonists
	Beta2 selective stimulants
	Butyrophenone neuroleptics
	Carbamate sedatives
	Carbazepine antiepileptics
	Central stimulants
	Chloral sedatives
	Corticosteroids
	Diphenylbutylpiperidine neuroleptics
	Dopaminergic antiparkinsonian agents
	Ergolines
	Flupenthixols
	Fluphenazine
	GABA related antiepileptics
	Haloperidols
	Hydrazine monoamine oxidase inhibiting antidepressants
	Monoamine oxidase inhibiting antidepressants
	Neuroleptics
	Organic iodinated contrast media
	Parasympathomimetics
	Phenothiazine neuroleptics
	Pilocarpine

Piperazine phenothiazine neuroleptics
Piperidine phenothiazine neuroleptics
Sedatives
Skeletal muscle relaxants
Thioxanthene neuroleptics
Thyroid agents
Tricyclic antidepressants
Zuclopenthixols

Agranulocytosis

4 Aminoquinoline antimalarials
4 Quinolones
ACE inhibitors
Aliphatic phenothiazine neuroleptics
Analgesics and anti-inflammatory drugs
Antibacterial agents
Antibiotic antifungals
Antidepressants
Antimalarials
Antithyroid agents
Antiulcer agents
Antivirals
Butyrophenone neuroleptics
Calcium antagonist vasodilators
Carbacephems
Carbamate sedatives
Carbazepine antiepileptics
Cephalosporins
Cephamycins
Chelating agents
Class I antiarrhythmics
Diphenylbutylpiperidine neuroleptics
Flupenthixols
Fluphenazine
Gastrointestinal agents
H1 antagonist antihistamines
Haloperidols
Histamine H2 antagonists
Hydantoin antiepileptics
Hydrazide antituberculous agents
Indanedione anticoagulants
Lincomycins
Neuroleptics
Nitrofuran antimicrobials
Oestrogen antagonist antineoplastics
Oral hypoglycaemics
Phenothiazine neuroleptics
Phenytoin
Piperazine phenothiazine neuroleptics
Piperidine phenothiazine neuroleptics
Skeletal muscle relaxants
Succinimide antiepileptics
Sulphonamides
Sulphone antileprotics
Sulphonylurea hypoglycaemics

	Tetracyclic antidepressants
	Thiouracil antithyroid agents
	Thiourea antithyroid agents
	Thioxanthene neuroleptics
	Tricyclic antidepressants
	Trimethoprim sulphonamide combinations
	Zuclopenthixols
Alcohol - toxic effect	Alcoholic disinfectants
	Antineoplastics
	Glycols
Alkaline phosphatase raised	Fat soluble vitamins
	Vitamin A substances
	Vitamins
Alkalosis	Expectorants
Allergic alveolitis	Antineoplastics
Allergic arthritis	Chelating agents
	Tetracyclic antidepressants
Allergic dermatitis	Alcohol metabolism modifiers
	Analgesics and anti-inflammatory drugs
	Gold salts
	Sulphone antileprotics
Allergic/hypersensitivity reaction	4 Quinolones
	ACE inhibitors
	Acetoglycerides
	Acridine disinfectant dyes
	Alcoholic disinfectants
	Alcoholic solvents
	Alkali metal soaps
	Alkyl gallates
	Alkyl sulphates
	Allantoin compounds
	Aluminium astringents
	Amide type anaesthetics
	Amidinopenicillins
	Amino acids
	Aminobenzoate sunscreen agents
	Aminoglycosides
	Aminopenicillanic derivatives
	Aminopenicillins
	Analgesics and anti-inflammatory drugs
	Animal desensitising agents
	Anionic and ampholytic surfactants
	Anionic surfactants
	Anthelmintics
	Antibacterial agents
	Antibiotic antineoplastics

Antibiotic antituberculous agents
Antidiarrhoeals
Antidiuretic hormones
Antidotes
Antiemetics
Antifungals
Antihypertensives
Antimalarials
Antimicrobial preservatives
Antineoplastics
Antioxidant preservatives
Antipseudomonal penicillins
Antisera
Aromatics
Azo colouring agents
Barbiturate antiepileptics
Barbiturate sedatives
Bases
Benzimidazole anthelmintics
Benzoates
Benzophenone sunscreen agents
Benzylpenicillin and derivatives
Beta lactamase inhibitors
Beta2 selective stimulants
Bioflavonoids
Bismuth salts
Bitters
Blood clotting factors
Blood products
Bromides
Bulk laxatives
Carbacephems
Carbapenems
Carboxypenicillins
Cardiac inotropic agents
Catechol O-methyl transferase inhibitors
Cellulose derived viscosity modifiers
Centrally acting antihypertensives
Cephalosporins
Cephamycins
Chloramphenicols
Cinchona antimalarials
Cinnamate sunscreen agents
Class I antiarrhythmics
Colony stimulating factors
Colouring agents
Contrast media
Cough suppressants
Coumarin anticoagulants
Cyanoacrylate adhesives
Cytoprotective agents
Dermatological agents
Dextrans
Diagnostic agents

Diagnostic dyes
Dibenzoylmethanes
Direct acting anticoagulants
Disinfectants
Docusate
Dopaminergic antiparkinsonian agents
Encephalitis vaccines
Ester type anaesthetics
Evening primrose oil
Fat and vegetable oil bases
Fatty alcohol bases
Fixed oils
Flavouring agents
Fluorescein colouring agents
Fluorescein diagnostic dyes
Fluorocarbon blood substitutes
Formaldehyde and related compounds
Gastrointestinal agents
Glucose tests
Glycerol
Glycerophosphates
Glycol and glycerol esters
Glycols
Gold salts
Gonad regulating hormones
Grass pollens
H1 antagonist antihistamines
Haemostatics
Heparinoids
Histamine H2 antagonists
HMG CoA reductase inhibitors
Hyaluronic acid
Hydrazide antituberculous agents
Hydroquinone dermatological agents
Hydroxybenzoates
Hydroxynaphthoquinones
Hydroxyquinoline antiprotozoals
Hypophosphites
Hypothalamic and pituitary hormones
Imidazole antifungals
Immunological agents
Immunosuppressants
Indanedione anticoagulants
Influenza vaccines
Insulin
Interleukins
Iodides
Iodine compounds
Iodophores
Isothiazolinones
Isoxazolyl penicillins
Laureths
Laxatives
Lecithin derivatives

Leech products
Lincomycins
Local anaesthetics
Low molecular weight heparins
Macrogol esters
Macrogol ethers
Macrolides
Measles vaccine
Medicinal enzymes
Mercurial dermatological agents
Mercurial diuretics
Metallic soaps
Mineral acids
Monobactams
Monoclonal antibodies
Mucolytics
Natural colouring agents
Natural penicillins
Neuroleptics
Nitrofuran antimicrobials
Nonionic surfactants
Nonoxinols
Nutritional agents
Octoxinols
Oestrogen antagonist antineoplastics
Oral hypoglycaemics
Organic acids
Organic iodinated contrast media
Organic mercurial disinfectants
Organic solvents
Osmotic diuretics
Oxacephalosporins
Oxytetracyclines
Paraffins
Penicillinase resistant penicillins
Permanganates
Pesticides
Petroleum distillate solvents
Phenothiazine antihistamines
Phenoxymethylpenicillin and derivatives
Phenoxypenicillins
Phenylmercuric salts
Plastics
Poliomyelitis vaccines
Poloxamers
Polyene antibiotics
Polymyxins
Polyoxyl stearates
Polysorbates
Posterior pituitary hormones
Preservatives
Product bases
Promethazines
Psoralen dermatological agents

Pyrethroid pesticides
Quaternary ammonium surfactants
Retinoic acid dermatological agents
Salicylate analgesics
Salicylate sunscreen agents
Sedatives
Selective serotonin reuptake inhibiting
    antidepressants
Serotonin and analogues
Siliceous viscosity modifiers
Sodium salts
Sorbates
Sorbitan derivatives
Streptogramins
Sulphated oils
Sulphites
Sulphonamides
Sulphonated anionic surfactants
Sulphonylurea hypoglycaemics
Sunscreen agents
Synthetic colouring agents
Tetracyclines
Thiazide diuretics
Thyrotrophic hormones
Toluidines
Trace elements
Tree pollens
Triazole antifungals
Trimethoprim and derivatives
Trimethoprim sulphonamide
    combinations
Triphenylmethane colouring agents
Triphenylmethane diagnostic dyes
Triphenylmethane disinfectant dyes
Typhoid vaccines
Ureido penicillins
Uricosuric agents
Vaccines
Vanillas
Vasopressins
Vegetable gums
Viscosity modifiers
Vitamin B substances
Vitamin B1 substances
Wax bases

Alopecia

4 Aminoquinoline antimalarials
ACE inhibitors
Alkyl sulphonate antineoplastics
Alkylating antineoplastics
Anabolics
Analgesics and anti-inflammatory drugs
Anthracycline antibiotic antineoplastics
Antibiotic antineoplastics

Antiepileptics
Antifolate antineoplastics
Antineoplastics
Antiulcer agents
Antivirals
Asparaginase antineoplastics
Benzimidazole anthelmintics
Biguanide antimalarials
Borates
Carbazepine antiepileptics
Clofibrate and analogues
Colchicum alkaloids
Coumarin anticoagulants
Direct acting anticoagulants
Ergot compounds
Ethyleneimine antineoplastics
Fluorouracil
Gold salts
H1 antagonist antihistamines
Heparinoids
Immunosuppressants
Indanedione anticoagulants
Low molecular weight heparins
Nitrofuran antimicrobials
Nitrogen mustards
Nitrosoureas
Norgestrels
Oestrogen antagonist antineoplastics
Progestogens
Purine antagonist antineoplastics
Pyrimidine antagonist antineoplastics
Retinoic acid dermatological agents
Selective serotonin reuptake inhibiting
    antidepressants
Sex hormones
Sulphur mustards
Thiouracil antithyroid agents
Thiourea antithyroid agents
Triazene antineoplastics
Vinca alkaloid antineoplastics
Xanthine oxidase inhibitors

Amblyopia	Antidepressants
	GABA related antiepileptics
	Pilocarpine
Amenorrhoea	Anabolics
	Antiepileptics
	Immunosuppressants
	Oestrogen antagonist antineoplastics
	Sex hormones
Anaemia	4 Quinolones
	Antibiotic antituberculous agents

Antineoplastics
Antivirals
Borates
Central stimulants
Colony stimulating factors
Diamidine antiprotozoals
Immunosuppressants
Organic iodinated contrast media
Polyene antibiotics
Pyrimidine antagonist antineoplastics
Retinoic acid dermatological agents
Sulphone antileprotics

Anal pain	Contrast media
	Gastrointestinal agents
	Laxatives
	Medicinal enzymes
Anal/rectal ulcer	Cation exchange resins
Anaphylactic shock	4 Quinolones
	Amidinopenicillins
	Aminopenicillanic derivatives
	Aminopenicillins
	Animal desensitising agents
	Antibacterial agents
	Antibiotic antituberculous agents
	Antineoplastics
	Antipseudomonal penicillins
	Antisera
	Asparaginase antineoplastics
	Bases
	Benzylpenicillin and derivatives
	Blood products
	Borates
	Carbacephems
	Carbapenems
	Carboxypenicillins
	Cephalosporins
	Cephamycins
	Chelating agents
	Class III antiarrhythmics
	Colony stimulating factors
	Contrast media
	Corticosteroids
	Corticotrophic hormones
	Dextrans
	Direct acting anticoagulants
	Erythropoietin
	Fluorocarbon blood substitutes
	Grass pollens
	H1 antagonist antihistamines
	Heparinoids
	Hyaluronic acid

Immunostimulants
Immunosuppressants
Iron compounds
Isoxazolyl penicillins
Low molecular weight heparins
Medicinal enzymes
Natural penicillins
Norgestrels
Oestrogen antagonist antineoplastics
Opioid analgesics
Organic iodinated contrast media
Parenteral anaesthetics
Penicillinase resistant penicillins
Phenothiazine antihistamines
Phenoxymethylpenicillin and derivatives
Phenoxypenicillins
Platelet activating factor antagonists
Polyene antibiotics
Progestogens
Promethazines
Pyrimidine antagonist antineoplastics
Sedatives
Sex hormones
Skeletal muscle relaxants
Specific immunoglobulins
Tree pollens
Triazole antifungals
Triphenylmethane diagnostic dyes
Ureido penicillins

Angina pectoris

Alpha blocking antihypertensives
Antiandrogens
Antidiuretic hormones
Beta1 selective stimulants
Central stimulants
Ergot compounds
HMG CoA reductase inhibitors
Lipid regulating agents
Nitrogen mustards
Posterior pituitary hormones
Serotonin and analogues
Thyroid agents
Vasopressins

Angioneurotic oedema

4 Quinolones
ACE inhibitors
Amidinopenicillins
Aminopenicillanic derivatives
Aminopenicillins
Angiotensin inhibiting antihypertensives
Antiepileptics
Antipseudomonal penicillins
Antiulcer agents
Benzylpenicillin and derivatives

Beta2 selective stimulants
Bisphosphonates
Calcium antagonist vasodilators
Carboxypenicillins
Cinchona antimalarials
Class I antiarrhythmics
Direct acting anticoagulants
H1 antagonist antihistamines
Heparinoids
Histamine H2 antagonists
HMG CoA reductase inhibitors
Isoxazolyl penicillins
Leukotriene inhibitors
Lipid regulating agents
Low molecular weight heparins
Medicinal enzymes
Natural penicillins
Nitrofuran antimicrobials
Nitrofuran antiprotozoals
Nitroimidazole antiprotozoals
Organic iodinated contrast media
Penicillinase resistant penicillins
Phenothiazine antihistamines
Phenoxymethylpenicillin and derivatives
Phenoxypenicillins
Promethazines
Skeletal muscle relaxants
Triazole antifungals
Ureido penicillins

Anosmia - loss of smell sense	4 Quinolones Disinfectants
Antibody formation	Somatotrophic hormones Specific immunoglobulins
Anxiety	Antituberculous agents
Anxiousness	4 Quinolones Amphetamines Antianginal vasodilators Antidepressants Antivirals Barbiturate antiepileptics Benzodiazepine antagonists Beta2 selective stimulants Central stimulants H1 antagonist antihistamines Lipid regulating agents Neuroleptics Opioid antagonists Prophylactic antiasthmatics Selective serotonin reuptake inhibiting antidepressants

Skeletal muscle relaxants
Sympathomimetics
Tricyclic antidepressants
Vasodilator antihypertensives

Apathy

Aliphatic phenothiazine neuroleptics
Butyrophenone neuroleptics
Diphenylbutylpiperidine neuroleptics
Flupenthixols
Fluphenazine
Haloperidols
Neuroleptics
Phenothiazine neuroleptics
Piperazine phenothiazine neuroleptics
Piperidine phenothiazine neuroleptics
Thioxanthene neuroleptics
Zuclopenthixols

Aplastic anaemia

4 Aminoquinoline antimalarials
Acetylurea antiepileptics
Analgesics and anti-inflammatory drugs
Antiepileptics
Antifungals
Antiprotozoals
Antithyroid agents
Carbacephems
Carbazepine antiepileptics
Cephalosporins
Cephamycins
Chelating agents
Chloramphenicols
Class I antiarrhythmics
Gastrointestinal agents
Histamine H2 antagonists
Hydantoin antiepileptics
Inorganic mercury compounds
Neuroleptics
Nitrofuran antimicrobials
Oral hypoglycaemics
Organic mercurial disinfectants
Oxazolidinedione antiepileptics
Phenytoin
Selective serotonin reuptake inhibiting
    antidepressants
Sulphonylurea hypoglycaemics
Tetracyclic antidepressants
Uricosuric agents

Apnoea

Benzodiazepine sedatives
Carbamate sedatives
Class III antiarrhythmics
E series prostaglandins
Inhalation anaesthetics
Polymyxins

Sedatives
Skeletal muscle relaxants

Appetite increased	Antiandrogens
	Antidepressants
	Antiepileptics
	H1 antagonist antihistamines
	Neuroleptics
	Skeletal muscle relaxants
	Tetracyclic antidepressants
	Tricyclic antidepressants

Appetite loss - anorexia	4 Methanolquinoline antimalarials
	4 Quinolones
	Amphetamines
	Anorectics
	Anthelmintics
	Antibiotic antituberculous agents
	Anticholinesterase parasympathomimetics
	Antidepressants
	Antiemetics
	Antiepileptics
	Antifungals
	Antimony antiprotozoals
	Antineoplastics
	Antituberculous agents
	Antiulcer agents
	Antivirals
	Benzimidazole anthelmintics
	Biguanide hypoglycaemics
	Borates
	Carbazepine antiepileptics
	Cardiac glycosides
	Catechol O-methyl transferase inhibitors
	Central stimulants
	Cephalosporins
	Chelating agents
	Clofibrate and analogues
	Colony stimulating factors
	Digitalis
	Dopaminergic antiparkinsonian agents
	Fat soluble vitamins
	HMG CoA reductase inhibitors
	Interleukins
	Lithium
	Nitrofuran antimicrobials
	Oestrogen antagonist antineoplastics
	Opioid antagonists
	Oxazolidinedione antiepileptics
	Polyene antibiotics
	Selective serotonin reuptake inhibiting antidepressants
	Skeletal muscle relaxants
	Somatotrophic hormones

Sulphone antileprotics
Sympathomimetics
Thiazide diuretics
Vaccines
Vasodilator antihypertensives
Vitamin D substances
Vitamins

Arthropathy	Histamine H2 antagonists
	Tetracyclic antidepressants

Asthenia	4 Quinolones
	Anticholinesterase parasympathomimetics
	Antihypertensives
	Antineoplastics
	Antituberculous agents
	Antiulcer agents
	Antivirals
	Cephalosporins
	H1 antagonist antihistamines
	HMG CoA reductase inhibitors
	Interleukins
	Neuroleptics
	Serotonin and analogues

Asthma	Gonad regulating hormones
	Organic iodinated contrast media

Ataxia	4 Methanolquinoline antimalarials
	4 Quinolones
	Alcoholic disinfectants
	Antidepressants
	Antiemetics
	Antiepileptics
	Antineoplastics
	Antivirals
	Barbiturate antiepileptics
	Barbiturate sedatives
	Benzodiazepine sedatives
	Carbamate sedatives
	Carbazepine antiepileptics
	Class I antiarrhythmics
	Class III antiarrhythmics
	GABA related antiepileptics
	Gastrointestinal agents
	H1 antagonist antihistamines
	Hydantoin antiepileptics
	Lithium
	Nitroimidazole antiprotozoals
	Oxazolidinedione antiepileptics
	Phenothiazine antihistamines
	Phenytoin
	Promethazines
	Sedatives

| | Skeletal muscle relaxants |
| | Succinimide antiepileptics |

| **Atony of bladder** | Organic solvents |

| **Atopic dermatitis and related** | Antituberculous agents |
| | Dermatological agents |

| **Atrophy of breast** | Progestogens |
| | Sex hormones |

Attention/concentration difficulty	Antiemetics
	Antiepileptics
	Antivirals
	Neuroleptics

| **Avascular necrosis, head-femur** | Corticosteroids |
| | Corticotrophic hormones |

Backache	ACE inhibitors
	Angiotensin inhibiting antihypertensives
	Antibacterial agents
	Antiulcer agents
	E series prostaglandins
	Gonad regulating hormones
	Progestogens
	Sex hormones

Bacterial infection	Antiulcer agents
	Antivirals
	Corticosteroids
	Corticotrophic hormones
	Immunosuppressants
	Interleukins
	Leech products
	Medicinal enzymes

| **Bacterial pneumonia** | Antivirals |

Behavioural disturbance	Antidepressants
	Ergot compounds
	GABA related antiepileptics
	Sedatives
	Skeletal muscle relaxants
	Tetracyclic antidepressants
	Tricyclic antidepressants

| **Benign neoplasm male breast** | Antiandrogens |

| **Biliary stasis** | 4 Quinolones |
| | Beta lactamase inhibitors |

Birth trauma/asphyxia/hypoxia	Oxytocic hormones
Bleeding time increased	Dermatological agents Salicylate analgesics
Blistering of skin	Retinoic acid dermatological agents
Blocked sinuses	Alpha blocking vasodilators
Blood disorders	4 Aminoquinoline antimalarials 4 Quinolones ACE inhibitors Aldosterone inhibitors Analgesics and anti-inflammatory drugs Antibacterial agents Antiepileptics Antifolate antineoplastics Antifungals Antineoplastics Antivirals Benzodiazepine sedatives Carbacephems Carbamate sedatives Carbapenems Cephalosporins Cephamycins Chelating agents Chloramphenicols Cinchona antimalarials Colchicum alkaloids Gastrointestinal agents Gold salts H1 antagonist antihistamines Histamine H2 antagonists Hydantoin antiepileptics Immunosuppressants Monobactams Nitrofuran antimicrobials Oxacephalosporins Phenothiazine antihistamines Phenytoin Polyene antibiotics Potassium sparing diuretics Promethazines Retinoic acid dermatological agents Skeletal muscle relaxants Succinimide antiepileptics Thiazide diuretics Uricosuric agents Vasodilator antihypertensives
Blood in urine - haematuria	Alpha blocking vasodilators Analgesics and anti-inflammatory drugs

Antivirals
Aromatics
Chelating agents
Colony stimulating factors
Gastrointestinal agents
Haemostatics
Salicylate analgesics
Skeletal muscle relaxants

Blood pressure changes	Oxazolidinedione antiepileptics
Blood pressure raised	Sympathomimetics
Blood urate raised	Antivirals Colony stimulating factors Immunosuppressants Loop diuretics Medicinal enzymes Nutritional carbohydrates Retinoic acid dermatological agents Thiazide diuretics Vasodilator antihypertensives
Blood urea raised	4 Quinolones ACE inhibitors Analgesics and anti-inflammatory drugs Antibiotic antineoplastics Antivirals Borates Erythropoietin Immunosuppressants Interleukin 2 Organic iodinated contrast media Vasodilator antihypertensives
Blurred vision	4 Aminoquinoline antimalarials 4 Methanolquinoline antimalarials 4 Quinolones Aliphatic phenothiazine neuroleptics Anabolics Analgesics and anti-inflammatory drugs Anthelmintics Antiandrogens Antidepressants Antiemetics Antiepileptics Antimuscarinics Antineoplastics Antiprotozoals Antiulcer agents Barbiturate antiepileptics Benzodiazepine sedatives Butyrophenone neuroleptics

Carbamate sedatives
Carbazepine antiepileptics
Carbonic anhydrase inhibitors
Cardiac glycosides
Central stimulants
Centrally acting antihypertensives
Chelating agents
Cholinesterase reactivators
Cinchona antimalarials
Class I antiarrhythmics
Clofibrate and analogues
Corticosteroids
Dermatological agents
Diagnostic agents
Digitalis
Diphenylbutylpiperidine neuroleptics
Dopaminergic antiparkinsonian agents
Flupenthixols
Fluphenazine
GABA related antiepileptics
Gonad regulating hormones
H1 antagonist antihistamines
Haloperidols
Hydantoin antiepileptics
Hydrazine monoamine oxidase inhibiting
    antidepressants
Immunosuppressants
Interleukins
Lithium
Monoamine oxidase inhibiting
    antidepressants
Neuroleptics
Oestrogen antagonist antineoplastics
Oral hypoglycaemics
Oxazolidinedione antiepileptics
Oxytetracyclines
Phenothiazine antihistamines
Phenothiazine neuroleptics
Phenytoin
Piperazine phenothiazine neuroleptics
Piperidine phenothiazine neuroleptics
Polymyxins
Progestogens
Promethazines
Retinoic acid dermatological agents
Salicylate analgesics
Sedatives
Serotonin and analogues
Sex hormones
Skeletal muscle relaxants
Smooth muscle relaxants
Tetracyclic antidepressants
Tetracyclines
Thioxanthene neuroleptics

	Tricyclic antidepressants
	Zuclopenthixols
Bone marrow suppression	ACE inhibitors
	Alkyl sulphonate antineoplastics
	Alkylating antineoplastics
	Anthracycline antibiotic antineoplastics
	Antibiotic antineoplastics
	Antifolate antineoplastics
	Antimalarials
	Antineoplastics
	Antivirals
	Asparaginase antineoplastics
	Ethyleneimine antineoplastics
	Fluorouracil
	Immunosuppressants
	Interleukin 2
	Loop diuretics
	Nitrogen mustards
	Nitrosoureas
	Oestrogen antagonist antineoplastics
	Purine antagonist antineoplastics
	Pyrimidine antagonist antineoplastics
	Sulphur mustards
	Triazene antineoplastics
	Trimethoprim and derivatives
	Trimethoprim sulphonamide combinations
	Vinca alkaloid antineoplastics
Bradycardia	4 Methanolquinoline antimalarials
	Alpha adrenoceptor stimulants
	Amide type anaesthetics
	Analgesics and anti-inflammatory drugs
	Antianginal vasodilators
	Antiarrhythmics
	Anticholinesterase parasympathomimetics
	Antidotes
	Antiemetics
	Antimuscarinics
	Antineoplastics
	Benzomorphan opioid analgesics
	Beta blockers
	Calcium antagonist vasodilators
	Calcium salts
	Cardioselective beta blockers
	Central stimulants
	Centrally acting antihypertensives
	Class I antiarrhythmics
	Class III antiarrhythmics
	Class IV antiarrhythmics
	Diagnostic agents
	Dopaminergic antiparkinsonian agents
	E series prostaglandins

Ergot alkaloids
Ergot compounds
Ester type anaesthetics
Gastrointestinal agents
Histamine H2 antagonists
I series prostaglandins
Inhalation anaesthetics
Local anaesthetics
Methadone and analogues
Morphinan opioid analgesics
Neuroleptics
Nutritional fats
Opioid analgesics
Opioid peptides
Opium alkaloid opioid analgesics
Opium poppy substances
Parasympathomimetics
Parenteral anaesthetics
Pethidine and analogues
Pilocarpine
Platelet activating factor antagonists
Rauwolfia antihypertensives
Respiratory stimulants
Selective serotonin reuptake inhibiting
   antidepressants
Serotonin and analogues
Skeletal muscle relaxants
Smooth muscle relaxants
Sympathomimetics
Vasodilators

Breath - smell of alcohol	Alcoholic disinfectants Alcoholic solvents Glycols
Breath-holding	Inhalation anaesthetics
Breathlessness	Antiandrogens Antibiotic antituberculous agents Antineoplastics
Bronchospasm	4 Quinolones Analgesics and anti-inflammatory drugs Anthelmintics Antiarrhythmics Antibacterial agents Antibiotic antituberculous agents Anticholinesterase parasympathomimetics Antiemetics Antineoplastics Antiulcer agents Beta blockers Beta2 selective stimulants

Blood products
Cardioselective beta blockers
Class III antiarrhythmics
Competitive muscle relaxants
Dermatological agents
Diagnostic agents
Diamidine antiprotozoals
F series prostaglandins
H1 antagonist antihistamines
Medicinal enzymes
Organic iodinated contrast media
Parasympathomimetics
Phenothiazine antihistamines
Pilocarpine
Polymyxins
Promethazines
Prophylactic antiasthmatics
Pyrimidine antagonist antineoplastics
Respiratory stimulants
Salicylate analgesics
Sulphites
Sympathomimetics
Thyrotrophic hormones
Vasodilators
Vinca alkaloid antineoplastics

Bullous eruption

Antiulcer agents
Sedatives

Burning or stinging

Aluminium astringents
Analgesics and anti-inflammatory drugs
Antifungals
Antivirals
Aromatics
Carbonic anhydrase inhibitors
Centrally acting antihypertensives
Chelating agents
Corticosteroids
Dermatological agents
Dithranols
Formaldehyde and related compounds
H1 antagonist antihistamines
Hydroquinone dermatological agents
Imidazole antifungals
Immunosuppressants
Medicinal enzymes
Prophylactic antiasthmatics
Psoralen dermatological agents
Pyrethroid pesticides
Retinoic acid dermatological agents
Serotonin and analogues
Triazole antifungals
Vitamin B substances
Vitamin D substances

Burns	Tannic acid and derivatives
Candidal vulvovaginitis	Cephalosporins
Candidiasis mouth/oesophagus/ gastrointestinal tra	Antiulcer agents Carbapenems
Capillary hyperpermeability	Colony stimulating factors
Carcinoma	Triphenylmethane disinfectant dyes
Cardiac arrest	Amide type anaesthetics Antibacterial agents Antiemetics Class IV antiarrhythmics E series prostaglandins Ester type anaesthetics Inhalation anaesthetics Local anaesthetics Medicinal enzymes Organic iodinated contrast media Peripheral and cerebral vasodilators
Cardiac conduction disorders	4 Methanolquinoline antimalarials Antiandrogens Antineoplastics Calcium antagonist vasodilators Carbazepine antiepileptics Class III antiarrhythmics
Cardiac dysrhythmias	ACE inhibitors Aliphatic phenothiazine neuroleptics Alpha blocking antihypertensives Amphetamines Antiandrogens Antiarrhythmics Antidepressants Antiemetics Antimalarials Antimuscarinics Antineoplastics Antivirals Beta adrenoceptor stimulants Beta sympathomimetic vasodilators Beta2 selective stimulants Butyrophenone neuroleptics Calcium salts Carbazepine antiepileptics Cardiac glycosides Cardiac inotropic agents Central stimulants Chelating agents Class I antiarrhythmics

Colony stimulating factors
Diamidine antiprotozoals
Digitalis
Diphenylbutylpiperidine neuroleptics
Dopaminergic antiparkinsonian agents
E series prostaglandins
Ergolines
Ester type anaesthetics
Flupenthixols
Fluphenazine
H1 antagonist antihistamines
Haloperidols
Hydantoin antiepileptics
Hydrazine monoamine oxidase inhibiting
    antidepressants
Inhalation anaesthetics
Interleukins
Iron compounds
Isoprenaline
Monoamine oxidase inhibiting
    antidepressants
Neuroleptics
Organic iodinated contrast media
Oxytocic hormones
Phenothiazine antihistamines
Phenothiazine neuroleptics
Phenytoin
Piperazine phenothiazine neuroleptics
Piperidine phenothiazine neuroleptics
Polyene antibiotics
Potassium salts
Promethazines
Respiratory stimulants
Serotonin and analogues
Skeletal muscle relaxants
Smooth muscle relaxants
Sympathomimetics
Tetracyclic antidepressants
Theophylline xanthines
Thioxanthene neuroleptics
Thyroid agents
Tricyclic antidepressants
Vasodilator antihypertensives
Vasodilators
Xanthine containing beverages
Xanthines
Zuclopenthixols

Cardiac murmur	Antineoplastics
Cardiomyopathy	Amphetamines
	Anorectics
	Anthracycline antibiotic antineoplastics
	Central stimulants

Cardiovascular symptoms	Antianginal vasodilators
	Antivirals
	Cinchona antimalarials
	Competitive muscle relaxants
	Expectorants
	Hydantoin antiepileptics
	Immunosuppressants
	Inhalation anaesthetics
	Lithium
	Nitrogen mustards
	Phenytoin
	Skeletal muscle relaxants

Cataract	Aliphatic phenothiazine neuroleptics
	Butyrophenone neuroleptics
	Chelating agents
	Corticosteroids
	Corticotrophic hormones
	Diphenylbutylpiperidine neuroleptics
	Flupenthixols
	Fluphenazine
	Haloperidols
	Neuroleptics
	Oestrogen antagonist antineoplastics
	Phenothiazine neuroleptics
	Piperazine phenothiazine neuroleptics
	Piperidine phenothiazine neuroleptics
	Retinoic acid dermatological agents
	Sex hormones
	Thioxanthene neuroleptics
	Zuclopenthixols

Cellulitis or abscess at site of injection	Aliphatic phenothiazine neuroleptics
	Antineoplastics
	Antivirals
	Butyrophenone neuroleptics
	Calcitonin
	Carbapenems
	Chelating agents
	Colony stimulating factors
	Diamidine antiprotozoals
	Diphenylbutylpiperidine neuroleptics
	Dopaminergic antiparkinsonian agents
	E series prostaglandins
	F series prostaglandins
	Flupenthixols
	Fluphenazine
	Gonad regulating hormones
	Haloperidols
	Hydantoin antiepileptics
	Imidazole antifungals
	Insulin
	Insulin zinc suspensions

Lincomycins
Neuroleptics
Oestrogen antagonist antineoplastics
Phenothiazine neuroleptics
Phenytoin
Piperazine phenothiazine neuroleptics
Piperidine phenothiazine neuroleptics
Sedatives
Thioxanthene neuroleptics
Vaccines
Zuclopenthixols

Cerebellar ataxia	Fluorouracil Pyrimidine antagonist antineoplastics
Cerebrovascular disorders	Colony stimulating factors
Change in bowel habit	Histamine H2 antagonists
Change in voice	ACE inhibitors Anabolics Medicinal enzymes Progestogens Sex hormones
Changes in breast size	Gonad regulating hormones
Chemical bronchitis/pneumonit.	Petroleum distillate solvents
Chest pain	Alpha blocking antihypertensives Antiandrogens Antiarrhythmics Antibacterial agents Antidotes Antiemetics Antimuscarinics Antiulcer agents Beta sympathomimetic vasodilators Beta2 selective stimulants Calcium antagonist vasodilators Cardiac inotropic agents Central stimulants Chelating agents Class I antiarrhythmics Colony stimulating factors Corticotrophic hormones E series prostaglandins Ergot alkaloids Ergot compounds HMG CoA reductase inhibitors Oestrogen antagonist antineoplastics Opioid antagonists Sedatives

	Serotonin and analogues
	Sympathomimetics
	Vasodilators

Chest tightness	Antiemetics
	Beta sympathomimetic vasodilators
	Beta2 selective stimulants
	Serotonin and analogues

| **Childhood hyperkinetic syndr.** | Respiratory stimulants |

Chills with fever	Alpha blocking vasodilators
	Antineoplastics
	Antiulcer agents
	Interleukins
	Triazole antifungals

Chloasma	Norgestrels
	Oestrogens
	Progestogens
	Sex hormones

| **Choking sensation** | Antiarrhythmics |
| | Vasodilators |

| **Cholangitis** | Pyrimidine antagonist antineoplastics |

| **Cholesterol gall stones** | Clofibrate and analogues |

Cholinergic urticaria	Anticholinesterase parasympathomimetics
	Parasympathomimetics
	Pilocarpine

| **Choreas** | Central stimulants |

| **Choreiform movement** | Ganglion blocking antihypertensives |

Chronic active hepatitis	Analgesics and anti-inflammatory drugs
	Centrally acting antihypertensives
	Hydrazide antituberculous agents
	Nitrofuran antimicrobials
	Nitrofuran antiprotozoals
	Retinoic acid dermatological agents
	Skeletal muscle relaxants
	Sulphonamides
	Tricyclic antidepressants

| **Chronic renal failure** | Inhalation anaesthetics |

| **Cirrhosis - non alcoholic** | Alcohol metabolism modifiers |

Cold extremities	Alpha adrenoceptor stimulants Sympathomimetics
Colicky abdominal pain	Anthelmintics Laxatives
Coma	Alcoholic disinfectants Anthelmintics Antianginal vasodilators Antivirals Aromatics Gases Lithium Organic iodinated contrast media Oxazolidinedione antiepileptics
Complete atrioventricular block	Calcium antagonist vasodilators Cardiac glycosides Class I antiarrhythmics Class IV antiarrhythmics Digitalis Histamine H2 antagonists
Complete epiphyseal arrest	Anabolics Androgens Sex hormones Testosterones
Confusion	4 Quinolones Aldosterone inhibitors Amide type anaesthetics Analgesics and anti-inflammatory drugs Anthelmintics Antibiotic antifungals Anticholinesterase parasympathomimetics Antidepressants Antidotes Antiemetics Antiepileptics Antifungals Antimuscarinics Antineoplastics Antiulcer agents Antivirals Barbiturate antiepileptics Barbiturate sedatives Benzodiazepine sedatives Borates Carbacephems Carbamate sedatives Carbapenems Carbazepine antiepileptics Cardiac glycosides

Catechol O-methyl transferase inhibitors
Cephalosporins
Cephamycins
Cinchona antimalarials
Class I antiarrhythmics
Colony stimulating factors
Digitalis
Dopaminergic antiparkinsonian agents
Ergolines
Ergot alkaloids
Ergot compounds
Ester type anaesthetics
GABA related antiepileptics
Ganglion blocking antihypertensives
Gases
Histamine H2 antagonists
Hydantoin antiepileptics
Hydrazine monoamine oxidase inhibiting
   antidepressants
Hydroxyquinoline antiprotozoals
Immunosuppressants
Local anaesthetics
Monoamine oxidase inhibiting
   antidepressants
Opioid analgesics
Organic iodinated contrast media
Osmotic diuretics
Phenytoin
Polymyxins
Potassium sparing diuretics
Respiratory stimulants
Salicylate analgesics
Sedatives
Selective serotonin reuptake inhibiting
   antidepressants
Skeletal muscle relaxants
Smooth muscle relaxants
Sympathomimetics
Tetracyclic antidepressants
Tricyclic antidepressants

Conjunct.vasc.disord.,/cysts	Centrally acting antihypertensives
Conjunctival blanching	Centrally acting antihypertensives
Conjunctival deposits	Aliphatic phenothiazine neuroleptics
	Butyrophenone neuroleptics
	Diphenylbutylpiperidine neuroleptics
	Flupenthixols
	Fluphenazine
	Haloperidols
	Neuroleptics
	Phenothiazine neuroleptics

Piperazine phenothiazine neuroleptics
Piperidine phenothiazine neuroleptics
Thioxanthene neuroleptics
Zuclopenthixols

Constipation	ACE inhibitors

Aliphatic phenothiazine neuroleptics
Analgesics and anti-inflammatory drugs
Anorectics
Antacid gastrointestinal agents
Antidepressants
Antidiarrhoeals
Antiemetics
Antimuscarinics
Antineoplastics
Antiulcer agents
Benzimidazole anthelmintics
Benzomorphan opioid analgesics
Bile acid binding resins
Bisphosphonates
Butyrophenone neuroleptics
Carbazepine antiepileptics
Catechol O-methyl transferase inhibitors
Centrally acting antihypertensives
Cephalosporins
Class I antiarrhythmics
Class IV antiarrhythmics
Contrast media
Cough suppressants
Dermatological agents
Diphenylbutylpiperidine neuroleptics
Dopaminergic antiparkinsonian agents
Ergolines
Ferric salts
Ferrous salts
Flupenthixols
Fluphenazine
Ganglion blocking antihypertensives
Gonad regulating hormones
Haloperidols
HMG CoA reductase inhibitors
Hydrazine monoamine oxidase inhibiting
    antidepressants
Interleukins
Iron compounds
Methadone and analogues
Monoamine oxidase inhibiting
    antidepressants
Morphinan cough suppressants
Morphinan opioid analgesics
Neuroleptics
Oestrogen antagonist antineoplastics
Opioid analgesics
Opioid antagonists

Opioid peptides
Opium alkaloid opioid analgesics
Opium poppy substances
Oral hypoglycaemics
Pethidine and analogues
Phenothiazine neuroleptics
Piperazine phenothiazine neuroleptics
Piperidine phenothiazine neuroleptics
Pyrimidine antagonist antineoplastics
Selective noradrenaline reuptake
  inhibiting antidepressants
Selective serotonin reuptake inhibiting
  antidepressants
Skeletal muscle relaxants
Smooth muscle relaxants
Tetracyclic antidepressants
Thiazide diuretics
Thioxanthene neuroleptics
Tricyclic antidepressants
Vinca alkaloid antineoplastics
Zuclopenthixols

Contact dermat.:dichromate	Dermatological agents
Contact dermat.:glycol	Glycols
Contact dermat.:mercurials	Inorganic mercury compounds Organic mercurial disinfectants
Contact dermatitis	Aliphatic phenothiazine neuroleptics Anthelmintics Butyrophenone neuroleptics Chlorinated phenol disinfectants Dermatological agents Diphenylbutylpiperidine neuroleptics Disinfectants Flupenthixols Fluphenazine Haloperidols Neuroleptics Phenothiazine neuroleptics Piperazine phenothiazine neuroleptics Piperidine phenothiazine neuroleptics Thioxanthene neuroleptics Vasodilator antihypertensives Zuclopenthixols
Contact dermatitis:solar rad.	Dermatological agents
Contact lens corneal oedema	Oestrogens Sex hormones
Convulsions	4 Methanolquinoline antimalarials 4 Quinolones

Aliphatic phenothiazine neuroleptics
Amide type anaesthetics
Analgesics and anti-inflammatory drugs
Anthelmintics
Antibiotic antituberculous agents
Antidepressants
Antidiuretic hormones
Antifungals
Antivirals
Aromatics
Benzimidazole anthelmintics
Benzodiazepine antagonists
Borates
Butyrophenone neuroleptics
Carbapenems
Central stimulants
Chelating agents
Class I antiarrhythmics
Colony stimulating factors
Diphenylbutylpiperidine neuroleptics
Dopaminergic antiparkinsonian agents
E series prostaglandins
Erythropoietin
Ester type anaesthetics
Flupenthixols
Fluphenazine
GABA related antiepileptics
Ganglion blocking antihypertensives
Gases
Gastrointestinal agents
Glycols
H1 antagonist antihistamines
Haloperidols
Hydrazide antituberculous agents
Hydrazine monoamine oxidase inhibiting
    antidepressants
Immunosuppressants
Lithium
Local anaesthetics
Monoamine oxidase inhibiting
    antidepressants
Neuroleptics
Nitroimidazole antiprotozoals
Opioid analgesics
Organic iodinated contrast media
Parenteral anaesthetics
Pethidine and analogues
Phenothiazine antihistamines
Phenothiazine neuroleptics
Piperazine phenothiazine neuroleptics
Piperidine phenothiazine neuroleptics
Polyene antibiotics
Posterior pituitary hormones
Promethazines

Respiratory stimulants
Retinoic acid dermatological agents
Salicylate analgesics
Selective serotonin reuptake inhibiting
  antidepressants
Skeletal muscle relaxants
Sympathomimetics
Tetracyclic antidepressants
Theophylline xanthines
Thioxanthene neuroleptics
Tricyclic antidepressants
Xanthine containing beverages
Xanthines
Zuclopenthixols

Coordination disorders (dyspraxia)	Antibiotic antifungals Antiemetics Antiepileptics H1 antagonist antihistamines Lithium Phenothiazine antihistamines Promethazines Sedatives
Corneal deposits	4 Aminoquinoline antimalarials Analgesics and anti-inflammatory drugs Antiprotozoals Class I antiarrhythmics Class III antiarrhythmics Dermatological agents Salicylate analgesics
Corneal disorders	Oestrogen antagonist antineoplastics Sex hormones
Corneal opacity	4 Aminoquinoline antimalarials Aliphatic phenothiazine neuroleptics Butyrophenone neuroleptics Diphenylbutylpiperidine neuroleptics Flupenthixols Fluphenazine Haloperidols Hydroquinone dermatological agents Neuroleptics Phenothiazine neuroleptics Piperazine phenothiazine neuroleptics Piperidine phenothiazine neuroleptics Retinoic acid dermatological agents Thioxanthene neuroleptics Zuclopenthixols
Coronary artery spasm	Ergot compounds

Corpus cavernosum haematoma	E series prostaglandins Papaverine and analogues
Corticoadrenal insufficiency	Parenteral anaesthetics
Cough	ACE inhibitors Anthelmintics Antimony antiprotozoals Antineoplastics Antiulcer agents Antivirals Aromatics GABA related antiepileptics Gases Inhalation anaesthetics Oestrogen antagonist antineoplastics Organic iodinated contrast media Prophylactic antiasthmatics Pyrimidine antagonist antineoplastics Respiratory stimulants
Cranial nerve palsy	4 Quinolones
Creatine kinase level raised	Central stimulants Clofibrate and analogues Depolarising muscle relaxants HMG CoA reductase inhibitors Neuroleptics
Crystalluria	4 Quinolones Gastrointestinal agents Skeletal muscle relaxants
Cushing's syndrome	Corticosteroids Corticotrophic hormones
Cyanide - toxic effects	Vasodilator antihypertensives
Cystitis	Analgesics and anti-inflammatory drugs Antibacterial agents Antineoplastics
Darkened tongue	Antidepressants Antidiarrhoeals Antiulcer agents Bismuth salts Histamine H2 antagonists Skeletal muscle relaxants Tetracyclic antidepressants Tricyclic antidepressants
Deafness	Antibacterial agents Antibiotic antituberculous agents

	Loop diuretics Macrolides Polyene antibiotics
Debility	Borates
Decreased sweating	Alpha blocking antihypertensives
Deformity	Dermatological agents
Degenerative skin disorders	Direct acting anticoagulants Heparinoids Low molecular weight heparins
Dehydration	Antifolate antineoplastics Interleukins
Delayed recovery from anaesthesia	Parenteral anaesthetics
Delirium	Cardiac glycosides Chloral sedatives Digitalis Inhalation anaesthetics Neuroleptics
Dental fluorosis	Fluorine compounds
Depression	4 Quinolones Aliphatic phenothiazine neuroleptics Alpha blocking antihypertensives Anabolics Analgesics and anti-inflammatory drugs Anorectics Antibiotic antituberculous agents Anticholinesterase parasympathomimetics Antidotes Antiemetics Antiepileptics Antineoplastics Antituberculous agents Antiulcer agents Antivirals Barbiturate antiepileptics Butyrophenone neuroleptics Calcium antagonist vasodilators Carbazepine antiepileptics Central stimulants Centrally acting antihypertensives Diphenylbutylpiperidine neuroleptics Dopaminergic antiparkinsonian agents Flupenthixols Fluphenazine GABA related antiepileptics

Gonad regulating hormones
H1 antagonist antihistamines
Haloperidols
Neuroleptics
Norgestrels
Oestrogens
Phenothiazine antihistamines
Phenothiazine neuroleptics
Piperazine phenothiazine neuroleptics
Piperidine phenothiazine neuroleptics
Progestogens
Promethazines
Rauwolfia antihypertensives
Retinoic acid dermatological agents
Salicylate analgesics
Sedatives
Sex hormones
Skeletal muscle relaxants
Succinimide antiepileptics
Thioxanthene neuroleptics
Zuclopenthixols

Dermatosis	Antiprotozoals
Desire to defaecate	Anticholinesterase parasympathomimetics Antidiuretic hormones Diagnostic agents Parasympathomimetics Pilocarpine Posterior pituitary hormones Vasopressins
Desire to micturate	Anticholinesterase parasympathomimetics Diagnostic agents Parasympathomimetics Pilocarpine Thyrotrophic hormones
Diabetes mellitus with ketoacidosis	Antivirals
Diarrhoea	4 Aminoquinoline antimalarials 4 Methanolquinoline antimalarials 4 Quinolones ACE inhibitors Adrenergic neurone blocking antihypertensives Alpha blocking antihypertensives Alpha blocking vasodilators Alpha glucosidase inhibitors Amidinopenicillins Amino acids Aminopenicillanic derivatives

Aminopenicillins
Anabolics
Analgesics and anti-inflammatory drugs
Anorectics
Antacid gastrointestinal agents
Anthelmintics
Antiandrogens
Antianginal vasodilators
Antibacterial agents
Antibiotic antituberculous agents
Anticholinesterase parasympathomimetics
Antiemetics
Antifungals
Antihypertensives
Antileprotics
Antimalarials
Antineoplastics
Antipseudomonal penicillins
Antituberculous agents
Antiulcer agents
Antivirals
Aspartic acid
Benzimidazole anthelmintics
Benzylpenicillin and derivatives
Beta blockers
Biguanide antimalarials
Biguanide hypoglycaemics
Bile acid binding resins
Bile acids and salts
Bisphosphonates
Borates
Carbacephems
Carbapenems
Carbazepine antiepileptics
Carboxypenicillins
Cardiac glycosides
Cardiac inotropic agents
Catechol O-methyl transferase inhibitors
Cation exchange resins
Central stimulants
Centrally acting antihypertensives
Cephalosporins
Cephamycins
Chloramphenicols
Class I antiarrhythmics
Colchicum alkaloids
Colony stimulating factors
Contrast media
Corticosteroids
Coumarin anticoagulants
Dermatological agents
Diagnostic agents
Digitalis
E series prostaglandins

Edetates
Ergolines
Essential amino acids
Expectorants
F series prostaglandins
Fat soluble vitamins
Ferric salts
Ferrous salts
Fixed oils
Gastrointestinal agents
Glucose tests
Glycerol
Glycol and glycerol esters
Gold salts
Gonad regulating hormones
H1 antagonist antihistamines
Haemostatics
HMG CoA reductase inhibitors
Hydroxynaphthoquinones
Hydroxyquinoline antiprotozoals
Immunosuppressants
Indanedione anticoagulants
Iron compounds
Isoxazolyl penicillins
Leukotriene inhibitors
Lincomycins
Lipid regulating agents
Lithium
Macrolides
Magnesium salts
Medicinal enzymes
Monobactams
Natural penicillins
Neuroleptics
Nitrofuran antimicrobials
Nutritional carbohydrates
Oestrogen antagonist antineoplastics
Opioid antagonists
Oral hypoglycaemics
Organic iodinated contrast media
Oxacephalosporins
Oxytetracyclines
Parasympathomimetics
Penicillinase resistant penicillins
Phenoxymethylpenicillin and derivatives
Phenoxypenicillins
Pilocarpine
Polyene antibiotics
Pyrimidine antagonist antineoplastics
Salicylate analgesics
Sedatives
Selective serotonin reuptake inhibiting
    antidepressants
Skeletal muscle relaxants

Smooth muscle relaxants
Somatotrophic hormones
Sulphonamides
Tetracyclines
Thiazide diuretics
Thyroid agents
Triazole antifungals
Trimethoprim sulphonamide
    combinations
Typhoid vaccines
Ureido penicillins
Vasodilators
Vitamin D substances
Vitamin E substances
Vitamins

Difficulty swallowing solids	Antimuscarinics
	Smooth muscle relaxants

Difficulty with micturition	Aliphatic phenothiazine neuroleptics
	Alkylating antineoplastics
	Antidepressants
	Antimuscarinics
	Benzomorphan opioid analgesics
	Beta blockers
	Butyrophenone neuroleptics
	Colony stimulating factors
	Diphenylbutylpiperidine neuroleptics
	Flupenthixols
	Fluphenazine
	Haloperidols
	Hydrazine monoamine oxidase inhibiting antidepressants
	Methadone and analogues
	Monoamine oxidase inhibiting antidepressants
	Morphinan opioid analgesics
	Neuroleptics
	Opioid analgesics
	Opioid peptides
	Opium alkaloid opioid analgesics
	Opium poppy substances
	Organic iodinated contrast media
	Pethidine and analogues
	Phenothiazine neuroleptics
	Piperazine phenothiazine neuroleptics
	Piperidine phenothiazine neuroleptics
	Skeletal muscle relaxants
	Smooth muscle relaxants
	Tetracyclic antidepressants
	Thioxanthene neuroleptics
	Tricyclic antidepressants
	Zuclopenthixols

Diplopia/double vision	Antiepileptics Ergolines GABA related antiepileptics Polyene antibiotics Sedatives Skeletal muscle relaxants
Direct Coombs test positive	Carbacephems Carbapenems Centrally acting antihypertensives Cephalosporins Cephamycins
Discolouration of teeth	Antibacterial agents Fluorine compounds Oxytetracyclines Tetracyclines Trimethoprim and derivatives Trimethoprim sulphonamide combinations
Disorders of calcium metabol.	Hydantoin antiepileptics Phenytoin
Disorders of conjunctiva	Interleukins
Disorientation	Antiemetics
Dizziness	4 Methanolquinoline antimalarials 4 Quinolones ACE inhibitors Alcoholic solvents Aldose reductase inhibitors Alpha blocking antihypertensives Alpha blocking vasodilators Amphetamines Anabolics Analgesics and anti-inflammatory drugs Angiotensin inhibiting antihypertensives Anorectics Anthelmintics Antiandrogens Antianginal vasodilators Antibacterial agents Antibiotic antifungals Antibiotic antituberculous agents Anticholinesterase parasympathomimetics Antidepressants Antidotes Antiemetics Antiepileptics Antihypertensives

Antineoplastics
Antiprotozoals
Antituberculous agents
Antiulcer agents
Antivirals
Barbiturate sedatives
Benzimidazole anthelmintics
Beta2 selective stimulants
Bisphosphonates
Calcium antagonist vasodilators
Carbacephems
Carbazepine antiepileptics
Catechol O-methyl transferase inhibitors
Central stimulants
Centrally acting antihypertensives
Cephalosporins
Cephamycins
Chelating agents
Cholinesterase reactivators
Class I antiarrhythmics
Class IV antiarrhythmics
Clofibrate and analogues
Contrast media
Cough suppressants
Cytoprotective agents
Dermatological agents
Diagnostic agents
Diamidine antiprotozoals
Dopaminergic antiparkinsonian agents
E series prostaglandins
Ergolines
Ergot alkaloids
Ergot compounds
F series prostaglandins
GABA related antiepileptics
Gases
Gonad regulating hormones
Haemostatics
Histamine H2 antagonists
HMG CoA reductase inhibitors
Hydantoin antiepileptics
Hydrazine monoamine oxidase inhibiting
    antidepressants
Immunosuppressants
Monoamine oxidase inhibiting
    antidepressants
Neuroleptics
Nitrofuran antiprotozoals
Nitroimidazole antiprotozoals
Oestrogen antagonist antineoplastics
Opioid antagonists
Organic iodinated contrast media
Oxazolidinedione antiepileptics
Peripheral and cerebral vasodilators

Phenytoin
Pilocarpine
Progestogens
Prophylactic antiasthmatics
Psoralen dermatological agents
Respiratory stimulants
Salicylate analgesics
Sedatives
Selective noradrenaline reuptake
    inhibiting antidepressants
Selective serotonin reuptake inhibiting
    antidepressants
Serotonin and analogues
Sex hormones
Skeletal muscle relaxants
Smooth muscle relaxants
Succinimide antiepileptics
Sympathomimetics
Tetracyclines
Thiazide diuretics
Thyrotrophic hormones
Triazole antifungals
Uricosuric agents
Vasodilator antihypertensives
Vitamin B substances

Drowsiness

4 Quinolones
Adrenergic neurone blocking
    antihypertensives
Alcohol metabolism modifiers
Alcoholic disinfectants
Alcoholic solvents
Aliphatic phenothiazine neuroleptics
Alpha blocking antihypertensives
Analgesics and anti-inflammatory drugs
Anorectics
Anthelmintics
Antiandrogens
Antibiotic antituberculous agents
Antidepressants
Antidiarrhoeals
Antiemetics
Antiepileptics
Antineoplastics
Antituberculous agents
Antiulcer agents
Antivirals
Asparaginase antineoplastics
Barbiturate antiepileptics
Barbiturate sedatives
Benzimidazole anthelmintics
Benzodiazepine sedatives
Benzomorphan opioid analgesics

Butyrophenone neuroleptics
Calcium antagonist vasodilators
Carbamate sedatives
Carbazepine antiepileptics
Cardiac glycosides
Central stimulants
Centrally acting antihypertensives
Cephalosporins
Chelating agents
Cholinesterase reactivators
Cough suppressants
Cytoprotective agents
Dermatological agents
Diagnostic agents
Digitalis
Diphenylbutylpiperidine neuroleptics
Dopaminergic antiparkinsonian agents
Ergolines
Ergot compounds
Flupenthixols
Fluphenazine
GABA related antiepileptics
Gonad regulating hormones
H1 antagonist antihistamines
Haloperidols
Histamine H2 antagonists
Hydrazine monoamine oxidase inhibiting
    antidepressants
Lithium
Methadone and analogues
Monoamine oxidase inhibiting
    antidepressants
Morphinan opioid analgesics
Neuroleptics
Nitrofuran antiprotozoals
Nitroimidazole antiprotozoals
Norgestrels
Oestrogen antagonist antineoplastics
Opioid analgesics
Opioid peptides
Opium alkaloid opioid analgesics
Opium poppy substances
Oxazolidinedione antiepileptics
Pethidine and analogues
Phenothiazine antihistamines
Phenothiazine neuroleptics
Piperazine phenothiazine neuroleptics
Piperidine phenothiazine neuroleptics
Progestogens
Promethazines
Prophylactic antiasthmatics
Pyrimidine antagonist antineoplastics
Retinoic acid dermatological agents
Salicylate analgesics

Sedatives
Selective serotonin reuptake inhibiting
    antidepressants
Serotonin and analogues
Sex hormones
Skeletal muscle relaxants
Succinimide antiepileptics
Sympathomimetics
Thioxanthene neuroleptics
Xanthine oxidase inhibitors
Zuclopenthixols

Drug dependence

Amphetamines
Anorectics
Benzodiazepine sedatives
Benzomorphan opioid analgesics
Carbamate sedatives
Central stimulants
Chloral sedatives
Methadone and analogues
Morphinan opioid analgesics
Opioid analgesics
Opioid peptides
Opium alkaloid opioid analgesics
Opium poppy substances
Pethidine and analogues
Sedatives
Skeletal muscle relaxants

Drug induced myelopathy

Hydroxyquinoline antiprotozoals

Drug psychoses

Alcohol metabolism modifiers
Amphetamines
Anorectics
Antiemetics
Antiprotozoals
Antituberculous agents
Antivirals
Central stimulants
Dopaminergic antiparkinsonian agents
Ergolines
Lithium
Parenteral anaesthetics
Sympathomimetics

Dry cough

ACE inhibitors

Dry eyes

Antimuscarinics
Beta blockers
Cardiac inotropic agents
Cardioselective beta blockers
Centrally acting antihypertensives
H1 antagonist antihistamines

	Retinoic acid dermatological agents
	Skeletal muscle relaxants

Dry hair	Fat soluble vitamins
	Vitamin A substances
	Vitamins

Dry mouth	Aliphatic phenothiazine neuroleptics
	Alpha blocking antihypertensives
	Alpha blocking vasodilators
	Amphetamines
	Analgesics and anti-inflammatory drugs
	Anorectics
	Antidepressants
	Antiemetics
	Antihypertensives
	Antimuscarinics
	Antiulcer agents
	Antivirals
	Aromatics
	Benzomorphan opioid analgesics
	Butyrophenone neuroleptics
	Catechol O-methyl transferase inhibitors
	Central stimulants
	Centrally acting antihypertensives
	Class I antiarrhythmics
	Dermatological agents
	Diphenylbutylpiperidine neuroleptics
	Ergolines
	Flupenthixols
	Fluphenazine
	H1 antagonist antihistamines
	Haloperidols
	Hydrazine monoamine oxidase inhibiting antidepressants
	Methadone and analogues
	Monoamine oxidase inhibiting antidepressants
	Morphinan opioid analgesics
	Neuroleptics
	Opioid analgesics
	Opioid peptides
	Opium alkaloid opioid analgesics
	Opium poppy substances
	Pethidine and analogues
	Phenothiazine antihistamines
	Phenothiazine neuroleptics
	Piperazine phenothiazine neuroleptics
	Piperidine phenothiazine neuroleptics
	Potassium sparing diuretics
	Promethazines
	Prophylactic antiasthmatics
	Rauwolfia antihypertensives
	Retinoic acid dermatological agents

Sedatives
Selective noradrenaline reuptake
    inhibiting antidepressants
Selective serotonin reuptake inhibiting
    antidepressants
Serotonin and analogues
Skeletal muscle relaxants
Smooth muscle relaxants
Sympathomimetics
Tetracyclic antidepressants
Thioxanthene neuroleptics
Tricyclic antidepressants
Zuclopenthixols

Dry skin

Antimuscarinics
Antivirals
Dermatological agents
Fat soluble vitamins
Gonad regulating hormones
Retinoic acid dermatological agents
Smooth muscle relaxants
Vitamin A substances
Vitamin B substances
Vitamins

Duodenal ulcer - (DU)

Analgesics and anti-inflammatory drugs

Dysarthria

Alcoholic disinfectants
Class I antiarrhythmics
GABA related antiepileptics
Ganglion blocking antihypertensives
Lithium

Dyskinesia

Aliphatic phenothiazine neuroleptics
Butyrophenone neuroleptics
Carbazepine antiepileptics
Catechol O-methyl transferase inhibitors
Central stimulants
Diphenylbutylpiperidine neuroleptics
Dopaminergic antiparkinsonian agents
Ergolines
Flupenthixols
Fluphenazine
Haloperidols
Hydantoin antiepileptics
Neuroleptics
Phenothiazine neuroleptics
Phenytoin
Piperazine phenothiazine neuroleptics
Piperidine phenothiazine neuroleptics
Selective serotonin reuptake inhibiting
    antidepressants
Succinimide antiepileptics

Thioxanthene neuroleptics
Tricyclic antidepressants
Zuclopenthixols

Dysmenorrhoea	Immunosuppressants

Dyspepsia	4 Quinolones
	ACE inhibitors
	Anabolics
	Analgesics and anti-inflammatory drugs
	Anticholinesterase parasympathomimetics
	Antidepressants
	Antimuscarinics
	Antiulcer agents
	Antivirals
	Catechol O-methyl transferase inhibitors
	Cephalosporins
	Corticosteroids
	Dermatological agents
	E series prostaglandins
	Ergolines
	Evening primrose oil
	GABA related antiepileptics
	Gastrointestinal agents
	H1 antagonist antihistamines
	HMG CoA reductase inhibitors
	Interleukins
	Neuroleptics
	Oestrogen antagonist antineoplastics
	Prophylactic antiasthmatics
	Salicylate analgesics
	Selective serotonin reuptake inhibiting antidepressants
	Smooth muscle relaxants
	Thiazide diuretics
	Triazole antifungals

Dysphagia	4 Quinolones
	Skeletal muscle relaxants

Dyspnoea	4 Quinolones
	Alkylating antineoplastics
	Analgesics and anti-inflammatory drugs
	Anthelmintics
	Antiarrhythmics
	Antibacterial agents
	Antidotes
	Antiemetics
	Antineoplastics
	Antivirals
	Class I antiarrhythmics
	Colony stimulating factors
	Corticotrophic hormones

	Diagnostic agents
	E series prostaglandins
	Ergolines
	Ergot alkaloids
	Ergot compounds
	F series prostaglandins
	Gases
	Immunosuppressants
	Interleukins
	Iron compounds
	Neuroleptics
	Oestrogen antagonist antineoplastics
	Organic iodinated contrast media
	Pyrimidine antagonist antineoplastics
	Respiratory stimulants
	Skeletal muscle relaxants
	Vasodilators
	Vinca alkaloid antineoplastics

Dysuria

Antivirals
Gonad regulating hormones
Selective noradrenaline reuptake
    inhibiting antidepressants

Ecchymoses

Hyaluronic acid
Interleukins
Selective serotonin reuptake inhibiting
    antidepressants
Skeletal muscle relaxants

Ectopic beats

Cardiac inotropic agents
Respiratory stimulants

Ectropion

Skeletal muscle relaxants

**Electrocardiogram (ECG)
abnormal**

4 Aminoquinoline antimalarials
Aliphatic phenothiazine neuroleptics
Butyrophenone neuroleptics
Calcium antagonist vasodilators
Diphenylbutylpiperidine neuroleptics
Edetates
Flupenthixols
Fluphenazine
Haloperidols
Lithium
Neuroleptics
Phenothiazine neuroleptics
Piperazine phenothiazine neuroleptics
Piperidine phenothiazine neuroleptics
Thioxanthene neuroleptics
Zuclopenthixols

**Electroencephalogram (EEG)
abnormal**

Aliphatic phenothiazine neuroleptics
Butyrophenone neuroleptics

	Diphenylbutylpiperidine neuroleptics
	Flupenthixols
	Fluphenazine
	Haloperidols
	Neuroleptics
	Phenothiazine neuroleptics
	Piperazine phenothiazine neuroleptics
	Piperidine phenothiazine neuroleptics
	Pulmonary surfactants
	Thioxanthene neuroleptics
	Zuclopenthixols
Electrolytes abnormal	Antibiotic antituberculous agents
	Antimalarials
	Antineoplastics
	Electrolytes
Emotional instability	Antiepileptics
	Oestrogen antagonist antineoplastics
Encephalitis-post plague vacc.	Vaccines
Encephalopathy	Antiandrogens
	Antiulcer agents
	Interleukin 2
Endocrine, nutritional, metabolic and immunity di	Immunosuppressants
Enteritis/colitis	Analgesics and anti-inflammatory drugs
	Gold salts
	Immunosuppressants
	Retinoic acid dermatological agents
Eosinophilia	4 Quinolones
	Antibacterial agents
	Antibiotic antituberculous agents
	Antidepressants
	Antivirals
	Carbacephems
	Carbapenems
	Cephalosporins
	Cephamycins
	Dopaminergic antiparkinsonian agents
	Lincomycins
	Neuroleptics
	Oxacephalosporins
	Skeletal muscle relaxants
	Sulphonamides
	Tetracyclic antidepressants
	Tricyclic antidepressants
	Trimethoprim sulphonamide combinations
	Xanthine oxidase inhibitors

Epididymitis

Class III antiarrhythmics

Epigastric pain

Alpha blocking vasodilators
Analgesics and anti-inflammatory drugs
Beta blockers
Ergolines
Ferric salts
Ferrous salts
Gastrointestinal agents
Iron compounds
Lipid regulating agents
Peripheral and cerebral vasodilators
Polyene antibiotics
Salicylate analgesics

Epileptic seizures - clonic

Anthelmintics
Erythropoietin

Epileptic seizures - tonic

Erythropoietin

Epileptiform seizures

Organic iodinated contrast media

Epiphora - excess lacrimation

Chelating agents
Edetates
Opioid antagonists
Organic iodinated contrast media
Pilocarpine
Prophylactic antiasthmatics
Skeletal muscle relaxants

Epistaxis

Analgesics and anti-inflammatory drugs
Angiotensin inhibiting antihypertensives
Antidiuretic hormones
Colony stimulating factors
Corticosteroids
Ergolines
Gold salts
Posterior pituitary hormones
Retinoic acid dermatological agents

Erythema

4 Methanolquinoline antimalarials
4 Quinolones
ACE inhibitors
Aliphatic phenothiazine neuroleptics
Analgesics and anti-inflammatory drugs
Antiandrogens
Antibacterial agents
Antibiotic antifungals
Antifungals
Antiulcer agents
Benzimidazole anthelmintics
Bisphosphonates

Borates
Butyrophenone neuroleptics
Calcium antagonist vasodilators
Carbacephems
Carbapenems
Carbazepine antiepileptics
Central stimulants
Centrally acting antihypertensives
Cephalosporins
Cephamycins
Chelating agents
Chloramphenicols
Class I antiarrhythmics
Class IV antiarrhythmics
Contrast media
Dermatological agents
Diphenylbutylpiperidine neuroleptics
E series prostaglandins
F series prostaglandins
Flupenthixols
Fluphenazine
Gastrointestinal agents
Haloperidols
Hyaluronic acid
Hydantoin antiepileptics
Hydrazide antituberculous agents
Hydroquinone dermatological agents
Lipid regulating agents
Medicinal enzymes
Neuroleptics
Nitrofuran antimicrobials
Oestrogens
Oral hypoglycaemics
Organic iodinated contrast media
Oxytetracyclines
Phenothiazine neuroleptics
Phenytoin
Piperazine phenothiazine neuroleptics
Piperidine phenothiazine neuroleptics
Psoralen dermatological agents
Pyrethroid pesticides
Pyrimidine antagonist antineoplastics
Retinoic acid dermatological agents
Rubefacient vasodilators
Sex hormones
Succinimide antiepileptics
Sulphonamides
Sulphonylurea hypoglycaemics
Tetracyclines
Thiazide diuretics
Thiouracil antithyroid agents
Thioxanthene neuroleptics
Trimethoprim sulphonamide
   combinations

	Vaccines
	Vasodilator antihypertensives
	Vitamin B substances
	Vitamin D substances
	Zuclopenthixols
Erythema multiforme	Antibacterial agents
	Antibiotic antifungals
	Central stimulants
	Oxazolidinedione antiepileptics
	Succinimide antiepileptics
Erythrocyte sedimentation rate (ESR) raised	Fat soluble vitamins
	Vitamin A substances
	Vitamins
Euphoria	Amphetamines
	Anabolics
	Analgesics and anti-inflammatory drugs
	Anorectics
	Antiemetics
	Central stimulants
	Centrally acting antihypertensives
	Corticosteroids
	Corticotrophic hormones
	Dopaminergic antiparkinsonian agents
	Prophylactic antiasthmatics
	Sedatives
	Skeletal muscle relaxants
	Succinimide antiepileptics
Exanthema	Analgesics and anti-inflammatory drugs
	Antidepressants
	Beta2 selective stimulants
	Oestrogen antagonist antineoplastics
	Typhoid vaccines
Excessive belching	Antidiuretic hormones
	Omega 3 triglycerides
	Posterior pituitary hormones
	Vasopressins
Excessive flatulence	Lipid regulating agents
Excessive salivation	Anticholinesterase parasympathomimetics
	Antiepileptics
	Antituberculous agents
	Benzodiazepine sedatives
	Blood products
	Calcium antagonist vasodilators
	Carbamate sedatives
	Inhalation anaesthetics
	Neuroleptics

Parasympathomimetics
Pilocarpine
Respiratory stimulants
Skeletal muscle relaxants

Excessive sweating

Amphetamines
Analgesics and anti-inflammatory drugs
Anorectics
Antianginal vasodilators
Anticholinesterase parasympathomimetics
Antidepressants
Antidotes
Benzomorphan opioid analgesics
Beta adrenoceptor stimulants
Beta sympathomimetic vasodilators
Beta2 selective stimulants
Catechol O-methyl transferase inhibitors
Central stimulants
Chelating agents
Colony stimulating factors
Diphenylbutylpiperidine neuroleptics
Dopaminergic antiparkinsonian agents
F series prostaglandins
Fat soluble vitamins
Gonad regulating hormones
H1 antagonist antihistamines
Histamine H2 antagonists
Hydrazine monoamine oxidase inhibiting
    antidepressants
I series prostaglandins
Isoprenaline
Methadone and analogues
Monoamine oxidase inhibiting
    antidepressants
Morphinan opioid analgesics
Opioid analgesics
Opioid antagonists
Opioid peptides
Opium alkaloid opioid analgesics
Opium poppy substances
Parasympathomimetics
Pethidine and analogues
Phenothiazine antihistamines
Pilocarpine
Promethazines
Retinoic acid dermatological agents
Sedatives
Selective serotonin reuptake inhibiting
    antidepressants
Skeletal muscle relaxants
Tetracyclic antidepressants
Thyroid agents
Tricyclic antidepressants
Vasodilator antihypertensives

Vitamin D substances
Vitamins

Excessive thirst

Antiandrogens
Antimuscarinics
Fat soluble vitamins
Opioid antagonists
Smooth muscle relaxants
Vitamin D substances
Vitamins

Exfoliative dermatitis

Amidinopenicillins
Aminoglycosides
Aminopenicillanic derivatives
Aminopenicillins
Antibacterial agents
Antipseudomonal penicillins
Benzylpenicillin and derivatives
Beta lactamase inhibitors
Carbapenems
Carboxypenicillins
Class IV antiarrhythmics
Dithranols
Gold salts
Isoxazolyl penicillins
Natural penicillins
Oxytetracyclines
Penicillinase resistant penicillins
Phenoxymethylpenicillin and derivatives
Phenoxypenicillins
Retinoic acid dermatological agents
Skeletal muscle relaxants
Sulphonamides
Tetracyclines
Theophylline xanthines
Tricyclic antidepressants
Ureido penicillins

Exfoliative erythema

Retinoic acid dermatological agents

Extrapyramidal symptoms

Aliphatic phenothiazine neuroleptics
Alpha blocking antihypertensives
Antiemetics
Antihypertensives
Butyrophenone neuroleptics
Centrally acting antihypertensives
Diphenylbutylpiperidine neuroleptics
Flupenthixols
Fluphenazine
Gastrointestinal agents
H1 antagonist antihistamines
Haloperidols
Neuroleptics

	Phenothiazine antihistamines
	Phenothiazine neuroleptics
	Piperazine phenothiazine neuroleptics
	Piperidine phenothiazine neuroleptics
	Promethazines
	Selective serotonin reuptake inhibiting antidepressants
	Thioxanthene neuroleptics
	Vasodilator antihypertensives
	Zuclopenthixols
Eye pain	Calcium antagonist vasodilators
Eye symptoms	Centrally acting antihypertensives
Eyelid entropion/trichiasis	Skeletal muscle relaxants
Faecal impaction	Ferric salts
	Ferrous salts
	Iron compounds
Faeces colour: dark	Antidiarrhoeals
	Antiulcer agents
	Bismuth salts
	Histamine H2 antagonists
Falls	Dopaminergic antiparkinsonian agents
	Sedatives
Fatigue	ACE inhibitors
	Alcohol metabolism modifiers
	Alpha blocking antihypertensives
	Analgesics and anti-inflammatory drugs
	Angiotensin inhibiting antihypertensives
	Antiandrogens
	Antibiotic antifungals
	Antidepressants
	Antidotes
	Antiemetics
	Antiepileptics
	Antineoplastics
	Antivirals
	Beta blockers
	Calcium antagonist vasodilators
	Cardiac glycosides
	Cardioselective beta blockers
	Central stimulants
	Class I antiarrhythmics
	Class III antiarrhythmics
	Class IV antiarrhythmics
	Clofibrate and analogues
	Colony stimulating factors
	Digitalis

Dopaminergic antiparkinsonian agents
GABA related antiepileptics
Gonad regulating hormones
H1 antagonist antihistamines
Histamine H2 antagonists
HMG CoA reductase inhibitors
Hydrazine monoamine oxidase inhibiting
   antidepressants
Immunosuppressants
Leukotriene inhibitors
Lipid regulating agents
Monoamine oxidase inhibiting
   antidepressants
Neuroleptics
Oestrogen antagonist antineoplastics
Opioid antagonists
Sedatives
Serotonin and analogues
Skeletal muscle relaxants
Thiazide diuretics
Trace elements
Vaccines

Feels hot/feverish	Antineoplastics
	Aromatics
	Serotonin and analogues
Female genital organ symptoms	Gonad regulating hormones
Feminising effects	Oestrogens
	Sex hormones
Fertility problems	Alkyl sulphonate antineoplastics
	Alkylating antineoplastics
	Anabolics
	Carbazepine antiepileptics
	Ethyleneimine antineoplastics
	Nitrogen mustards
	Nitrosoureas
	Sulphur mustards
	Triazene antineoplastics
Fever	4 Quinolones
	Anthelmintics
	Antifolate antineoplastics
	Antineoplastics
	Antithyroid agents
	Antiulcer agents
	Antivirals
	Cardiac inotropic agents
	Edetates
	Gonad regulating hormones
	Leech products

	Platelet activating factor antagonists Triazole antifungals
Fibrosing alveolitis	Class I antiarrhythmics Class III antiarrhythmics Gastrointestinal agents
Fibrosis of penis	E series prostaglandins Papaverine and analogues
Flatulence/wind	4 Quinolones Alpha glucosidase inhibitors Analgesics and anti-inflammatory drugs Antacid gastrointestinal agents Antimuscarinics Antiulcer agents Antivirals Aromatics Bile acid binding resins Bulk laxatives Cephalosporins Chloral sedatives Corticosteroids Dichloroacetamide antiprotozoals E series prostaglandins HMG CoA reductase inhibitors Hypoglycaemics Laxatives Lipid regulating agents Nutritional carbohydrates Somatotrophic hormones Sweetening agents Triazole antifungals
Fluid retention	Adrenergic neurone blocking antihypertensives Anabolics Analgesics and anti-inflammatory drugs Androgens Antidiuretic hormones Antineoplastics Antiulcer agents Centrally acting antihypertensives Corticosteroids Corticotrophic hormones Liquorice Norgestrels Oestrogen antagonist antineoplastics Oestrogens Posterior pituitary hormones Progestogens Rauwolfia antihypertensives Salicylate analgesics

	Sex hormones
	Testosterones
	Uricosuric agents
	Vasodilator antihypertensives

Fluid/electrolyte/acid-base	Neuroleptics

Flushing	ACE inhibitors
	Alpha blocking vasodilators
	Analgesics and anti-inflammatory drugs
	Angiotensin inhibiting antihypertensives
	Antiandrogens
	Antianginal vasodilators
	Antiarrhythmics
	Antibacterial agents
	Antibiotic antituberculous agents
	Antidepressants
	Antidotes
	Antiemetics
	Antihypertensives
	Antimuscarinics
	Antineoplastics
	Antivirals
	Benzodiazepine antagonists
	Benzomorphan opioid analgesics
	Beta sympathomimetic vasodilators
	Beta2 selective stimulants
	Calcitonin
	Calcium antagonist vasodilators
	Cinchona antimalarials
	Class IV antiarrhythmics
	Competitive muscle relaxants
	Corticotrophic hormones
	Cytoprotective agents
	Diagnostic agents
	Diamidine antiprotozoals
	Dopaminergic antiparkinsonian agents
	E series prostaglandins
	Ergolines
	Ergot compounds
	F series prostaglandins
	Gonad regulating hormones
	Hyaluronic acid
	I series prostaglandins
	Inhalation anaesthetics
	Iron compounds
	Lipid regulating agents
	Magnesium salts
	Methadone and analogues
	Morphinan opioid analgesics
	Oestrogen antagonist antineoplastics
	Opioid analgesics
	Opioid peptides
	Opium alkaloid opioid analgesics

Opium poppy substances
Organic iodinated contrast media
Peripheral and cerebral vasodilators
Pethidine and analogues
Progestogens
Rubefacient vasodilators
Serotonin and analogues
Sex hormones
Smooth muscle relaxants
Somatotrophic hormones
Sulphonylurea hypoglycaemics
Thyroid agents
Thyrotrophic hormones
Uricosuric agents
Vasodilators
Vitamin B substances

Folate-deficiency anaemia	Barbiturate antiepileptics
	Gastrointestinal agents
	Hydantoin antiepileptics
	Phenytoin
Frostbite	Local anaesthetics
Fructose in urine	Nutritional carbohydrates
Full blood count abnormal	Analgesics and anti-inflammatory drugs
	Vasodilator antihypertensives
Galactorrhoe	Aliphatic phenothiazine neuroleptics
	Antiandrogens
	Antiemetics
	Butyrophenone neuroleptics
	Carbazepine antiepileptics
	Diphenylbutylpiperidine neuroleptics
	Flupenthixols
	Fluphenazine
	Haloperidols
	Neuroleptics
	Phenothiazine neuroleptics
	Piperazine phenothiazine neuroleptics
	Piperidine phenothiazine neuroleptics
	Selective serotonin reuptake inhibiting antidepressants
	Thioxanthene neuroleptics
	Tricyclic antidepressants
	Zuclopenthixols
Gall stones	Somatotrophic hormones
Gallbladder disorders incl Cholestasis	ACE inhibitors
	Aliphatic phenothiazine neuroleptics
	Analgesics and anti-inflammatory drugs

Antiandrogens
Antibacterial agents
Antibiotic antifungals
Beta lactamase inhibitors
Chelating agents
Coumarin anticoagulants
Gold salts
Histamine H2 antagonists
Hydantoin antiepileptics
Immunosuppressants
Indanedione anticoagulants
Isoxazolyl penicillins
Macrolides
Methadone and analogues
Neuroleptics
Nitrofuran antimicrobials
Oestrogen antagonist antineoplastics
Oral hypoglycaemics
Phenytoin
Sex hormones
Skeletal muscle relaxants
Sulphonamides
Sulphonylurea hypoglycaemics
Thiouracil antithyroid agents
Thiourea antithyroid agents
Tricyclic antidepressants
Trimethoprim sulphonamide
  combinations

Gangrene	Ergot alkaloids
	Ergot compounds
Gastric ulcer - (GU)	Analgesics and anti-inflammatory drugs
	Medicinal enzymes
Gastritis	Analgesics and anti-inflammatory drugs
	Antiepileptics
	Antiulcer agents
	Chloral sedatives
	Ergolines
Gastrointestinal disturbances	4 Aminoquinoline antimalarials
	Alcohol metabolism modifiers
	Aldosterone inhibitors
	Alkylating antineoplastics
	Alpha blocking antihypertensives
	Amphetamines
	Anabolics
	Anorectics
	Anthelmintics
	Antiandrogens
	Antibacterial agents
	Antibiotic antituberculous agents

Anticholinesterase parasympathomimetics
Antidepressants
Antidotes
Antiepileptics
Antifolate antineoplastics
Antineoplastics
Antiprotozoals
Antituberculous agents
Antiulcer agents
Antivirals
Benzodiazepine sedatives
Beta blockers
Biguanide antimalarials
Bisphosphonates
Borates
Calcium antagonist vasodilators
Calcium salts
Carbamate sedatives
Cardiac inotropic agents
Cardioselective beta blockers
Central stimulants
Centrally acting antihypertensives
Chelating agents
Class I antiarrhythmics
Clofibrate and analogues
Corticosteroids
Cough suppressants
Diagnostic agents
Dopaminergic antiparkinsonian agents
Ergot compounds
Expectorants
Ferric salts
Ferrous salts
GABA related antiepileptics
Gonad regulating hormones
H1 antagonist antihistamines
Haemostatics
Hydrazine monoamine oxidase inhibiting
    antidepressants
Immunosuppressants
Inhalation anaesthetics
Iron compounds
Lipid regulating agents
Lithium
Loop diuretics
Medicinal enzymes
Mercurial diuretics
Monoamine oxidase inhibiting
    antidepressants
Mucolytics
Neuroleptics
Nitroimidazole antiprotozoals
Norgestrels
Oestrogen antagonist antineoplastics

Oral hypoglycaemics
Parasympathomimetics
Pesticides
Phenothiazine antihistamines
Pilocarpine
Potassium sparing diuretics
Progestogens
Promethazines
Sedatives
Sex hormones
Skeletal muscle relaxants
Somatotrophic hormones
Succinimide antiepileptics
Sulphonylurea hypoglycaemics
Sympathomimetics
Theophylline xanthines
Thiazide diuretics
Trace elements
Uricosuric agents
Vasodilator antihypertensives
Vegetable astringents
Xanthine containing beverages
Xanthine oxidase inhibitors
Xanthines

Gastrointestinal haemorrhage	Alpha blocking vasodilators
	Analgesics and anti-inflammatory drugs
	Antivirals
	Colchicum alkaloids
	Dopaminergic antiparkinsonian agents
	Selective serotonin reuptake inhibiting antidepressants
	Uricosuric agents
Gastrojejunal ulcer (GJU)	Analgesics and anti-inflammatory drugs
Giddiness	Antileprotics
	Haemostatics
	Lithium
Gilles de la Tourette's disorder	Central stimulants
Gingival hyperplasia	Calcium antagonist vasodilators
	Class IV antiarrhythmics
	Hydantoin antiepileptics
	Immunosuppressants
	Phenytoin
Gingivitis	Lipid regulating agents
Glossitis	Gold salts
	Macrolides
	Sulphonamides

Trimethoprim sulphonamide
combinations

Glucose tolerance test impaired	Somatotrophic hormones
Goitre	Analgesics and anti-inflammatory drugs Antithyroid agents Iodides Iodine compounds Iodine radiopharmaceuticals Iodophores Lithium
Goodpasture's syndrome	Chelating agents
Gout	Loop diuretics Thiazide diuretics
Granulomatous hepatitis	Analgesics and anti-inflammatory drugs Carbazepine antiepileptics Centrally acting antihypertensives Cinchona antimalarials Class I antiarrhythmics Hydantoin antiepileptics Oral hypoglycaemics Phenytoin Sulphonamides Sulphonylurea hypoglycaemics Vasodilator antihypertensives Xanthine oxidase inhibitors
Granulomatous lesions	Retinoic acid dermatological agents
Griping pain	Anthraquinone glycosides Docusate Laxatives Picosulphate
Growth retardation in children	Amphetamines Anorectics Central stimulants Corticosteroids Corticotrophic hormones
Guillain-Barre syndrome	Medicinal enzymes
Gynaecomastia	Aldosterone inhibitors Aliphatic phenothiazine neuroleptics Anorectics Antiandrogens Antiemetics Antiepileptics Antiulcer agents Butyrophenone neuroleptics

Carbazepine antiepileptics
Class IV antiarrhythmics
Diphenylbutylpiperidine neuroleptics
Flupenthixols
Fluphenazine
Gonad regulating hormones
Gonadotrophic hormones
Haloperidols
Histamine H2 antagonists
Hydrazide antituberculous agents
Imidazole antifungals
Immunosuppressants
Neuroleptics
Nitrogen mustards
Phenothiazine neuroleptics
Piperazine phenothiazine neuroleptics
Piperidine phenothiazine neuroleptics
Thioxanthene neuroleptics
Zuclopenthixols

Haematemesis	Analgesics and anti-inflammatory drugs Salicylate analgesics
Haematocrit - PCV - low	Antivirals Coumarin anticoagulants Indanedione anticoagulants Interleukins
Haematology result abnormal	Analgesics and anti-inflammatory drugs
Haemoglobin estimation	Angiotensin inhibiting antihypertensives
Haemoglobin low	Antivirals GABA related antiepileptics Interleukins
Haemolysis, haemoglobinuria	Antidotes Dermatological agents
Haemolytic anaemia	4 Quinolones 8 Aminoquinoline antimalarials Aliphatic phenothiazine neuroleptics Analgesics and anti-inflammatory drugs Antiandrogens Antibacterial agents Antibiotic antituberculous agents Antimalarials Butyrophenone neuroleptics Carbacephems Centrally acting antihypertensives Cephalosporins Cephamycins Chelating agents

Diphenylbutylpiperidine neuroleptics
Dopaminergic antiparkinsonian agents
Flupenthixols
Fluphenazine
Haloperidols
Neuroleptics
Phenothiazine neuroleptics
Piperazine phenothiazine neuroleptics
Piperidine phenothiazine neuroleptics
Selective serotonin reuptake inhibiting
    antidepressants
Thioxanthene neuroleptics
Vasodilator antihypertensives
Zuclopenthixols

Haemolytic-uraemic syndrome	Immunosuppressants Pyrimidine antagonist antineoplastics
Haemorrhage	Analgesics and anti-inflammatory drugs Antidepressants Coumarin anticoagulants Direct acting anticoagulants Gold salts Heparinoids Hydrazide antituberculous agents Indanedione anticoagulants Leech products Low molecular weight heparins Platelet activating factor antagonists Skeletal muscle relaxants Sulphonamides Tetracyclic antidepressants Thiouracil antithyroid agents Tricyclic antidepressants Trimethoprim sulphonamide combinations
Haemorrhage of rectum and anus	Analgesics and anti-inflammatory drugs Contrast media Salicylate analgesics
Haemorrhagic bullae	4 Quinolones
Haemorrhagic cystitis	Antineoplastics Nitrogen mustards
Haemorrhagic disorder	Medicinal enzymes
Halitosis	Alcohol metabolism modifiers
Hallucinations	4 Quinolones Analgesics and anti-inflammatory drugs Anorectics Anthelmintics

Antidepressants
Antiemetics
Antifungals
Antimuscarinics
Antineoplastics
Antiulcer agents
Antivirals
Aromatics
Benzomorphan opioid analgesics
Cardiac glycosides
Catechol O-methyl transferase inhibitors
Central stimulants
Class I antiarrhythmics
Digitalis
Dopaminergic antiparkinsonian agents
Ergolines
Hydrazine monoamine oxidase inhibiting
    antidepressants
Methadone and analogues
Monoamine oxidase inhibiting
    antidepressants
Morphinan opioid analgesics
Opioid analgesics
Opioid peptides
Opium alkaloid opioid analgesics
Opium poppy substances
Parenteral anaesthetics
Pethidine and analogues
Respiratory stimulants
Sedatives
Skeletal muscle relaxants
Smooth muscle relaxants

Has a sore throat	Antineoplastics
Has numbness	Sedatives
Headache	4 Aminoquinoline antimalarials
	4 Methanolquinoline antimalarials
	4 Quinolones
	ACE inhibitors
	Adrenergic neurone blocking
	antihypertensives
	Alcoholic solvents
	Aldosterone inhibitors
	Alpha adrenoceptor stimulants
	Alpha blocking antihypertensives
	Alpha blocking vasodilators
	Amphetamines
	Anabolics
	Analgesics and anti-inflammatory drugs
	Angiotensin inhibiting antihypertensives
	Anorectics
	Anthelmintics

Antiandrogens
Antianginal vasodilators
Antibiotic antifungals
Antibiotic antituberculous agents
Anticholinesterase parasympathomimetics
Antidepressants
Antidiuretic hormones
Antidotes
Antiemetics
Antiepileptics
Antifolate antineoplastics
Antifungals
Antihypertensives
Antileprotics
Antimuscarinics
Antineoplastics
Antiprotozoals
Antituberculous agents
Antiulcer agents
Antivirals
Barbiturate sedatives
Benzimidazole anthelmintics
Benzodiazepine sedatives
Benzomorphan opioid analgesics
Beta adrenoceptor stimulants
Beta blockers
Beta2 selective stimulants
Bisphosphonates
Calcium antagonist vasodilators
Carbacephems
Carbamate sedatives
Carbapenems
Carbazepine antiepileptics
Carbonic anhydrase inhibitors
Cardiac glycosides
Cardiac inotropic agents
Catechol O-methyl transferase inhibitors
Central stimulants
Centrally acting antihypertensives
Cephalosporins
Cephamycins
Chelating agents
Chloral sedatives
Cholinesterase reactivators
Cinchona antimalarials
Class I antiarrhythmics
Class III antiarrhythmics
Class IV antiarrhythmics
Clofibrate and analogues
Colony stimulating factors
Contrast media
Corticosteroids
Cough suppressants
Dermatological agents

Diagnostic agents
Digitalis
Dopaminergic antiparkinsonian agents
E series prostaglandins
Edetates
Ergolines
Ergot alkaloids
Ergot compounds
Evening primrose oil
F series prostaglandins
Fat soluble vitamins
GABA related antiepileptics
Gases
Gastrointestinal agents
Gonad regulating hormones
Gonadotrophic hormones
H1 antagonist antihistamines
Haemostatics
Histamine H2 antagonists
HMG CoA reductase inhibitors
Hyaluronic acid
Hydantoin antiepileptics
Hydrazine monoamine oxidase inhibiting
    antidepressants
Hydroxynaphthoquinones
I series prostaglandins
Imidazole antifungals
Immunosuppressants
Inhalation anaesthetics
Isoprenaline
Leukotriene inhibitors
Lipid regulating agents
Macrolides
Methadone and analogues
Monoamine oxidase inhibiting
    antidepressants
Morphinan opioid analgesics
Mucolytics
Neuroleptics
Nitrofuran antiprotozoals
Nitroimidazole antiprotozoals
Oestrogen antagonist antineoplastics
Oestrogens
Opioid analgesics
Opioid antagonists
Opioid peptides
Opium alkaloid opioid analgesics
Opium poppy substances
Oral hypoglycaemics
Organic iodinated contrast media
Osmotic diuretics
Oxazolidinedione antiepileptics
Oxytetracyclines
Pethidine and analogues

Phenothiazine antihistamines
Phenytoin
Polyene antibiotics
Posterior pituitary hormones
Progestogens
Promethazines
Prophylactic antiasthmatics
Psoralen dermatological agents
Retinoic acid dermatological agents
Salicylate analgesics
Sedatives
Selective serotonin reuptake inhibiting
  antidepressants
Sex hormones
Skeletal muscle relaxants
Smooth muscle relaxants
Succinimide antiepileptics
Sulphone antileprotics
Sulphonylurea hypoglycaemics
Sympathomimetics
Tetracyclines
Theophylline xanthines
Thiazide diuretics
Thiouracil antithyroid agents
Thiourea antithyroid agents
Thyroid agents
Triazole antifungals
Uricosuric agents
Vaccines
Vasodilator antihypertensives
Vasodilators
Vitamin B substances
Vitamin D substances
Vitamins
Xanthine containing beverages
Xanthine oxidase inhibitors
Xanthines

Hearing difficulty	Chelating agents
	Retinoic acid dermatological agents
Hearing symptoms	4 Quinolones
Heart failure	Anabolics
	Anthelmintics
	Antiandrogens
	Antiulcer agents
	Beta blockers
	Cardioselective beta blockers
	Class I antiarrhythmics
	Colony stimulating factors
	Liquorice

Heartburn	Antibacterial agents
	Bile acid binding resins
	Ergot compounds
	Gastrointestinal agents
	Lipid regulating agents

| **Heinz-body anaemia** | Gastrointestinal agents |

| **Hemianopia** | Ergolines |

| **Hepatic coma** | Anabolics |

Hepatomegaly	Antituberculous agents
	Antivirals
	Fat soluble vitamins
	Vitamin A substances
	Vitamins

Hiccough	Barbiturate anaesthetics
	Cytoprotective agents
	Oxazolidinedione antiepileptics
	Succinimide antiepileptics

Hirsutism	Anabolics
	Corticosteroids
	Corticotrophic hormones
	Hydantoin antiepileptics
	Immunosuppressants
	Norgestrels
	Oestrogen antagonist antineoplastics
	Phenytoin
	Progestogens
	Sex hormones
	Vasodilator antihypertensives

| **Hoarseness** | Retinoic acid dermatological agents |

Hyperactivity	Carbacephems
	Cephalosporins
	Cephamycins

Hyperaemia of conjunctiva	Alpha blocking vasodilators
	Centrally acting antihypertensives
	F series prostaglandins
	H1 antagonist antihistamines

| **Hyperaesthesia** | Antivirals |

| **Hyperammonaemia** | Antiepileptics |
| | Expectorants |

Hypercalcaemia	Anabolics
	Androgens
	Antacid gastrointestinal agents
	Calcium salts
	Fat soluble vitamins
	Gonad regulating hormones
	Sex hormones
	Testosterones
	Thiazide diuretics
	Vitamin A substances
	Vitamin D substances
	Vitamins
Hypercalcinuria	Fat soluble vitamins
	Vitamin D substances
	Vitamins
Hyperfibrinogenaemia	Blood clotting factors
Hyperglycaemia	Analgesics and anti-inflammatory drugs
	Antidepressants
	Antivirals
	Asparaginase antineoplastics
	Diamidine antiprotozoals
	Glucose tests
	HMG CoA reductase inhibitors
	Hydrazide antituberculous agents
	Immunosuppressants
	Loop diuretics
	Neuroleptics
	Progestogens
	Sex hormones
	Skeletal muscle relaxants
	Somatotrophic hormones
	Tetracyclic antidepressants
	Thiazide diuretics
	Tricyclic antidepressants
	Vasodilator antihypertensives
Hyperkalaemia	ACE inhibitors
	Aldosterone inhibitors
	Analgesics and anti-inflammatory drugs
	Angiotensin inhibiting antihypertensives
	Depolarising muscle relaxants
	Diamidine antiprotozoals
	Erythropoietin
	Immunosuppressants
	Potassium salts
	Potassium sparing diuretics
Hyperkinesia	Barbiturate antiepileptics
	Ergolines
	Neuroleptics

Hyperphosphataemia	Electrolyte anions
	Erythropoietin
	Fat soluble vitamins
	Vitamin D substances
	Vitamins
Hyperpigmentation	Antineoplastics
	Tetracyclines
Hyperpyrexia	Borates
Hyperreflexia	Lithium
Hypertension	Alpha adrenoceptor stimulants
	Amphetamines
	Analgesics and anti-inflammatory drugs
	Anorectics
	Antidepressants
	Antineoplastics
	Antiulcer agents
	Antivirals
	Benzodiazepine antagonists
	Beta adrenoceptor stimulants
	Beta1 selective stimulants
	Central stimulants
	Chelating agents
	Corticosteroids
	Corticotrophic hormones
	Dopaminergic antiparkinsonian agents
	Ergot alkaloids
	Ergot compounds
	Erythropoietin
	F series prostaglandins
	Gases
	Gonad regulating hormones
	Immunosuppressants
	Inhalation anaesthetics
	Liquorice
	Neuroleptics
	Opioid analgesics
	Oxytocic hormones
	Parenteral anaesthetics
	Pilocarpine
	Platelet activating factor antagonists
	Respiratory stimulants
	Salicylate analgesics
	Serotonin and analogues
	Skeletal muscle relaxants
	Sympathomimetics
	Thyrotrophic hormones
	Xanthine oxidase inhibitors
Hypertensive encephalopathy	Erythropoietin

Hypertonic uterus	E series prostaglandins
	F series prostaglandins
Hypertrophic cardiomyopathy	Immunosuppressants
Hypertrophy of breast	Oestrogens
	Sex hormones
	Tricyclic antidepressants
Hypertrophy of clitoris	Progestogens
	Sex hormones
Hypertrophy of salivary gland	Beta sympathomimetic vasodilators
	Beta2 selective stimulants
Hyperventilation	Cholinesterase reactivators
Hypervitaminosis A	Retinoic acid dermatological agents
Hypocalcaemia	Antineoplastics
	Antivirals
	Bisphosphonates
	Cytoprotective agents
	Diamidine antiprotozoals
	Loop diuretics
Hypochloraemia	Loop diuretics
	Thiazide diuretics
Hypoglycaemia	4 Quinolones
	Alcoholic disinfectants
	Antidepressants
	Antituberculous agents
	Antivirals
	Cinchona antimalarials
	Class I antiarrhythmics
	Diamidine antiprotozoals
	HMG CoA reductase inhibitors
	Insulin
	Insulin zinc suspensions
	Oral hypoglycaemics
	Skeletal muscle relaxants
	Tetracyclic antidepressants
	Tricyclic antidepressants
Hypokalaemia	Antineoplastics
	Antiulcer agents
	Beta blockers
	Beta2 selective stimulants
	Carbonic anhydrase inhibitors
	Carboxypenicillins
	Corticosteroids
	Corticotrophic hormones

Diphenylbutylpiperidine neuroleptics
E series prostaglandins
Glucose tests
Interleukins
Liquorice
Lithium
Loop diuretics
Penicillinase resistant penicillins
Polyene antibiotics
Thiazide diuretics

Hypomagnesaemia	Aminoglycosides
	Antibacterial agents
	Antineoplastics
	Bisphosphonates
	Cation exchange resins
	Immunosuppressants
	Loop diuretics
	Polyene antibiotics
	Thiazide diuretics
Hypomania	Antidepressants
	Barbiturate antiepileptics
	Dopaminergic antiparkinsonian agents
	Hydrazine monoamine oxidase inhibiting antidepressants
	Monoamine oxidase inhibiting antidepressants
	Selective serotonin reuptake inhibiting antidepressants
	Skeletal muscle relaxants
	Tetracyclic antidepressants
	Tricyclic antidepressants
Hypoparathyroidism	Iodine radiopharmaceuticals
Hypophosphataemia	Antineoplastics
Hyposmolality/hyponatraemia	ACE inhibitors
	Aldosterone inhibitors
	Analgesics and anti-inflammatory drugs
	Antidepressants
	Antidiuretic hormones
	Carbazepine antiepileptics
	Hydrazine monoamine oxidase inhibiting antidepressants
	Loop diuretics
	Monoamine oxidase inhibiting antidepressants
	Posterior pituitary hormones
	Potassium sparing diuretics
	Selective serotonin reuptake inhibiting antidepressants

	Skeletal muscle relaxants
	Sulphonylurea hypoglycaemics
	Tetracyclic antidepressants
	Thiazide diuretics
	Tricyclic antidepressants
	Vinca alkaloid antineoplastics
Hypotension	4 Quinolones
	ACE inhibitors
	Alcoholic disinfectants
	Aliphatic phenothiazine neuroleptics
	Alpha blocking antihypertensives
	Amide type anaesthetics
	Anorectics
	Antianginal vasodilators
	Antibacterial agents
	Anticholinesterase parasympathomimetics
	Antidiarrhoeals
	Antidotes
	Antiemetics
	Antineoplastics
	Antivirals
	Benzodiazepine sedatives
	Benzomorphan opioid analgesics
	Beta adrenoceptor stimulants
	Beta sympathomimetic vasodilators
	Beta2 selective stimulants
	Butyrophenone neuroleptics
	Calcium antagonist vasodilators
	Carbamate sedatives
	Cardiac inotropic agents
	Central stimulants
	Centrally acting antihypertensives
	Chelating agents
	Class I antiarrhythmics
	Class II antiarrhythmics
	Class IV antiarrhythmics
	Colony stimulating factors
	Competitive muscle relaxants
	Corticotrophic hormones
	Cytoprotective agents
	Diagnostic agents
	Diamidine antiprotozoals
	Diphenylbutylpiperidine neuroleptics
	Dopaminergic antiparkinsonian agents
	E series prostaglandins
	Edetates
	Ergolines
	Ester type anaesthetics
	Flupenthixols
	Fluphenazine
	H1 antagonist antihistamines
	Haloperidols
	Hydantoin antiepileptics

I series prostaglandins
Immunosuppressants
Inhalation anaesthetics
Interleukin 2
Isoprenaline
Local anaesthetics
Loop diuretics
Medicinal enzymes
Mercurial diuretics
Methadone and analogues
Morphinan opioid analgesics
Neuroleptics
Opioid analgesics
Opioid peptides
Opium alkaloid opioid analgesics
Opium poppy substances
Organic iodinated contrast media
Parasympathomimetics
Peripheral and cerebral vasodilators
Pethidine and analogues
Phenothiazine antihistamines
Phenothiazine neuroleptics
Phenytoin
Pilocarpine
Piperazine phenothiazine neuroleptics
Piperidine phenothiazine neuroleptics
Potassium sparing diuretics
Promethazines
Pyrimidine antagonist antineoplastics
Sedatives
Selective noradrenaline reuptake
    inhibiting antidepressants
Selective serotonin reuptake inhibiting
    antidepressants
Skeletal muscle relaxants
Sympathomimetics
Thioxanthene neuroleptics
Triazole antifungals
Vasodilator antihypertensives
Vasodilators
Zuclopenthixols

Hypothermia

Aliphatic phenothiazine neuroleptics
Benzomorphan opioid analgesics
Butyrophenone neuroleptics
Diphenylbutylpiperidine neuroleptics
Flupenthixols
Fluphenazine
Haloperidols
Methadone and analogues
Morphinan opioid analgesics
Neuroleptics
Opioid analgesics
Opioid peptides

	Opium alkaloid opioid analgesics
	Opium poppy substances
	Pethidine and analogues
	Phenothiazine neuroleptics
	Piperazine phenothiazine neuroleptics
	Piperidine phenothiazine neuroleptics
	Thioxanthene neuroleptics
	Zuclopenthixols
Impotence	ACE inhibitors
	Aldosterone inhibitors
	Aliphatic phenothiazine neuroleptics
	Anorectics
	Antiandrogens
	Antidepressants
	Antiulcer agents
	Butyrophenone neuroleptics
	Carbazepine antiepileptics
	Centrally acting antihypertensives
	Clofibrate and analogues
	Diphenylbutylpiperidine neuroleptics
	Flupenthixols
	Fluphenazine
	Gonad regulating hormones
	Haloperidols
	Histamine H2 antagonists
	HMG CoA reductase inhibitors
	Neuroleptics
	Opioid antagonists
	Phenothiazine neuroleptics
	Piperazine phenothiazine neuroleptics
	Piperidine phenothiazine neuroleptics
	Selective noradrenaline reuptake inhibiting antidepressants
	Thiazide diuretics
	Thioxanthene neuroleptics
	Zuclopenthixols
Inappropriate ADH secretion syndrome	Antidepressants
	Carbazepine antiepileptics
	Lithium
	Skeletal muscle relaxants
	Sulphonylurea hypoglycaemics
	Tetracyclic antidepressants
	Tricyclic antidepressants
	Vinca alkaloid antineoplastics
Incontinence of urine	Alpha blocking antihypertensives
	Neuroleptics
	Skeletal muscle relaxants
Incontinent of faeces	Lipid regulating agents

Increased growth	Androgens Sex hormones Testosterones
Increased menstrual loss	Gonad regulating hormones
Indirect Coombs test positive	Carbapenems Centrally acting antihypertensives
Induration of skin at site of injection	Aliphatic phenothiazine neuroleptics Butyrophenone neuroleptics Carbapenems Diphenylbutylpiperidine neuroleptics Flupenthixols Fluphenazine Haloperidols Lincomycins Neuroleptics Phenothiazine neuroleptics Piperazine phenothiazine neuroleptics Piperidine phenothiazine neuroleptics Thioxanthene neuroleptics Vaccines Vinca alkaloid antineoplastics Zuclopenthixols
Infection	Antifolate antineoplastics Antineoplastics Immunosuppressants
Inflammation of eyelids	Beta2 selective stimulants H1 antagonist antihistamines Skeletal muscle relaxants
Influenza-like syndrome	Antibiotic antituberculous agents Antiepileptics Antiulcer agents Antivirals Chelating agents Erythropoietin Leukotriene inhibitors Lipid regulating agents Tetracyclic antidepressants
Inhibited female orgasm	Antidepressants
Inhibited male orgasm	Adrenergic neurone blocking antihypertensives Alpha blocking antihypertensives Antidepressants Centrally acting antihypertensives Opioid antagonists

Insomnia

4 Quinolones
ACE inhibitors
Aliphatic phenothiazine neuroleptics
Amphetamines
Anabolics
Analgesics and anti-inflammatory drugs
Anorectics
Anthelmintics
Antiandrogens
Anticholinesterase parasympathomimetics
Antidepressants
Antiemetics
Antiepileptics
Antihypertensives
Antimalarials
Antiulcer agents
Antivirals
Beta blockers
Beta2 selective stimulants
Butyrophenone neuroleptics
Calcium antagonist vasodilators
Carbacephems
Cardiac inotropic agents
Cardioselective beta blockers
Catechol O-methyl transferase inhibitors
Central stimulants
Centrally acting antihypertensives
Cephalosporins
Cephamycins
Class III antiarrhythmics
Corticosteroids
Diphenylbutylpiperidine neuroleptics
Dopaminergic antiparkinsonian agents
Ergolines
Ergot compounds
Flupenthixols
Fluphenazine
Ganglion blocking antihypertensives
Gonad regulating hormones
H1 antagonist antihistamines
Haloperidols
HMG CoA reductase inhibitors
Hydantoin antiepileptics
Hydroxynaphthoquinones
Monoamine oxidase inhibiting
    antidepressants
Neuroleptics
Norgestrels
Opioid antagonists
Oxazolidinedione antiepileptics
Phenothiazine antihistamines
Phenothiazine neuroleptics
Phenytoin
Piperazine phenothiazine neuroleptics

Piperidine phenothiazine neuroleptics
Progestogens
Promethazines
Pyrimidine antagonist antineoplastics
Salicylate analgesics
Selective noradrenaline reuptake
    inhibiting antidepressants
Selective serotonin reuptake inhibiting
    antidepressants
Sex hormones
Skeletal muscle relaxants
Sulphone antileprotics
Sympathomimetics
Theophylline xanthines
Thioxanthene neuroleptics
Xanthine containing beverages
Xanthines
Zuclopenthixols

Interstitial lung disease	Antiandrogens
Interstitial nephritis	4 Quinolones
	ACE inhibitors
	Amidinopenicillins
	Aminopenicillanic derivatives
	Aminopenicillins
	Antibacterial agents
	Antibiotic antituberculous agents
	Antipseudomonal penicillins
	Antituberculous agents
	Antiulcer agents
	Barbiturate antiepileptics
	Benzylpenicillin and derivatives
	Beta lactamase inhibitors
	Carbacephems
	Carboxypenicillins
	Centrally acting antihypertensives
	Cephalosporins
	Cephamycins
	Gastrointestinal agents
	Histamine H2 antagonists
	Hydantoin antiepileptics
	Hydrazide antituberculous agents
	Immunosuppressants
	Isoxazolyl penicillins
	Loop diuretics
	Macrolides
	Natural penicillins
	Penicillinase resistant penicillins
	Phenoxymethylpenicillin and derivatives
	Phenoxypenicillins
	Phenytoin
	Sulphonamides
	Tetracyclines

	Thiazide diuretics
	Ureido penicillins
	Xanthine oxidase inhibitors
Interstitial pneumonia	Antifolate antineoplastics
	Chelating agents
	Class III antiarrhythmics
	Gastrointestinal agents
	Gold salts
	Nitrofuran antimicrobials
	Nitrofuran antiprotozoals
Intestinal obstruction	Bulk laxatives
	Hypoglycaemics
Intracerebral haemorrhage	Sympathomimetics
Intravascular coagulation	Cinchona antimalarials
Involuntary movements	Barbiturate anaesthetics
	Dopaminergic antiparkinsonian agents
	Parenteral anaesthetics
	Selective serotonin reuptake inhibiting antidepressants
Iritis	Analgesics and anti-inflammatory drugs
	F series prostaglandins
Irritability	Amphetamines
	Anorectics
	Antidotes
	Antiepileptics
	Aromatics
	Central stimulants
	GABA related antiepileptics
	Opioid antagonists
	Respiratory stimulants
	Sedatives
Ischaemic heart disease	Serotonin and analogues
Itching	4 Quinolones
	Analgesics and anti-inflammatory drugs
	Anthelmintics
	Antifungals
	Antineoplastics
	Antiulcer agents
	Antivirals
	Calcium antagonist vasodilators
	Central stimulants
	Cephalosporins
	Cough suppressants

Dermatological agents
Hyaluronic acid
Imidazole antifungals
Leukotriene inhibitors
Lipid regulating agents
Oestrogens
Oral hypoglycaemics
Prophylactic antiasthmatics
Psoralen dermatological agents
Retinoic acid dermatological agents
Sex hormones
Triazole antifungals
Vitamin D substances

Itchy eyes

H1 antagonist antihistamines
Organic iodinated contrast media

Jaundice

4 Quinolones
ACE inhibitors
Aliphatic phenothiazine neuroleptics
Anabolics
Androgens
Antiandrogens
Antibacterial agents
Antibiotic antituberculous agents
Antidepressants
Antiepileptics
Antifungals
Antituberculous agents
Benzodiazepine sedatives
Beta lactamase inhibitors
Borates
Butyrophenone neuroleptics
Carbamate sedatives
Carbazepine antiepileptics
Carbonic anhydrase inhibitors
Chelating agents
Class I antiarrhythmics
Diphenylbutylpiperidine neuroleptics
Flupenthixols
Fluphenazine
Haloperidols
HMG CoA reductase inhibitors
Hydrazine monoamine oxidase inhibiting
    antidepressants
Inhalation anaesthetics
Leukotriene inhibitors
Lincomycins
Macrolides
Monoamine oxidase inhibiting
    antidepressants
Neuroleptics
Nitrofuran antimicrobials
Nitrofuran antiprotozoals

Norgestrels
Oestrogen antagonist antineoplastics
Oestrogens
Oral hypoglycaemics
Phenothiazine neuroleptics
Piperazine phenothiazine neuroleptics
Piperidine phenothiazine neuroleptics
Progestogens
Retinoic acid dermatological agents
Sedatives
Sex hormones
Skeletal muscle relaxants
Sulphonamides
Sulphonylurea hypoglycaemics
Tetracyclic antidepressants
Thiazide diuretics
Thiouracil antithyroid agents
Thiourea antithyroid agents
Thioxanthene neuroleptics
Tricyclic antidepressants
Trimethoprim sulphonamide
  combinations
Uricosuric agents
Zuclopenthixols

Keratitis	Skeletal muscle relaxants
Ketonuria	Chloral sedatives
L-eye completely blind	Hydroxyquinoline antiprotozoals
Lactic acidosis	Antivirals Biguanide hypoglycaemics Nutritional carbohydrates
Lactose intolerance	Nutritional carbohydrates
Lagophthalmos	Skeletal muscle relaxants
Laryngeal oedema	Medicinal enzymes Organic iodinated contrast media
Laryngospasm	Inhalation anaesthetics Respiratory stimulants
Lens opacity	Antineoplastics
Leucocytosis	Aliphatic phenothiazine neuroleptics Antibiotic antituberculous agents Antiulcer agents Butyrophenone neuroleptics Diphenylbutylpiperidine neuroleptics E series prostaglandins

F series prostaglandins
Flupenthixols
Fluphenazine
Haloperidols
Neuroleptics
Phenothiazine neuroleptics
Piperazine phenothiazine neuroleptics
Piperidine phenothiazine neuroleptics
Thioxanthene neuroleptics
Zuclopenthixols

Leucopenia

4 Methanolquinoline antimalarials
4 Quinolones
Aliphatic phenothiazine neuroleptics
Amidinopenicillins
Aminopenicillanic derivatives
Aminopenicillins
Analgesics and anti-inflammatory drugs
Antibacterial agents
Antibiotic antifungals
Antibiotic antituberculous agents
Antidepressants
Antiepileptics
Antifungals
Antipseudomonal penicillins
Antithyroid agents
Antiulcer agents
Antivirals
Benzimidazole anthelmintics
Benzylpenicillin and derivatives
Beta sympathomimetic vasodilators
Beta2 selective stimulants
Butyrophenone neuroleptics
Carbazepine antiepileptics
Carboxypenicillins
Central stimulants
Chelating agents
Diamidine antiprotozoals
Diphenylbutylpiperidine neuroleptics
Dopaminergic antiparkinsonian agents
Flupenthixols
Fluphenazine
Gastrointestinal agents
H1 antagonist antihistamines
Haloperidols
Hydantoin antiepileptics
Hydrazine monoamine oxidase inhibiting
   antidepressants
Immunosuppressants
Indanedione anticoagulants
Inhalation anaesthetics
Isoxazolyl penicillins
Monoamine oxidase inhibiting
   antidepressants

Natural penicillins
Neuroleptics
Nitroimidazole antiprotozoals
Organic iodinated contrast media
Oxacephalosporins
Penicillinase resistant penicillins
Phenothiazine neuroleptics
Phenoxymethylpenicillin and derivatives
Phenoxypenicillins
Phenytoin
Piperazine phenothiazine neuroleptics
Piperidine phenothiazine neuroleptics
Progestogens
Pyrimidine antagonist antineoplastics
Sex hormones
Skeletal muscle relaxants
Succinimide antiepileptics
Sulphonamides
Tetracyclic antidepressants
Thioxanthene neuroleptics
Tricyclic antidepressants
Trimethoprim sulphonamide
    combinations
Ureido penicillins
Zuclopenthixols

Leukorrhoea	Cephalosporins
Lichenified skin	Beta blockers
Lid retraction or lag	Centrally acting antihypertensives
Light-headedness	Analgesics and anti-inflammatory drugs Anthelmintics Antiarrhythmics Antidepressants Antivirals Benzodiazepine sedatives Calcium antagonist vasodilators Carbamate sedatives Dopaminergic antiparkinsonian agents Gastrointestinal agents Oestrogen antagonist antineoplastics Sedatives Sex hormones Skeletal muscle relaxants Vasodilators
Liver enzymes abnormal	4 Quinolones Angiotensin inhibiting antihypertensives Anthelmintics Antiandrogens Antibiotic antituberculous agents

Antidepressants
Antiemetics
Antifolate antineoplastics
Antimalarials
Antineoplastics
Antiulcer agents
Antivirals
Bile acids and salts
Calcium antagonist vasodilators
Carbapenems
Central stimulants
Cephalosporins
Chelating agents
Colony stimulating factors
Dopaminergic antiparkinsonian agents
H1 antagonist antihistamines
Leukotriene inhibitors
Low molecular weight heparins
Mucolytics
Oestrogen antagonist antineoplastics
Oral hypoglycaemics
Parasympathomimetics
Pyrimidine antagonist antineoplastics
Retinoic acid dermatological agents
Sedatives
Sex hormones
Skeletal muscle relaxants
Sulphonylurea hypoglycaemics
Uricosuric agents

Liver function tests abnormal	4 Methanolquinoline antimalarials
	Acetylurea antiepileptics
	Aldosterone inhibitors
	Aliphatic phenothiazine neuroleptics
	Alkylating antineoplastics
	Alpha blocking vasodilators
	Anabolics
	Analgesics and anti-inflammatory drugs
	Angiotensin inhibiting antihypertensives
	Anthelmintics
	Antiandrogens
	Antibacterial agents
	Antibiotic antituberculous agents
	Antiepileptics
	Antifungals
	Antineoplastics
	Antituberculous agents
	Antiulcer agents
	Antivirals
	Aromatics
	Asparaginase antineoplastics
	Beta blockers
	Bile acids and salts
	Borates

Butyrophenone neuroleptics
Calcium antagonist vasodilators
Cardiac inotropic agents
Catechol O-methyl transferase inhibitors
Central stimulants
Centrally acting antihypertensives
Cephalosporins
Coumarin anticoagulants
Diamidine antiprotozoals
Diphenylbutylpiperidine neuroleptics
Flupenthixols
Fluphenazine
GABA related antiepileptics
H1 antagonist antihistamines
Haloperidols
Histamine H2 antagonists
HMG CoA reductase inhibitors
Immunosuppressants
Indanedione anticoagulants
Inhalation anaesthetics
Interleukin 2
Laxatives
Methadone and analogues
Neuroleptics
Nitrogen mustards
Oestrogens
Opioid antagonists
Parasympathomimetics
Peripheral and cerebral vasodilators
Phenothiazine antihistamines
Phenothiazine neuroleptics
Piperazine phenothiazine neuroleptics
Piperidine phenothiazine neuroleptics
Polyene antibiotics
Promethazines
Pyrimidine antagonist antineoplastics
Selective noradrenaline reuptake
    inhibiting antidepressants
Selective serotonin reuptake inhibiting
    antidepressants
Serotonin and analogues
Sex hormones
Skeletal muscle relaxants
Somatotrophic hormones
Succinimide antiepileptics
Tannic acid and derivatives
Tetracyclines
Thioxanthene neuroleptics
Triazole antifungals
Uricosuric agents
Vitamin B substances
Xanthine oxidase inhibitors
Zuclopenthixols

Liver moderately enlarged	Leukotriene inhibitors

Local irritation	4 Quinolones
	Aldehyde disinfectants
	Aluminium astringents
	Antifungals
	Aromatic solvents
	Aromatics
	Biguanide disinfectants
	Carbamate pesticides
	Carbonic anhydrase inhibitors
	Cellulose derived viscosity modifiers
	Chlorinated pesticides
	Chlorine releasing substances
	Dermatological agents
	Disinfectants
	Dithranols
	F series prostaglandins
	Formaldehyde and related compounds
	Glycols
	H1 antagonist antihistamines
	Hydroquinone dermatological agents
	Hydroxyquinoline antiprotozoals
	Magnesium salts
	Medicinal enzymes
	Organic solvents
	Organophosphate pesticides
	Pesticides
	Phenol disinfectants
	Podophyllums
	Prophylactic antiasthmatics
	Pyrethroid pesticides
	Retinoic acid dermatological agents
	Rubefacient vasodilators
	Tars
	Triphenylmethane disinfectant dyes
	Vitamin B substances

Locomotor impairment	H1 antagonist antihistamines
	Organic iodinated contrast media
	Phenothiazine antihistamines
	Promethazines

Loss of libido	Alcohol metabolism modifiers
	Anorectics
	Antiandrogens
	Antidepressants
	Antiemetics
	Benzodiazepine sedatives
	Carbamate sedatives
	Gonad regulating hormones
	Hydrazine monoamine oxidase inhibiting antidepressants

	Monoamine oxidase inhibiting antidepressants
	Norgestrels
	Progestogens
	Selective serotonin reuptake inhibiting antidepressants
	Sex hormones
	Skeletal muscle relaxants
	Tetracyclic antidepressants
	Tricyclic antidepressants

Lung disease	Nitrofuran antimicrobials
	Nitrofuran antiprotozoals

Lupus erythematosus	Hydrazide antituberculous agents

Lymphadenopathy	Anthelmintics
	Antiepileptics
	Carbazepine antiepileptics
	Hydantoin antiepileptics
	Oxazolidinedione antiepileptics
	Phenytoin
	Xanthine oxidase inhibitors

Lymphoedema	Antiandrogens
	Somatotrophic hormones

Lymphopenia	Bisphosphonates
	Immunosuppressants

Malaise/lethargy	4 Aminoquinoline antimalarials
	Aldosterone inhibitors
	Alpha blocking antihypertensives
	Anorectics
	Anthelmintics
	Antiandrogens
	Anticholinesterase parasympathomimetics
	Antidotes
	Antiepileptics
	Antifolate antineoplastics
	Antineoplastics
	Antiulcer agents
	Antivirals
	Barbiturate antiepileptics
	Calcium antagonist vasodilators
	Central stimulants
	Chelating agents
	Edetates
	Encephalitis vaccines
	Ergolines
	Fat soluble vitamins
	Influenza vaccines
	Leukotriene inhibitors
	Lipid regulating agents

Measles vaccine
Oestrogen antagonist antineoplastics
Opioid antagonists
Oxazolidinedione antiepileptics
Pesticides
Poliomyelitis vaccines
Pyrimidine antagonist antineoplastics
Retinoic acid dermatological agents
Sedatives
Skeletal muscle relaxants
Specific immunoglobulins
Typhoid vaccines
Vaccines
Vitamin D substances
Vitamins
Xanthine oxidase inhibitors

Malignant hyperpyrexia	Aliphatic phenothiazine neuroleptics
	Butyrophenone neuroleptics
	Competitive muscle relaxants
	Depolarising muscle relaxants
	Diphenylbutylpiperidine neuroleptics
	Flupenthixols
	Fluphenazine
	Haloperidols
	Inhalation anaesthetics
	Neuroleptics
	Parenteral anaesthetics
	Phenothiazine neuroleptics
	Piperazine phenothiazine neuroleptics
	Piperidine phenothiazine neuroleptics
	Thioxanthene neuroleptics
	Zuclopenthixols
Malignant neoplasm of thyroid gland	Iodine radiopharmaceuticals
Mastodynia - pain in breast	Antiandrogens
	Gonad regulating hormones
	Norgestrels
	Oestrogens
	Progestogens
	Sex hormones
	Vasodilator antihypertensives
Megaloblastic anaemia	Antibiotic antituberculous agents
	Trimethoprim and derivatives
	Trimethoprim sulphonamide combinations
Melaena	Analgesics and anti-inflammatory drugs
	Salicylate analgesics
Memory loss - amnesia	Antimuscarinics
	Benzodiazepine sedatives

	Carbamate sedatives
	GABA related antiepileptics
	Hydroxyquinoline antiprotozoals
	Sedatives
	Skeletal muscle relaxants
	Smooth muscle relaxants
Meningism	Benzimidazole anthelmintics
	Organic iodinated contrast media
Meningitis- aseptic	Analgesics and anti-inflammatory drugs
	Salicylate analgesics
Menopause	Gonad regulating hormones
Menorrhagia	E series prostaglandins
	Gold salts
Menstrual disorders	Aldosterone inhibitors
	Aliphatic phenothiazine neuroleptics
	Antibiotic antituberculous agents
	Borates
	Butyrophenone neuroleptics
	Corticosteroids
	Diphenylbutylpiperidine neuroleptics
	Flupenthixols
	Fluphenazine
	Gonad regulating hormones
	Haloperidols
	Lipid regulating agents
	Neuroleptics
	Norgestrels
	Phenothiazine neuroleptics
	Piperazine phenothiazine neuroleptics
	Piperidine phenothiazine neuroleptics
	Progestogens
	Retinoic acid dermatological agents
	Sex hormones
	Thioxanthene neuroleptics
	Tricyclic antidepressants
	Zuclopenthixols
Mercury - toxic effect	Inorganic mercury compounds
	Mercurial dermatological agents
	Organic mercurial disinfectants
Metabolic acidosis	4 Quinolones
	Alcoholic disinfectants
	Nutritional carbohydrates
Metabolic alkalosis	Electrolyte anions
	Loop diuretics
	Thiazide diuretics

Methaemoglobinaemia	8 Aminoquinoline antimalarials
	Amide type anaesthetics
	Antianginal vasodilators
	Antidotes
	Dermatological agents
	Disinfectants
Microangiopathic haemol.anaem.	Pyrimidine antagonist antineoplastics
Micturition frequency	Pilocarpine
Migraine	Anabolics
	Gonad regulating hormones
Mild memory disturbance	GABA related antiepileptics
	Sedatives
Mood changes	ACE inhibitors
	Benzomorphan opioid analgesics
	Gases
	Gonad regulating hormones
	Gonadotrophic hormones
	Methadone and analogues
	Morphinan opioid analgesics
	Opioid analgesics
	Opioid peptides
	Opium alkaloid opioid analgesics
	Opium poppy substances
	Pethidine and analogues
	Retinoic acid dermatological agents
	Sedatives
Multiple pregnancy	Gonadotrophic hormones
Muscle cramps	ACE inhibitors
	Aldosterone inhibitors
	Anabolics
	Antiulcer agents
	Beta2 selective stimulants
	Calcium antagonist vasodilators
	Carbonic anhydrase inhibitors
	Central stimulants
	Corticosteroids
	Diagnostic agents
	Diuretics
	Edetates
	Ergolines
	Ergot compounds
	Histamine H2 antagonists
	HMG CoA reductase inhibitors
	Immunosuppressants
	Loop diuretics
	Mercurial diuretics

Oestrogen antagonist antineoplastics
Osmotic diuretics
Potassium sparing diuretics
Sympathomimetics
Thiazide diuretics
Thyroid agents

Muscle hypertonia

Carbacephems
Cephalosporins
Cephamycins
Parenteral anaesthetics

Muscle hypotonia

Antiepileptics

Muscle spasm

Progestogens
Sex hormones

Muscle weakness

4 Methanolquinoline antimalarials
4 Quinolones
Alpha blocking antihypertensives
Antibiotic antituberculous agents
Anticholinesterase parasympathomimetics
Antidepressants
Antiulcer agents
Beta blockers
Carbamate sedatives
Cholinesterase reactivators
E series prostaglandins
Hydrazine monoamine oxidase inhibiting
   antidepressants
Immunosuppressants
Liquorice
Lithium
Monoamine oxidase inhibiting
   antidepressants
Parasympathomimetics
Pilocarpine
Polymyxins
Sedatives
Serotonin and analogues
Skeletal muscle relaxants

Muscular fasciculation

Antianginal vasodilators
Anticholinesterase parasympathomimetics
Depolarising muscle relaxants
Gases
Parasympathomimetics
Pilocarpine
Respiratory stimulants
Skeletal muscle relaxants

Muscular incoordination

Anthelmintics

Musculoskeletal pain	Antibiotic antituberculous agents
	Antifolate antineoplastics
	Antineoplastics
	Antivirals
	Bisphosphonates
	Colony stimulating factors
	Depolarising muscle relaxants
	Gonad regulating hormones
	Immunosuppressants
	Oestrogen antagonist antineoplastics
	Opioid antagonists
	Polyene antibiotics
	Skeletal muscle relaxants
Myalgia	4 Methanolquinoline antimalarials
	4 Quinolones
	Analgesics and anti-inflammatory drugs
	Anthelmintics
	Antidepressants
	Antifungals
	Antineoplastics
	Antiulcer agents
	Antivirals
	Beta2 selective stimulants
	Clofibrate and analogues
	Colony stimulating factors
	Depolarising muscle relaxants
	Edetates
	Gonad regulating hormones
	H1 antagonist antihistamines
	Histamine H2 antagonists
	Interleukins
	Loop diuretics
	Phenothiazine antihistamines
	Promethazines
	Retinoic acid dermatological agents
	Sex hormones
	Thiourea antithyroid agents
Myalgia/myositis	Cardiac inotropic agents
	Clofibrate and analogues
	HMG CoA reductase inhibitors
Myasthenia gravis	Oxazolidinedione antiepileptics
Myasthenic syndrome	Aminoglycosides
	Antibacterial agents
	Chelating agents
	Clofibrate and analogues
Mycoses	Antivirals
	Corticosteroids

	Corticotrophic hormones Immunosuppressants
Myoclonus	Carbapenems Class I antiarrhythmics
Myoglobinuria	Clofibrate and analogues HMG CoA reductase inhibitors
Myopathy	Antibiotic antituberculous agents Antivirals Class III antiarrhythmics Clofibrate and analogues Expectorants Haemostatics HMG CoA reductase inhibitors Immunosuppressants
Myopia	Thiazide diuretics
Nail disorders	Antineoplastics
Nasal congestion	Adrenergic neurone blocking antihypertensives Aliphatic phenothiazine neuroleptics Alpha adrenoceptor stimulants Alpha blocking antihypertensives Butyrophenone neuroleptics Centrally acting antihypertensives Cough suppressants Diphenylbutylpiperidine neuroleptics Dopaminergic antiparkinsonian agents Edetates Ergot compounds Flupenthixols Fluphenazine Haemostatics Haloperidols Neuroleptics Phenothiazine neuroleptics Piperazine phenothiazine neuroleptics Piperidine phenothiazine neuroleptics Rauwolfia antihypertensives Sedatives Smooth muscle relaxants Thioxanthene neuroleptics Zuclopenthixols
Nasal symptoms	Antivirals
Nausea	4 Aminoquinoline antimalarials 4 Methanolquinoline antimalarials 4 Quinolones

8 Aminoquinoline antimalarials
ACE inhibitors
Alcohol metabolism modifiers
Aldosterone inhibitors
Alkyl sulphonate antineoplastics
Alkylating antineoplastics
Alpha blocking antihypertensives
Alpha blocking vasodilators
Amino acids
Aminopenicillins
Anabolics
Analgesics and anti-inflammatory drugs
Angiotensin inhibiting antihypertensives
Anthelmintics
Anthracycline antibiotic antineoplastics
Antiandrogens
Antianginal vasodilators
Antiarrhythmics
Antibacterial agents
Antibiotic antifungals
Antibiotic antineoplastics
Antibiotic antituberculous agents
Anticholinesterase parasympathomimetics
Antidepressants
Antidiarrhoeals
Antidiuretic hormones
Antidotes
Antiemetics
Antiepileptics
Antifolate antineoplastics
Antifungals
Antihypertensives
Antileprotics
Antimalarials
Antineoplastics
Antiprotozoals
Antithyroid agents
Antituberculous agents
Antiulcer agents
Antivirals
Aromatics
Asparaginase antineoplastics
Aspartic acid
Barbiturate antiepileptics
Benzimidazole anthelmintics
Benzodiazepine antagonists
Benzomorphan opioid analgesics
Beta blockers
Beta sympathomimetic vasodilators
Beta1 selective stimulants
Beta2 selective stimulants
Biguanide hypoglycaemics
Bile acid binding resins
Bismuth salts

Bisphosphonates
Blood products
Calcitonin
Calcium antagonist vasodilators
Carbacephems
Carbapenems
Carbazepine antiepileptics
Cardiac glycosides
Cardiac inotropic agents
Catechol O-methyl transferase inhibitors
Central stimulants
Centrally acting antihypertensives
Cephalosporins
Cephamycins
Chelating agents
Chloramphenicols
Cholinesterase reactivators
Cinchona antimalarials
Class I antiarrhythmics
Class II antiarrhythmics
Class III antiarrhythmics
Class IV antiarrhythmics
Clofibrate and analogues
Colchicum alkaloids
Colony stimulating factors
Contrast media
Corticosteroids
Cough suppressants
Coumarin anticoagulants
Cytoprotective agents
Dermatological agents
Diagnostic agents
Diamidine antiprotozoals
Digitalis
Dopaminergic antiparkinsonian agents
E series prostaglandins
Edetates
Ergolines
Ergot alkaloids
Ergot compounds
Essential amino acids
Ethyleneimine antineoplastics
Evening primrose oil
Expectorants
F series prostaglandins
Fat soluble vitamins
Ferric salts
Ferrous salts
Fluorouracil
GABA related antiepileptics
Gases
Gastrointestinal agents
Glucose tests
Glycol and glycerol esters

Glycols
Gonad regulating hormones
H1 antagonist antihistamines
Haemostatics
Histamine H2 antagonists
HMG CoA reductase inhibitors
Hydantoin antiepileptics
Hydrazide antituberculous agents
Hydroxynaphthoquinones
Imidazole antifungals
Immunosuppressants
Indanedione anticoagulants
Inhalation anaesthetics
Iron compounds
Laxatives
Leukotriene inhibitors
Lincomycins
Lipid regulating agents
Loop diuretics
Macrolides
Medicinal enzymes
Methadone and analogues
Monoamine oxidase inhibiting
    antidepressants
Monobactams
Morphinan opioid analgesics
Neuroleptics
Nitrofuran antimicrobials
Nitrofuran antiprotozoals
Nitrogen mustards
Nitroimidazole antiprotozoals
Nitrosoureas
Oestrogen antagonist antineoplastics
Oestrogens
Omega 3 triglycerides
Opioid analgesics
Opioid antagonists
Opioid peptides
Opium alkaloid opioid analgesics
Opium poppy substances
Oral hypoglycaemics
Organic iodinated contrast media
Oxazolidinedione antiepileptics
Oxytetracyclines
Parasympathomimetics
Peripheral and cerebral vasodilators
Pethidine and analogues
Phenytoin
Pilocarpine
Platelet activating factor antagonists
Polyene antibiotics
Posterior pituitary hormones
Progestogens
Prophylactic antiasthmatics

Purine antagonist antineoplastics
Pyrimidine antagonist antineoplastics
Respiratory stimulants
Retinoic acid dermatological agents
Salicylate analgesics
Sedatives
Selective serotonin reuptake inhibiting
    antidepressants
Serotonin and analogues
Sex hormones
Skeletal muscle relaxants
Somatotrophic hormones
Sulphonamides
Sulphone antileprotics
Sulphur mustards
Sympathomimetics
Tetracyclic antidepressants
Tetracyclines
Theophylline xanthines
Thiazide diuretics
Thiouracil antithyroid agents
Thiourea antithyroid agents
Thyrotrophic hormones
Triazene antineoplastics
Triazole antifungals
Tricyclic antidepressants
Trimethoprim and derivatives
Trimethoprim sulphonamide
    combinations
Triphenylmethane diagnostic dyes
Typhoid vaccines
Uricosuric agents
Vaccines
Vasodilator antihypertensives
Vasodilators
Vasopressins
Vinca alkaloid antineoplastics
Vitamin B substances
Vitamin D substances
Vitamins
Xanthine containing beverages
Xanthines

Neoplasms	Immunosuppressants
Nephritis, nephrosis	Organic iodinated contrast media
Nephrotic syndrome	Antithyroid agents
	Chelating agents
	Gastrointestinal agents
	Mercurial dermatological agents
	Oxazolidinedione antiepileptics
	Uricosuric agents

Nerves - nervousness	4 Quinolones
	ACE inhibitors
	Amphetamines
	Analgesics and anti-inflammatory drugs
	Anorectics
	Antidepressants
	Antimuscarinics
	Antiulcer agents
	Antivirals
	Beta2 selective stimulants
	Carbacephems
	Central stimulants
	Cephalosporins
	Cephamycins
	Dopaminergic antiparkinsonian agents
	GABA related antiepileptics
	Gonad regulating hormones
	Hydantoin antiepileptics
	Hydrazine monoamine oxidase inhibiting antidepressants
	Interleukins
	Monoamine oxidase inhibiting antidepressants
	Neuroleptics
	Opioid antagonists
	Phenytoin
	Progestogens
	Sedatives
	Selective serotonin reuptake inhibiting antidepressants
	Sex hormones
	Skeletal muscle relaxants
Neurological symptoms	Antiepileptics
	Antivirals
	Gastrointestinal agents
	Glycols
	Immunosuppressants
	Organic iodinated contrast media
Neutropenia	8 Aminoquinoline antimalarials
	ACE inhibitors
	Angiotensin inhibiting antihypertensives
	Antibacterial agents
	Antineoplastics
	Antivirals
	Carbapenems
	Central stimulants
	Chelating agents
	Gastrointestinal agents
	H1 antagonist antihistamines
	Lincomycins
	Macrolides
	Monobactams

	Neuroleptics
	Oxazolidinedione antiepileptics
	Retinoic acid dermatological agents
	Thiazide diuretics
	Thiourea antithyroid agents
Newborn disseminated intravascular coagulation	E series prostaglandins
Night blindness	Retinoic acid dermatological agents
Night terrors	Amphetamines
	Anorectics
	Central stimulants
Nightmares	Aliphatic phenothiazine neuroleptics
	Antivirals
	Butyrophenone neuroleptics
	Calcium antagonist vasodilators
	Class III antiarrhythmics
	Diphenylbutylpiperidine neuroleptics
	Flupenthixols
	Fluphenazine
	Haloperidols
	Neuroleptics
	Phenothiazine neuroleptics
	Piperazine phenothiazine neuroleptics
	Piperidine phenothiazine neuroleptics
	Sedatives
	Thioxanthene neuroleptics
	Zuclopenthixols
Non-alcoholic fatty liver	Antivirals
	Oestrogen antagonist antineoplastics
	Sex hormones
Numbness	Analgesics and anti-inflammatory drugs
	Organic iodinated contrast media
Nystagmus	Alcoholic disinfectants
	Anticholinesterase parasympathomimetics
	Class I antiarrhythmics
	GABA related antiepileptics
	Hydantoin antiepileptics
	Parasympathomimetics
	Phenytoin
	Pilocarpine
	Skeletal muscle relaxants
Obstetric trauma	Oxytocic hormones
Oedema	4 Quinolones
	Alpha blocking antihypertensives

Anabolics
Analgesics and anti-inflammatory drugs
Androgens
Anthelmintics
Antiandrogens
Antibiotic antituberculous agents
Antidepressants
Antiepileptics
Antifolate antineoplastics
Antineoplastics
Antiulcer agents
Antivirals
Calcium antagonist vasodilators
Carbazepine antiepileptics
Class IV antiarrhythmics
Colony stimulating factors
Dermatological agents
Dopaminergic antiparkinsonian agents
E series prostaglandins
Ergot compounds
Gonad regulating hormones
Gonadotrophic hormones
Hydrazine monoamine oxidase inhibiting antidepressants
Immunosuppressants
Interleukins
Lithium
Monoamine oxidase inhibiting antidepressants
Neuroleptics
Oestrogen antagonist antineoplastics
Organic iodinated contrast media
Progestogens
Pyrethroid pesticides
Pyrimidine antagonist antineoplastics
Salicylate analgesics
Sex hormones
Testosterones
Vasodilator antihypertensives

Oedema of eyelid	Centrally acting antihypertensives Erythropoietin
Oedema of glottis	Phenol disinfectants
Oedema of larynx	Phenol disinfectants
Oesophagitis	Amidinopenicillins Analgesics and anti-inflammatory drugs Antimuscarinics Bisphosphonates Salicylate analgesics Tetracyclines

Oligospermia	Gastrointestinal agents
Oliguria	Alpha blocking vasodilators Cardiac inotropic agents Lithium
Onycholysis	ACE inhibitors
Optic neuritis	Antituberculous agents Chloramphenicols Class III antiarrhythmics Hydrazide antituberculous agents Retinoic acid dermatological agents
Oral aphthae	Analgesics and anti-inflammatory drugs Antibiotic antineoplastics Antifolate antineoplastics Antivirals Biguanide antimalarials Fluorouracil Gold salts Monobactams Pyrimidine antagonist antineoplastics
Organic psychotic conditions	Aromatics
Orofacial dyskinesia	Central stimulants Dopaminergic antiparkinsonian agents H1 antagonist antihistamines
Osteomalacia	Aldosterone inhibitors Antacid gastrointestinal agents Barbiturate sedatives Bisphosphonates Hydantoin antiepileptics Phenytoin
Osteoporosis	Antiandrogens Bisphosphonates Corticosteroids Corticotrophic hormones Direct acting anticoagulants Gonad regulating hormones Heparinoids Low molecular weight heparins Thyroid agents
Other penile inflammatory disorders	E series prostaglandins
Ototoxicity - deafness	Aminoglycosides Antibacterial agents Antineoplastics

Ovarian cysts	Gonad regulating hormones
Ovarian hyperstimulation	Sex hormones
Pain	Antifolate antineoplastics Antivirals Central stimulants Interleukins Medicinal enzymes
Pain at injection site	Alpha blocking vasodilators Antidotes Antivirals Cardiac inotropic agents Contrast media H1 antagonist antihistamines Hyaluronic acid Leech products Medicinal enzymes Penicillinase resistant penicillins Phenothiazine antihistamines Vinca alkaloid antineoplastics
Pain in joints – arthralgia	4 Quinolones Amidinopenicillins Aminopenicillanic derivatives Aminopenicillins Anthelmintics Antidotes Antifungals Antineoplastics Antipseudomonal penicillins Antituberculous agents Antiulcer agents Antivirals Benzylpenicillin and derivatives Carbacephems Carbazepine antiepileptics Carboxypenicillins Central stimulants Cephalosporins Cephamycins Class I antiarrhythmics Gastrointestinal agents Histamine H2 antagonists Hydrazide antituberculous agents Isoxazolyl penicillins Natural penicillins Nitrofuran antimicrobials Oestrogen antagonist antineoplastics Penicillinase resistant penicillins Phenoxymethylpenicillin and derivatives

Phenoxypenicillins
Polyene antibiotics
Prophylactic antiasthmatics
Retinoic acid dermatological agents
Tetracyclic antidepressants
Thiouracil antithyroid agents
Thiourea antithyroid agents
Ureido penicillins
Vaccines
Xanthine oxidase inhibitors

Pain in testicle	E series prostaglandins
Painful extremities	Antidotes
	Cardiac inotropic agents
	Clofibrate and analogues
Painful swallowing	Antineoplastics
Painful urination	Analgesics and anti-inflammatory drugs
	Organic iodinated contrast media
Pallor	Aliphatic phenothiazine neuroleptics
	Analgesics and anti-inflammatory drugs
	Antidiuretic hormones
	Butyrophenone neuroleptics
	Diphenylbutylpiperidine neuroleptics
	Dopaminergic antiparkinsonian agents
	Flupenthixols
	Fluphenazine
	Haloperidols
	I series prostaglandins
	Neuroleptics
	Phenothiazine neuroleptics
	Piperazine phenothiazine neuroleptics
	Piperidine phenothiazine neuroleptics
	Posterior pituitary hormones
	Thioxanthene neuroleptics
	Vasopressins
	Zuclopenthixols
Palpitations	ACE inhibitors
	Alpha adrenoceptor stimulants
	Alpha blocking antihypertensives
	Amphetamines
	Analgesics and anti-inflammatory drugs
	Anorectics
	Antianginal vasodilators
	Antidepressants
	Antimuscarinics
	Benzomorphan opioid analgesics
	Beta sympathomimetic vasodilators
	Beta2 selective stimulants

Calcium antagonist vasodilators
Central stimulants
Centrally acting antihypertensives
Class I antiarrhythmics
Corticosteroids
E series prostaglandins
Ergolines
Ergot alkaloids
Ergot compounds
Gases
Gonad regulating hormones
H1 antagonist antihistamines
Methadone and analogues
Morphinan opioid analgesics
Opioid analgesics
Opioid peptides
Opium alkaloid opioid analgesics
Opium poppy substances
Pethidine and analogues
Phenothiazine antihistamines
Promethazines
Sedatives
Selective serotonin reuptake inhibiting
    antidepressants
Serotonin and analogues
Smooth muscle relaxants
Sympathomimetics
Theophylline xanthines
Vasodilator antihypertensives
Vitamin B substances
Xanthine containing beverages
Xanthines

Pancreatic steatorrhoea	Somatotrophic hormones
Pancytopenia	4 Quinolones Antibacterial agents Antithyroid agents Antivirals Benzimidazole anthelmintics Oxazolidinedione antiepileptics Selective serotonin reuptake inhibiting antidepressants
Papilloedema	Interleukins Retinoic acid dermatological agents
Paraesthesia	4 Methanolquinoline antimalarials 4 Quinolones ACE inhibitors Antidepressants Antiepileptics Antimuscarinics

Antiulcer agents
Antivirals
Carbamate sedatives
Carbapenems
Carbamazepine antiepileptics
Carbonic anhydrase inhibitors
Central stimulants
Class I antiarrhythmics
Colony stimulating factors
Ergot compounds
Gonad regulating hormones
H1 antagonist antihistamines
HMG CoA reductase inhibitors
Hydroxyquinoline antiprotozoals
Immunosuppressants
Interleukins
Neuroleptics
Organic iodinated contrast media
Oxazolidinedione antiepileptics
Phenothiazine antihistamines
Polymyxins
Promethazines
Selective noradrenaline reuptake
    inhibiting antidepressants
Serotonin and analogues
Skeletal muscle relaxants
Thiazide diuretics
Vitamin D substances
Xanthine oxidase inhibitors

Paralysis

Antianginal vasodilators
Antibiotic antituberculous agents
Anticholinesterase parasympathomimetics
Chelating agents
Organic iodinated contrast media
Parasympathomimetics
Pilocarpine
Skeletal muscle relaxants

Paralytic ileus

Antidepressants
Calcium antagonist vasodilators
Skeletal muscle relaxants
Tetracyclic antidepressants
Tricyclic antidepressants
Vinca alkaloid antineoplastics

Paronychia of finger

Retinoic acid dermatological agents

Paronychia of toe

Retinoic acid dermatological agents

Parotid swelling

Encephalitis vaccines
Influenza vaccines
Measles vaccine

	Organic iodinated contrast media Poliomyelitis vaccines Typhoid vaccines Vaccines
Parotitis	Analgesics and anti-inflammatory drugs
Paroxysmal choreo-athetosis	Central stimulants
Paroxysmal nocturnal haemoglobinuria	Chloramphenicols
Paroxysmal supravent.tachycard	Anthracycline antibiotic antineoplastics H1 antagonist antihistamines
Paroxysmal ventric. tachycard.	Antimalarials Beta blockers Inhalation anaesthetics Lipid regulating agents
Partial atrioventricular block	Calcium antagonist vasodilators Cardiac glycosides Class I antiarrhythmics Class IV antiarrhythmics Digitalis Histamine H2 antagonists
Patches of alopecia	Alkylating antineoplastics Analgesics and anti-inflammatory drugs Antibacterial agents Antifolate antineoplastics Antineoplastics Antituberculous agents Gonad regulating hormones HMG CoA reductase inhibitors Interleukins Oestrogen antagonist antineoplastics Oxazolidinedione antiepileptics Pyrimidine antagonist antineoplastics
Peeling skin	Retinoic acid dermatological agents
Pellagra	Antituberculous agents Hydrazide antituberculous agents
Pemphigus	Chelating agents
Peptic ulcer	Analgesics and anti-inflammatory drugs Antineoplastics Corticosteroids Corticotrophic hormones Salicylate analgesics Uricosuric agents

Peptic ulcer symptoms	Central stimulants
Peri-op haemorrhage/ haematoma	Analgesics and anti-inflammatory drugs
Perineal pain	4 Quinolones Corticosteroids E series prostaglandins Oestrogens Respiratory stimulants
Peripheral autonomic neuropathy	Antineoplastics Antivirals HMG CoA reductase inhibitors Vinca alkaloid antineoplastics
Peripheral enthesopathies	4 Quinolones Interleukins
Peripheral neuritis or neuropathy	4 Aminoquinoline antimalarials 4 Quinolones Alcohol metabolism modifiers Analgesics and anti-inflammatory drugs Antibiotic antifungals Antidepressants Antineoplastics Antituberculous agents Antivirals Chloramphenicols Class I antiarrhythmics Class III antiarrhythmics Colchicum alkaloids Dermatological agents Dopaminergic antiparkinsonian agents Gold salts Hydantoin antiepileptics Hydrazide antituberculous agents Hydrazine monoamine oxidase inhibiting antidepressants Immunosuppressants Monoamine oxidase inhibiting antidepressants Nitrofuran antimicrobials Nitroimidazole antiprotozoals Phenytoin Polyene antibiotics Salicylate analgesics Sulphone antileprotics Vasodilator antihypertensives Vinca alkaloid antineoplastics Xanthine oxidase inhibitors
Peripheral neuropathy	Antituberculous agents

| | Dermatological agents |
| | Vitamin B6 substances |

Peripheral vascular symptoms	Beta blockers
	Cardioselective beta blockers
	Platelet activating factor antagonists
	Respiratory stimulants

Persistent miosis	Alpha blocking antihypertensives
	Anticholinesterase parasympathomimetics
	Aromatics
	Benzomorphan opioid analgesics
	Methadone and analogues
	Morphinan opioid analgesics
	Opioid analgesics
	Opioid peptides
	Opium alkaloid opioid analgesics
	Opium poppy substances
	Parasympathomimetics
	Pethidine and analogues
	Pilocarpine

Persistent mydriasis	Antimuscarinics
	Aromatics
	Centrally acting antihypertensives
	Ganglion blocking antihypertensives
	Neuroleptics
	Smooth muscle relaxants

Personality disorders	Acetylurea antiepileptics
	Central stimulants
	Dopaminergic antiparkinsonian agents
	Oxazolidinedione antiepileptics

Petechiae	4 Quinolones
	Organic iodinated contrast media
	Skeletal muscle relaxants

Phlebitis and thrombophlebitis	4 Quinolones
	Antibacterial agents
	Antibiotic antituberculous agents
	Antivirals
	Benzodiazepine sedatives
	Carbamate sedatives
	Carbapenems
	Gonad regulating hormones
	Haemostatics
	Immunosuppressants
	Lincomycins
	Macrolides
	Oestrogen antagonist antineoplastics
	Osmotic diuretics
	Penicillinase resistant penicillins

	Sedatives Skeletal muscle relaxants Vasodilator antihypertensives
Phocomelia limb unspecified	Dermatological agents
Phocomelia upper limb NOS	Dermatological agents
Photophobia	Centrally acting antihypertensives Neuroleptics Oxazolidinedione antiepileptics Retinoic acid dermatological agents Skeletal muscle relaxants Succinimide antiepileptics
Photosensitiveness	4 Quinolones Aliphatic phenothiazine neuroleptics Aminobenzoate sunscreen agents Analgesics and anti-inflammatory drugs Anthelmintics Antibiotic antifungals Antiepileptics Antifungals Antineoplastics Antituberculous agents Antiulcer agents Aromatics Benzophenone sunscreen agents Carbazepine antiepileptics Chlorinated phenol disinfectants Cinnamate sunscreen agents Class I antiarrhythmics Class III antiarrhythmics Dibenzoylmethanes Diphenylbutylpiperidine neuroleptics Disinfectants Flupenthixols Fluphenazine Gastrointestinal agents H1 antagonist antihistamines Loop diuretics Neuroleptics Oxytetracyclines Phenothiazine antihistamines Phenothiazine neuroleptics Piperazine phenothiazine neuroleptics Piperidine phenothiazine neuroleptics Potassium sparing diuretics Promethazines Retinoic acid dermatological agents Salicylate sunscreen agents Sulphonylurea hypoglycaemics Sunscreen agents

Tars
Tetracyclines
Thiazide diuretics
Thioxanthene neuroleptics
Tricyclic antidepressants
Vegetable astringents
Zuclopenthixols

Pleural effusion
Colony stimulating factors
Ergolines
Skeletal muscle relaxants

Pneumonitis
Antifolate antineoplastics
Antivirals
Class I antiarrhythmics
Thiazide diuretics

Pneumothorax
Antivirals

Polyarteritis nodosa
Hydantoin antiepileptics
Phenytoin

Polydipsia
Lithium

Polyuria
Alkylating antineoplastics
Alpha blocking antihypertensives
Calcium antagonist vasodilators
Fat soluble vitamins
Lithium
Skeletal muscle relaxants
Uricosuric agents
Vitamin D substances
Vitamins

Post operative UTI
Haemostatics

Post-operative haematoma formation
Analgesics and anti-inflammatory drugs
Platelet activating factor antagonists

Postmenopausal bleeding
E series prostaglandins

Postural hypotension
Adrenergic neurone blocking antihypertensives
Aliphatic phenothiazine neuroleptics
Alpha blocking antihypertensives
Alpha blocking vasodilators
Angiotensin inhibiting antihypertensives
Anthelmintics
Antianginal vasodilators
Antidepressants
Antineoplastics
Antituberculous agents

	Benzomorphan opioid analgesics
	Beta blockers
	Centrally acting antihypertensives
	Class I antiarrhythmics
	Dopaminergic antiparkinsonian agents
	Ergolines
	Ergot compounds
	Hydrazine monoamine oxidase inhibiting antidepressants
	Methadone and analogues
	Monoamine oxidase inhibiting antidepressants
	Morphinan opioid analgesics
	Neuroleptics
	Opioid analgesics
	Opioid peptides
	Opium alkaloid opioid analgesics
	Opium poppy substances
	Peripheral and cerebral vasodilators
	Pethidine and analogues
	Potassium sparing diuretics
	Rauwolfia antihypertensives
	Skeletal muscle relaxants
	Tetracyclic antidepressants
	Thiazide diuretics
	Tricyclic antidepressants
	Vasodilator antihypertensives
Premature ejaculation	Antidepressants
Premenstrual tension syndrome	Norgestrels
	Oestrogens
	Progestogens
	Sex hormones
Priapism	Alpha blocking vasodilators
	Androgens
	Antidepressants
	E series prostaglandins
	Neuroleptics
	Papaverine and analogues
	Testosterones
Primary malignant neoplasm of liver	Anabolics
Primary pulmonary hypertension	Anorectics
Prolactin level increased	Antiemetics
	Neuroleptics
Proteinuria	Analgesics and anti-inflammatory drugs
	Antineoplastics

Antivirals
Carbazepine antiepileptics
Chelating agents
Colony stimulating factors
Gastrointestinal agents
Gold salts

Prothrombin time increased	4 Quinolones Class III antiarrhythmics Oxacephalosporins
Proximal myopathy	Corticosteroids Corticotrophic hormones
Pruritus	4 Methanolquinoline antimalarials 4 Quinolones Anabolics Anthelmintics Antiandrogens Antibacterial agents Antifungals Antimalarials Antineoplastics Antiulcer agents Antivirals Benzimidazole anthelmintics Benzomorphan opioid analgesics Beta2 selective stimulants Bile acids and salts Blood products Calcium antagonist vasodilators Carbacephems Carbapenems Central stimulants Cephalosporins Cephamycins Class IV antiarrhythmics Clofibrate and analogues Colony stimulating factors Dichloroacetamide antiprotozoals Fluorocarbon blood substitutes Gold salts Gonad regulating hormones HMG CoA reductase inhibitors Imidazole antifungals Immunosuppressants Methadone and analogues Morphinan opioid analgesics Nitrofuran antimicrobials Oestrogen antagonist antineoplastics Opioid analgesics Opioid peptides Opium alkaloid opioid analgesics

Opium poppy substances
Organic iodinated contrast media
Pethidine and analogues
Pyrethroid pesticides
Pyrimidine antagonist antineoplastics
Retinoic acid dermatological agents
Skeletal muscle relaxants
Thiouracil antithyroid agents
Thiourea antithyroid agents
Triazole antifungals
Trimethoprim and derivatives
Trimethoprim sulphonamide
    combinations
Vitamin B substances

Pruritus ani	Analgesics and anti-inflammatory drugs Salicylate analgesics
Pruritus of genital organs	Oestrogen antagonist antineoplastics Sex hormones
Pseudomembranous Colitis - ***Clostridium difficile***	4 Quinolones Aminoglycosides Antibacterial agents Antibiotic antituberculous agents Carbacephems Carbapenems Cephalosporins Cephamycins Lincomycins Macrolides Oxytetracyclines Sulphonamides Tetracyclines Trimethoprim sulphonamide combinations
Psoriasiform rash	Antivirals Lithium
Psychiatric disturbances	4 Aminoquinoline antimalarials 4 Methanolquinoline antimalarials 4 Quinolones Acetylurea antiepileptics Analgesics and anti-inflammatory drugs Anorectics Antibiotic antituberculous agents Antidepressants Antiepileptics Antimuscarinics Carbapenems Carbazepine antiepileptics Class I antiarrhythmics

Corticosteroids
Corticotrophic hormones
Dopaminergic antiparkinsonian agents
Ergot compounds
GABA related antiepileptics
Hydrazide antituberculous agents
Opioid analgesics
Polymyxins
Salicylate analgesics
Smooth muscle relaxants
Succinimide antiepileptics

Ptosis	Alpha blocking vasodilators
	Skeletal muscle relaxants
Pulmonary eosinophilia	Selective serotonin reuptake inhibiting antidepressants
Pulmonary fibrosis	Alkyl sulphonate antineoplastics
	Analgesics and anti-inflammatory drugs
	Antibiotic antineoplastics
	Class I antiarrhythmics
	Class III antiarrhythmics
	Gastrointestinal agents
	Gold salts
	Nitrofuran antimicrobials
	Nitrofuran antiprotozoals
	Nitrogen mustards
	Nitrosoureas
Pulmonary haemorrhage	Pulmonary surfactants
Pulmonary oedema	Analgesics and anti-inflammatory drugs
	Beta sympathomimetic vasodilators
	Beta2 selective stimulants
	Colony stimulating factors
	Ergot alkaloids
	Ergot compounds
	F series prostaglandins
	Glycols
	Haloperidols
	Interleukin 2
	Morphinan opioid analgesics
	Nitrofuran antiprotozoals
	Opioid antagonists
	Organic iodinated contrast media
	Oxytocic hormones
	Polyene antibiotics
	Sympathomimetics
	Thiazide diuretics
Punctate keratitis	Anthelmintics

Pyrexia

4 Quinolones
Aliphatic phenothiazine neuroleptics
Amidinopenicillins
Aminopenicillanic derivatives
Aminopenicillins
Anthelmintics
Antibacterial agents
Antibiotic antituberculous agents
Antiepileptics
Antimuscarinics
Antineoplastics
Antipseudomonal penicillins
Antituberculous agents
Antiulcer agents
Antivirals
Benzimidazole anthelmintics
Benzylpenicillin and derivatives
Bisphosphonates
Butyrophenone neuroleptics
Carbacephems
Carbapenems
Carbazepine antiepileptics
Carboxypenicillins
Central stimulants
Cephalosporins
Cephamycins
Chelating agents
Class I antiarrhythmics
Colony stimulating factors
Diphenylbutylpiperidine neuroleptics
E series prostaglandins
Encephalitis vaccines
F series prostaglandins
Flupenthixols
Fluphenazine
Gastrointestinal agents
Gold salts
Haloperidols
Hydantoin antiepileptics
Hydrazide antituberculous agents
Hydroxynaphthoquinones
Indanedione anticoagulants
Influenza vaccines
Inhalation anaesthetics
Isoxazolyl penicillins
Macrogol ethers
Measles vaccine
Natural penicillins
Neuroleptics
Norgestrels
Oral hypoglycaemics
Penicillinase resistant penicillins
Phenothiazine neuroleptics
Phenoxymethylpenicillin and derivatives

Phenoxypenicillins
Phenytoin
Piperazine phenothiazine neuroleptics
Piperidine phenothiazine neuroleptics
Poliomyelitis vaccines
Polyene antibiotics
Progestogens
Selective serotonin reuptake inhibiting
   antidepressants
Sex hormones
Smooth muscle relaxants
Sulphonylurea hypoglycaemics
Thioxanthene neuroleptics
Typhoid vaccines
Ureido penicillins
Vaccines
Vasodilator antihypertensives
Vitamin B substances
Xanthine oxidase inhibitors
Zuclopenthixols

R-eye completely blind	Hydroxyquinoline antiprotozoals
Raised intracranial pressure	4 Quinolones Anthelmintics Class III antiarrhythmics Colony stimulating factors Oxytetracyclines Progestogens Retinoic acid dermatological agents Sex hormones Tetracyclines
Raised intraocular pressure	Antianginal vasodilators Antimuscarinics Ganglion blocking antihypertensives Hyaluronic acid Smooth muscle relaxants
Rash	4 Methanolquinoline antimalarials 4 Quinolones ACE inhibitors Aldosterone inhibitors Aliphatic phenothiazine neuroleptics Alkylating antineoplastics Aminopenicillins Anabolics Analgesics and anti-inflammatory drugs Angiotensin inhibiting antihypertensives Anorectics Anthelmintics Antiandrogens Antibacterial agents Antibiotic antifungals

Antibiotic antituberculous agents
Antidepressants
Antidotes
Antiemetics
Antiepileptics
Antifolate antineoplastics
Antifungals
Antimalarials
Antineoplastics
Antithyroid agents
Antiulcer agents
Antivirals
Aromatics
Barbiturate antiepileptics
Benzimidazole anthelmintics
Benzodiazepine sedatives
Beta blockers
Bisphosphonates
Butyrophenone neuroleptics
Calcium antagonist vasodilators
Carbacephems
Carbamate sedatives
Carbapenems
Carbonic anhydrase inhibitors
Cardioselective beta blockers
Central stimulants
Centrally acting antihypertensives
Cephalosporins
Cephamycins
Chelating agents
Chloral sedatives
Cinchona antimalarials
Class I antiarrhythmics
Class III antiarrhythmics
Clofibrate and analogues
Colchicum alkaloids
Colony stimulating factors
Competitive muscle relaxants
Corticosteroids
Cough suppressants
Coumarin anticoagulants
Dermatological agents
Diamidine antiprotozoals
Diphenylbutylpiperidine neuroleptics
Dopaminergic antiparkinsonian agents
E series prostaglandins
Edetates
Encephalitis vaccines
Ergolines
Ergot compounds
F series prostaglandins
Flupenthixols
Fluphenazine
Gastrointestinal agents

Gonad regulating hormones
H1 antagonist antihistamines
Haemostatics
Haloperidols
Histamine H2 antagonists
HMG CoA reductase inhibitors
Hyaluronic acid
Hydantoin antiepileptics
Hydrazine monoamine oxidase inhibiting
    antidepressants
Hydroxynaphthoquinones
Imidazole antifungals
Immunosuppressants
Indanedione anticoagulants
Influenza vaccines
Inorganic mercury compounds
Interleukins
Leukotriene inhibitors
Lincomycins
Lipid regulating agents
Loop diuretics
Macrolides
Measles vaccine
Medicinal enzymes
Monoamine oxidase inhibiting
    antidepressants
Monobactams
Mucolytics
Neuroleptics
Nitrofuran antimicrobials
Nitrofuran antiprotozoals
Nitroimidazole antiprotozoals
Oestrogen antagonist antineoplastics
Oestrogens
Opioid antagonists
Oral hypoglycaemics
Organic iodinated contrast media
Organic mercurial disinfectants
Oxazolidinedione antiepileptics
Pesticides
Phenothiazine antihistamines
Phenothiazine neuroleptics
Phenytoin
Piperazine phenothiazine neuroleptics
Piperidine phenothiazine neuroleptics
Poliomyelitis vaccines
Polyene antibiotics
Potassium sparing diuretics
Progestogens
Promethazines
Prophylactic antiasthmatics
Pyrethroid pesticides
Pyrimidine antagonist antineoplastics
Retinoic acid dermatological agents

Salicylate analgesics
Sedatives
Sex hormones
Skeletal muscle relaxants
Smooth muscle relaxants
Succinimide antiepileptics
Sulphonamides
Sulphonylurea hypoglycaemics
Sympathomimetics
Tetracyclic antidepressants
Tetracyclines
Thiazide diuretics
Thiouracil antithyroid agents
Thiourea antithyroid agents
Thioxanthene neuroleptics
Triazole antifungals
Tricyclic antidepressants
Trimethoprim and derivatives
Trimethoprim sulphonamide
   combinations
Typhoid vaccines
Uricosuric agents
Vaccines
Vasodilator antihypertensives
Vasodilators
Vitamin B substances
Xanthine oxidase inhibitors
Zuclopenthixols

Rate of respiration changes	Gases
Raynaud's phenomenon	Antibiotic antineoplastics Centrally acting antihypertensives Ergolines
RBCs - reticulocytes present	Antivirals
Reactive confusion	Opioid analgesics
Rectal discharge	Lipid regulating agents
Rectal pain	Analgesics and anti-inflammatory drugs Lipid regulating agents Salicylate analgesics Sedatives
Recurrent erosion of cornea	Centrally acting antihypertensives F series prostaglandins
Recurrent manic episodes	Central stimulants Selective serotonin reuptake inhibiting antidepressants

Recurrent URTI	Angiotensin inhibiting antihypertensives
Red blood cell aplasia and hypoplasia	Antiepileptics Carbonic anhydrase inhibitors
Red/green colour blindness	Antituberculous agents
Redness of eye	Sympathomimetics
Reduced sebum production	Antiandrogens
Reflux oesophagitis	Antivirals

Renal function tests abnormal	ACE inhibitors
	Acetylurea antiepileptics
	Alkylating antineoplastics
	Antibacterial agents
	Antibiotic antituberculous agents
	Antiepileptics
	Antineoplastics
	Antiulcer agents
	Beta2 selective stimulants
	Borates
	Chloral sedatives
	Clofibrate and analogues
	Colchicum alkaloids
	HMG CoA reductase inhibitors
	Immunosuppressants
	Liquorice
	Lithium
	Oxytetracyclines
	Polyene antibiotics
	Pyrimidine antagonist antineoplastics
	Selective noradrenaline reuptake
	   inhibiting antidepressants
	Somatotrophic hormones
	Tetracyclines
	Thiazide diuretics
	Trimethoprim and derivatives
	Trimethoprim sulphonamide
	   combinations

Renal stones	Antiepileptics Antivirals
Repeated rapid eye movement sleep interruptions	Anticholinesterase parasympathomimetics Parasympathomimetics Pilocarpine
Resorcinol hypothyroidism	Dermatological agents
Respiratory arrest	Organic iodinated contrast media

Respiratory depression	Amide type anaesthetics
	Anthelmintics
	Antidiarrhoeals
	Antiepileptics
	Antivirals
	Barbiturate anaesthetics
	Barbiturate antiepileptics
	Barbiturate sedatives
	Benzomorphan opioid analgesics
	Competitive muscle relaxants
	Cough suppressants
	Depolarising muscle relaxants
	Ester type anaesthetics
	Ganglion blocking antihypertensives
	Inhalation anaesthetics
	Local anaesthetics
	Methadone and analogues
	Morphinan cough suppressants
	Morphinan opioid analgesics
	Opioid analgesics
	Opioid peptides
	Opium alkaloid opioid analgesics
	Opium poppy substances
	Pethidine and analogues
	Sedatives
	Skeletal muscle relaxants
Respiratory distress	Hydantoin antiepileptics
	Phenytoin
Respiratory symptoms	ACE inhibitors
	Antibiotic antituberculous agents
	Hydantoin antiepileptics
	Phenytoin
Restlessness	4 Quinolones
	Amphetamines
	Anorectics
	Antianginal vasodilators
	Antiemetics
	Antivirals
	Barbiturate antiepileptics
	Central stimulants
	Diphenylbutylpiperidine neuroleptics
	Dopaminergic antiparkinsonian agents
	Monoamine oxidase inhibiting antidepressants
	Respiratory stimulants
	Sedatives
	Skeletal muscle relaxants
	Sympathomimetics
	Thyroid agents

Retinal damage	4 Aminoquinoline antimalarials
Retinal detachments & defects	Antivirals
Retinal exudate or deposits	Aliphatic phenothiazine neuroleptics Butyrophenone neuroleptics Diphenylbutylpiperidine neuroleptics Flupenthixols Fluphenazine Haloperidols Neuroleptics Phenothiazine neuroleptics Piperazine phenothiazine neuroleptics Piperidine phenothiazine neuroleptics Thioxanthene neuroleptics Zuclopenthixols
Retinopathy	Antineoplastics Chelating agents Gases Oestrogen antagonist antineoplastics Sex hormones
Retroperitoneal fibrosis	Beta blockers Cardioselective beta blockers Ergolines Ergot alkaloids Ergot compounds Haloperidols Morphinan opioid analgesics Salicylate analgesics
Retrosternal pain	Antianginal vasodilators Antimony antiprotozoals Vasodilator antihypertensives
Rhabdomyolysis	4 Quinolones Aliphatic phenothiazine neuroleptics Barbiturate anaesthetics Barbiturate antiepileptics Barbiturate sedatives Benzodiazepine sedatives Benzomorphan opioid analgesics Clofibrate and analogues Colchicum alkaloids Dopaminergic antiparkinsonian agents Fluphenazine Histamine H2 antagonists HMG CoA reductase inhibitors Hydrazine monoamine oxidase inhibiting antidepressants Lithium Methadone and analogues

Monoamine oxidase inhibiting
antidepressants
Monoamine oxidase inhibiting
antihypertensives
Morphinan opioid analgesics
Neuroleptics
Opioid analgesics
Opioid peptides
Opium alkaloid opioid analgesics
Opium poppy substances
Pethidine and analogues
Phenothiazine antihistamines
Phenothiazine neuroleptics
Piperazine phenothiazine neuroleptics
Piperidine phenothiazine neuroleptics
Polyene antibiotics
Promethazines
Retinoic acid dermatological agents
Theophylline xanthines
Trimethoprim sulphonamide
combinations

Rhinitis	Antineoplastics
	Antiulcer agents
	Ergolines
	GABA related antiepileptics
	H1 antagonist antihistamines
	Neuroleptics
	Organic iodinated contrast media
	Pilocarpine
	Pyrimidine antagonist antineoplastics
Rhinorrhoea	Alpha blocking vasodilators
	Oestrogen antagonist antineoplastics
Rickets	Hydantoin antiepileptics
	Phenytoin
Right upper quadrant pain	Leukotriene inhibitors
Rigors	Colony stimulating factors
Ruptured uterus	E series prostaglandins
	Oxytocic hormones
Saliva – abnormal colouration	Antibiotic antituberculous agents
	Antiprotozoals
	Dopaminergic antiparkinsonian agents
Seborrhoea	Progestogens
	Sex hormones
Seborrhoeic dermatitis	Anabolics

Sedation	Aliphatic phenothiazine neuroleptics
	Alpha blocking antihypertensives
	Antidepressants
	Antifungals
	Antihypertensives
	Antineoplastics
	Butyrophenone neuroleptics
	Centrally acting antihypertensives
	Diphenylbutylpiperidine neuroleptics
	Dopaminergic antiparkinsonian agents
	Flupenthixols
	Fluphenazine
	GABA related antiepileptics
	Ganglion blocking antihypertensives
	Haloperidols
	Neuroleptics
	Pesticides
	Phenothiazine neuroleptics
	Piperazine phenothiazine neuroleptics
	Piperidine phenothiazine neuroleptics
	Rauwolfia antihypertensives
	Skeletal muscle relaxants
	Tetracyclic antidepressants
	Thioxanthene neuroleptics
	Tricyclic antidepressants
	Zuclopenthixols
Semen sample volume	Neuroleptics
Sensory symptoms	Diagnostic agents
	Organic iodinated contrast media
	Serotonin and analogues
Serum bicarbonate abnormal	Antivirals
Serum bilirubin raised	Angiotensin inhibiting antihypertensives
	Anthelmintics
	Antibacterial agents
	Antivirals
	Carbapenems
Serum cholesterol raised	Anabolics
	Antidepressants
	Antivirals
	Loop diuretics
	Retinoic acid dermatological agents
	Thiazide diuretics
Serum creatinine abnormal	Cephalosporins
Serum creatinine raised	4 Quinolones
	ACE inhibitors
	Analgesics and anti-inflammatory drugs

Angiotensin inhibiting antihypertensives
Antibacterial agents
Antibiotic antineoplastics
Antivirals
Borates
Erythropoietin
Immunosuppressants
Interleukin 2
Organic iodinated contrast media
Vasodilator antihypertensives

Serum lipids high	Asparaginase antineoplastics

Serum sickness	Carbacephems
	Cephalosporins
	Cephamycins

Serum sodium level abnormal	Sulphonylurea hypoglycaemics

Serum triglycerides raised	Anabolics
	Antivirals
	Loop diuretics
	Retinoic acid dermatological agents
	Thiazide diuretics

Severe uterine contractions	Anthelmintics
	E series prostaglandins
	F series prostaglandins

Sexual dysfunction	Adrenergic neurone blocking antihypertensives
	Alpha blocking antihypertensives
	Antidepressants
	Centrally acting antihypertensives
	Opioid antagonists
	Piperidine phenothiazine neuroleptics

Sexual precocity	Androgens
	Gonadotrophic hormones
	Testosterones

Shivering	Alpha blocking vasodilators
	Anabolics
	Antibacterial agents
	Antibiotic antineoplastics
	Antibiotic antituberculous agents
	Antidepressants
	Antivirals
	Blood clotting factors
	Blood products
	Cardiac inotropic agents
	Contrast media
	Cytoprotective agents

E series prostaglandins
F series prostaglandins
Immunosuppressants
Opioid antagonists
Osmotic diuretics
Pilocarpine
Skeletal muscle relaxants
Specific immunoglobulins

Sideroblastic anaemia	Antituberculous agents
Sinoatrial block	Calcium antagonist vasodilators Class I antiarrhythmics
Sinus tachycardia	Respiratory stimulants
Skeletal hyperostosis	Interleukins Retinoic acid dermatological agents
Skin and finger nail pigmentation	4 Aminoquinoline antimalarials Aliphatic phenothiazine neuroleptics Antibiotic antineoplastics Antileprotics Antiprotozoals Antivirals Butyrophenone neuroleptics Cardiac inotropic agents Dermatological agents Diphenylbutylpiperidine neuroleptics F series prostaglandins Flupenthixols Fluphenazine Haloperidols Hydroquinone dermatological agents Hydroxyquinoline antiprotozoals Neuroleptics Phenothiazine neuroleptics Piperazine phenothiazine neuroleptics Piperidine phenothiazine neuroleptics Retinoic acid dermatological agents Sulphonamides Thioxanthene neuroleptics Zuclopenthixols
Skin disorders/reactions	4 Aminoquinoline antimalarials Alcohol metabolism modifiers Analgesics and anti-inflammatory drugs Antibiotic antineoplastics Antineoplastics Biguanide antimalarials Bisphosphonates Borates Chelating agents

| | Erythropoietin |
| | Thiazide diuretics |

| **Skin nodules** | Dopaminergic antiparkinsonian agents |

| **Skin pigmented over lesions** | Antileprotics |

| **Skin scaling** | Retinoic acid dermatological agents |

| **Skin ulceration** | Dopaminergic antiparkinsonian agents |
| | Pyrimidine antagonist antineoplastics |

Slurred speech	Hydantoin antiepileptics
	Phenytoin
	Polymyxins

| **Sneezing** | Cytoprotective agents |
| | Edetates |

| **Soiling - encopresis** | Lipid regulating agents |

Somnolence	Anticholinesterase parasympathomimetics
	Antiepileptics
	Antimuscarinics
	Antiulcer agents
	Antivirals
	Central stimulants
	Dermatological agents
	Dopaminergic antiparkinsonian agents
	Inhalation anaesthetics
	Neuroleptics
	Serotonin and analogues

| **Sore gums** | Gold salts |

Sore mouth	Antineoplastics
	Antivirals
	Oestrogen antagonist antineoplastics
	Phenol disinfectants

Sore throat	ACE inhibitors
	Anthelmintics
	Antiulcer agents
	Antivirals
	Centrally acting antihypertensives
	Corticosteroids
	Gold salts
	Oestrogen antagonist antineoplastics
	Prophylactic antiasthmatics

| **Spasm of sphincter of Oddi** | Benzomorphan opioid analgesics |
| | Methadone and analogues |

	Morphinan opioid analgesics
	Opioid analgesics
	Opioid peptides
	Opium alkaloid opioid analgesics
	Opium poppy substances
	Pethidine and analogues
Spasmodic torticollis	Skeletal muscle relaxants
Speech problems	Dopaminergic antiparkinsonian agents
	Skeletal muscle relaxants
Sperm absent - azoospermia	Anabolics
	Androgens
	Antiandrogens
	Antivirals
	Testosterones
Sperm morphology affected	Antibiotic antifungals
Sperm no./cc v.low: 0-10 mill.	Antivirals
Splenomegaly	Colony stimulating factors
Spontaneous bruising	Gold salts
	Low molecular weight heparins
	Skeletal muscle relaxants
Steroid acne	Corticosteroids
	Corticotrophic hormones
Steroid facies	Anabolics
	Androgens
	Corticosteroids
	Corticotrophic hormones
	Norgestrels
	Oestrogens
	Progestogens
	Sex hormones
	Testosterones
Steroid induced diabetes	Anabolics
	Androgens
	Corticosteroids
	Corticotrophic hormones
	Norgestrels
	Oestrogens
	Progestogens
	Sex hormones
	Testosterones
Steroid-induced glaucoma	Anabolics
	Androgens

Corticosteroids
Corticotrophic hormones
Norgestrels
Oestrogens
Progestogens
Sex hormones
Testosterones

Stevens-Johnson syndrome	4 Methanolquinoline antimalarials
	4 Quinolones
	Analgesics and anti-inflammatory drugs
	Anthelmintics
	Antibacterial agents
	Antiepileptics
	Antifungals
	Antivirals
	Carbazepine antiepileptics
	Chelating agents
	Class I antiarrhythmics
	Gastrointestinal agents
	Hydantoin antiepileptics
	Phenytoin
	Polyene antibiotics
	Sulphonamides
	Triazole antifungals
	Trimethoprim sulphonamide combinations
	Xanthine oxidase inhibitors
Stomatitis	ACE inhibitors
	Analgesics and anti-inflammatory drugs
	Antibiotic antineoplastics
	Antifolate antineoplastics
	Antineoplastics
	Antiulcer agents
	Beta2 selective stimulants
	Biguanide antimalarials
	Chelating agents
	Colony stimulating factors
	Expectorants
	Fluorouracil
	Macrolides
	Medicinal enzymes
	Polyene antibiotics
	Pyrimidine antagonist antineoplastics
Striae atrophicae	Corticosteroids
	Corticotrophic hormones
Stricture of intestine	Medicinal enzymes
Stroke and cerebrovascular accident	ACE inhibitors
	Ergot alkaloids

	Ergot compounds Selective serotonin reuptake inhibiting antidepressants
Subacute confusional state	Opioid analgesics
Subacute hepatitis-noninfect.	Retinoic acid dermatological agents
Subarachnoid haemorrhage	Oxytocic hormones
Subcutaneous sclerotic plaques	Antibiotic antineoplastics
Sudden death	Antiandrogens Antianginal vasodilators Lithium Mercurial diuretics
Suicidal	Retinoic acid dermatological agents
Suicidal ideation	Rauwolfia antihypertensives Selective serotonin reuptake inhibiting antidepressants
Sulphuric acid - toxic effect	Mineral acids
Supraventricular ectopic beats	Anthracycline antibiotic antineoplastics
Sweating	Alpha blocking vasodilators Antifolate antineoplastics Antiulcer agents Oestrogen antagonist antineoplastics Pilocarpine Pyrimidine antagonist antineoplastics Respiratory stimulants Selective noradrenaline reuptake inhibiting antidepressants
Swelling at site of injection	Hyaluronic acid Organic iodinated contrast media
Syncope	Analgesics and anti-inflammatory drugs Antianginal vasodilators Antibiotic antituberculous agents Antidepressants Antiemetics Benzimidazole anthelmintics Catechol O-methyl transferase inhibitors Colony stimulating factors Contrast media Corticotrophic hormones Cytoprotective agents Diamidine antiprotozoals

Dopaminergic antiparkinsonian agents
E series prostaglandins
Ergolines
H1 antagonist antihistamines
Lithium
Neuroleptics
Papaverine and analogues
Salicylate analgesics
Sedatives
Skeletal muscle relaxants
Tetracyclic antidepressants
Tricyclic antidepressants

Synovitis and tenosynovitis	4 Quinolones
Systemic lupus erythematosus	Aliphatic phenothiazine neuroleptics
	Centrally acting antihypertensives
	Class I antiarrhythmics
	Gastrointestinal agents
	Neuroleptics
	Sex hormones
	Tetracyclines
	Thiouracil antithyroid agents
	Vasodilator antihypertensives
Tachycardia	4 Quinolones
	ACE inhibitors
	Aliphatic phenothiazine neuroleptics
	Alpha adrenoceptor stimulants
	Alpha blocking antihypertensives
	Alpha blocking vasodilators
	Amphetamines
	Analgesics and anti-inflammatory drugs
	Anorectics
	Antianginal vasodilators
	Antidepressants
	Antiemetics
	Antimuscarinics
	Antineoplastics
	Aromatics
	Benzodiazepine antagonists
	Beta adrenoceptor stimulants
	Beta sympathomimetic vasodilators
	Beta1 selective stimulants
	Beta2 selective stimulants
	Butyrophenone neuroleptics
	Calcium antagonist vasodilators
	Central stimulants
	Chelating agents
	Cholinesterase reactivators
	Diagnostic agents
	Diphenylbutylpiperidine neuroleptics
	Dopaminergic antiparkinsonian agents
	E series prostaglandins

Edetates
Ergolines
Ergot compounds
Flupenthixols
Fluphenazine
Ganglion blocking antihypertensives
Glycols
H1 antagonist antihistamines
Haloperidols
Immunosuppressants
Inhalation anaesthetics
Interleukins
Isoprenaline
Lipid regulating agents
Neuroleptics
Parenteral anaesthetics
Peripheral and cerebral vasodilators
Phenothiazine neuroleptics
Piperazine phenothiazine neuroleptics
Piperidine phenothiazine neuroleptics
Respiratory stimulants
Sedatives
Selective noradrenaline reuptake
    inhibiting antidepressants
Serotonin and analogues
Skeletal muscle relaxants
Smooth muscle relaxants
Sulphone antileprotics
Sympathomimetics
Tetracyclic antidepressants
Theophylline xanthines
Thioxanthene neuroleptics
Thyroid agents
Thyrotrophic hormones
Tricyclic antidepressants
Vasodilator antihypertensives
Xanthine containing beverages
Xanthines
Zuclopenthixols

Tachypnoea	Antivirals
Taste disturbance	4 Quinolones
	ACE inhibitors
	Angiotensin inhibiting antihypertensives
	Antifolate antineoplastics
	Antifungals
	Antineoplastics
	Antituberculous agents
	Antiulcer agents
	Antivirals
	Beta2 selective stimulants
	Bisphosphonates
	Calcitonin

Carbapenems
Carbonic anhydrase inhibitors
Centrally acting antihypertensives
Cephalosporins
Chelating agents
Class I antiarrhythmics
Class III antiarrhythmics
Contrast media
Diamidine antiprotozoals
Disinfectants
Gold salts
H1 antagonist antihistamines
Macrolides
Monobactams
Nitroimidazole antiprotozoals
Organic iodinated contrast media
Prophylactic antiasthmatics
Sedatives
Skeletal muscle relaxants
Thyrotrophic hormones
Vasodilator antihypertensives
Xanthine oxidase inhibitors

Telangiectasia	Calcium antagonist vasodilators
Temporary blindness	Cinchona antimalarials
Temporary worsening of symptoms	Fluorouracil Oestrogen antagonist antineoplastics Pyrimidine antagonist antineoplastics Retinoic acid dermatological agents Sex hormones
Throat irritation	Corticosteroids
Throat pain	Chelating agents Serotonin and analogues
Thrombocythaemia	Carbapenems Erythropoietin Pyrimidine antagonist antineoplastics Retinoic acid dermatological agents
Thrombocytopenia	4 Aminoquinoline antimalarials 4 Methanolquinoline antimalarials 4 Quinolones ACE inhibitors Alpha blocking vasodilators Amidinopenicillins Aminopenicillanic derivatives Aminopenicillins Analgesics and anti-inflammatory drugs Antiandrogens

Antibacterial agents
Antibiotic antituberculous agents
Antidepressants
Antiepileptics
Antifungals
Antineoplastics
Antipseudomonal penicillins
Antiulcer agents
Antivirals
Benzylpenicillin and derivatives
Calcium antagonist vasodilators
Carbacephems
Carbapenems
Carbazepine antiepileptics
Carboxypenicillins
Cardiac inotropic agents
Central stimulants
Cephalosporins
Cephamycins
Chelating agents
Cinchona antimalarials
Class I antiarrhythmics
Class III antiarrhythmics
Dermatological agents
Diagnostic agents
Diamidine antiprotozoals
Direct acting anticoagulants
Gastrointestinal agents
Heparinoids
Histamine H2 antagonists
Hydantoin antiepileptics
Imidazole antifungals
Immunosuppressants
Isoxazolyl penicillins
Lincomycins
Low molecular weight heparins
Monobactams
Natural penicillins
Nitrofuran antimicrobials
Oestrogen antagonist antineoplastics
Opioid antagonists
Oral hypoglycaemics
Organic iodinated contrast media
Oxacephalosporins
Oxazolidinedione antiepileptics
Penicillinase resistant penicillins
Phenoxymethylpenicillin and derivatives
Phenoxypenicillins
Phenytoin
Platelet activating factor antagonists
Progestogens
Pyrimidine antagonist antineoplastics
Retinoic acid dermatological agents
Salicylate analgesics

Sedatives
Selective serotonin reuptake inhibiting
    antidepressants
Sex hormones
Skeletal muscle relaxants
Sulphonamides
Sulphonylurea hypoglycaemics
Tetracyclic antidepressants
Thiazide diuretics
Tricyclic antidepressants
Trimethoprim sulphonamide
    combinations
Ureido penicillins
Vasodilator antihypertensives

Thromboembolism	Carbazepine antiepileptics
	Direct acting anticoagulants
Thrombosis of arterio-venous surgical shunt	Erythropoietin
Thyroid hormone tests high	Antineoplastics
	Antivirals
	Dermatological agents
	Interleukin 2
Thyroid hormone tests low	Antineoplastics
	Antivirals
	Dermatological agents
	Interleukin 2
Thyroid swelling	Thyrotrophic hormones
Thyrotoxicosis	Class III antiarrhythmics
	Iodides
	Iodine compounds
	Iodophores
Tics	Central stimulants
Tightening pain	Serotonin and analogues
Tingling sensation	Alpha adrenoceptor stimulants
	Alpha blocking vasodilators
	Antivirals
	Beta blockers
	Calcitonin
	Carbonic anhydrase inhibitors
	Chelating agents
	Diagnostic agents
	H1 antagonist antihistamines
	HMG CoA reductase inhibitors

Oestrogen antagonist antineoplastics
Serotonin and analogues
Sympathomimetics

Tinnitus symptoms

4 Quinolones
Analgesics and anti-inflammatory drugs
Antibacterial agents
Antibiotic antituberculous agents
Antineoplastics
Benzimidazole anthelmintics
Calcium antagonist vasodilators
Cinchona antimalarials
Dermatological agents
Ergot alkaloids
Ergot compounds
Haemostatics
Mucolytics
Salicylate analgesics

Tiredness

ACE inhibitors
Alpha blocking antihypertensives
Alpha blocking vasodilators
Antiandrogens
Antianginal vasodilators
Antidepressants
Antiepileptics
Antifolate antineoplastics
Antineoplastics
Antivirals
Beta blockers
Bisphosphonates
Calcium antagonist vasodilators
Colony stimulating factors
Ergolines
GABA related antiepileptics
Gonadotrophic hormones
Histamine H2 antagonists
Oestrogen antagonist antineoplastics
Pilocarpine
Sedatives
Selective serotonin reuptake inhibiting
    antidepressants

Tissue necrosis

Alkyl sulphonate antineoplastics
Alkylating antineoplastics
Anthracycline antibiotic antineoplastics
Antibiotic antineoplastics
Antifolate antineoplastics
Antineoplastics
Asparaginase antineoplastics
Class II antiarrhythmics
Diamidine antiprotozoals
Ethyleneimine antineoplastics
Fluorouracil

Immunostimulants
Immunosuppressants
Interleukin 2
Nitrogen mustards
Nitrosoureas
Organic iodinated contrast media
Purine antagonist antineoplastics
Pyrimidine antagonist antineoplastics
Sulphur mustards
Triazene antineoplastics
Vinca alkaloid antineoplastics

Toxic encephalitis due to mercury	Mercurial dermatological agents Organic mercurial disinfectants
Toxic epidermal necrolysis	4 Quinolones ACE inhibitors Analgesics and anti-inflammatory drugs Antibiotic antifungals Antiepileptics Antifungals Antivirals Carbacephems Carbapenems Carbazepine antiepileptics Cephalosporins Cephamycins HMG CoA reductase inhibitors Hydantoin antiepileptics Phenytoin Sulphonamides Thiazide diuretics Trimethoprim sulphonamide combinations Xanthine oxidase inhibitors
Toxic optic neuropathy	Antituberculous agents
Tremor	4 Quinolones Amphetamines Analgesics and anti-inflammatory drugs Anorectics Anthelmintics Antibiotic antituberculous agents Anticholinesterase parasympathomimetics Antidepressants Antiemetics Antiepileptics Antivirals Barbiturate anaesthetics Beta adrenoceptor stimulants Beta1 selective stimulants Beta2 selective stimulants

Central stimulants
Class I antiarrhythmics
Class III antiarrhythmics
Corticosteroids
Dopaminergic antiparkinsonian agents
GABA related antiepileptics
Ganglion blocking antihypertensives
Gastrointestinal agents
H1 antagonist antihistamines
Hydantoin antiepileptics
Hydrazine monoamine oxidase inhibiting
    antidepressants
Immunosuppressants
Isoprenaline
Lithium
Monoamine oxidase inhibiting
    antidepressants
Phenothiazine antihistamines
Phenytoin
Promethazines
Respiratory stimulants
Sedatives
Selective serotonin reuptake inhibiting
    antidepressants
Skeletal muscle relaxants
Sympathomimetics
Tetracyclic antidepressants
Tricyclic antidepressants

Ulcer of oesophagus	Analgesics and anti-inflammatory drugs
	Bisphosphonates
	Medicinal enzymes

Unspecified cell type leukaemia	Alkyl sulphonate antineoplastics

Uraemia	Organic iodinated contrast media

Urinary retention	Analgesics and anti-inflammatory drugs
	Antimuscarinics
	Benzodiazepine sedatives
	Carbamate sedatives
	Cardiac inotropic agents
	Class I antiarrhythmics
	H1 antagonist antihistamines
	Haemostatics
	Neuroleptics
	Phenothiazine antihistamines
	Promethazines
	Selective noradrenaline reuptake inhibiting antidepressants
	Skeletal muscle relaxants

Urinary system symptoms	Skeletal muscle relaxants

Urinary tract infection	Anticholinesterase parasympathomimetics
	Antiulcer agents
	Lipid regulating agents
	Smooth muscle relaxants

Urine - abnormal colouration	4 Quinolones
	Analgesics and anti-inflammatory drugs
	Anthraquinone glycosides
	Antibiotic antituberculous agents
	Antileprotics
	Antiprotozoals
	Carbapenems
	Dopaminergic antiparkinsonian agents
	Gastrointestinal agents
	Indanedione anticoagulants
	Nitroimidazole antiprotozoals

Urine albumin	Aromatics

Urine colour abnormal	Anthelmintics

Urine looks dark	Nitrofuran antiprotozoals

Urine protein abnormal	Anthelmintics

Urine urate raised	Antivirals
	Medicinal enzymes

Urticaria	4 Methanolquinoline antimalarials
	ACE inhibitors
	Amidinopenicillins
	Aminopenicillanic derivatives
	Aminopenicillins
	Analgesics and anti-inflammatory drugs
	Anthelmintics
	Antibacterial agents
	Antibiotic antituberculous agents
	Antiemetics
	Antifungals
	Antineoplastics
	Antipseudomonal penicillins
	Antituberculous agents
	Antiulcer agents
	Antivirals
	Benzomorphan opioid analgesics
	Benzylpenicillin and derivatives
	Beta2 selective stimulants
	Carbacephems
	Carbapenems
	Carboxypenicillins
	Central stimulants
	Cephalosporins

Cephamycins
Clofibrate and analogues
Dichloroacetamide antiprotozoals
Direct acting anticoagulants
Gastrointestinal agents
Gold salts
Gonad regulating hormones
Heparinoids
Histamine H2 antagonists
Imidazole antifungals
Immunosuppressants
Isoxazolyl penicillins
Laxatives
Leukotriene inhibitors
Low molecular weight heparins
Macrolides
Medicinal enzymes
Methadone and analogues
Monobactams
Morphinan opioid analgesics
Mucolytics
Natural penicillins
Nitrofuran antimicrobials
Nitroimidazole antiprotozoals
Norgestrels
Opioid analgesics
Opioid peptides
Opium alkaloid opioid analgesics
Opium poppy substances
Organic iodinated contrast media
Penicillinase resistant penicillins
Pethidine and analogues
Phenoxymethylpenicillin and derivatives
Phenoxypenicillins
Polyene antibiotics
Progestogens
Sedatives
Sex hormones
Skeletal muscle relaxants
Thyrotrophic hormones
Triazole antifungals
Typhoid vaccines
Ureido penicillins

Uterus rupture in/after labour	Oxytocic hormones
Uveitis	Antibiotic antituberculous agents Beta blockers F series prostaglandins
Vaginal discharge	Gonad regulating hormones Oestrogen antagonist antineoplastics Sex hormones

Vaginitis and vulvovaginitis	Cephalosporins
Vasculitis	Cardiac inotropic agents
Vasodilatation	Contrast media Organic iodinated contrast media
Venous embolus/thrombus	Haemostatics Oestrogens Sex hormones
Ventricular ectopic beats	Antimalarials Beta1 selective stimulants H1 antagonist antihistamines
Ventricular fibrillat./flutter	Antianginal vasodilators Antimalarials Beta blockers Calcium antagonist vasodilators H1 antagonist antihistamines Inhalation anaesthetics Lipid regulating agents
Vertigo	Alpha blocking antihypertensives Analgesics and anti-inflammatory drugs Anthelmintics Antibiotic antituberculous agents Antiemetics Antifungals Antiulcer agents Benzodiazepine sedatives Benzomorphan opioid analgesics Carbamate sedatives Class III antiarrhythmics Clofibrate and analogues Dermatological agents Fat soluble vitamins Gases Gonad regulating hormones Methadone and analogues Morphinan opioid analgesics Opioid analgesics Opioid peptides Opium alkaloid opioid analgesics Opium poppy substances Pethidine and analogues Polymyxins Salicylate analgesics Sedatives Skeletal muscle relaxants Tetracyclines Vitamin D substances

	Vitamins Xanthine oxidase inhibitors
Vesicles	Antifungals
Vesicular eruption	Pyrimidine antagonist antineoplastics
Vestibular disorders	Aminoglycosides Antibacterial agents
Viral/chlamydial infection	Antivirals Corticosteroids Corticotrophic hormones Immunosuppressants Oestrogen antagonist antineoplastics
Virilism	Anabolics Androgens Medicinal enzymes Sex hormones Testosterones
Visual disturbances	Antiulcer agents Barbiturate antiepileptics
Visual symptoms	Antiandrogens Oxazolidinedione antiepileptics
Vitamin B12 deficiency anaemia	Biguanide hypoglycaemics Inhalation anaesthetics
Vitamin K deficiency	Bile acid binding resins
Voice disturbance	Gases
Vomiting	4 Aminoquinoline antimalarials 4 Methanolquinoline antimalarials 4 Quinolones 8 Aminoquinoline antimalarials ACE inhibitors Alcoholic disinfectants Aldosterone inhibitors Alkyl sulphonate antineoplastics Alkylating antineoplastics Alpha adrenoceptor stimulants Alpha blocking antihypertensives Alpha blocking vasodilators Amino acids Anabolics Analgesics and anti-inflammatory drugs Anthelmintics Anthracycline antibiotic antineoplastics

Antiandrogens
Antianginal vasodilators
Antibacterial agents
Antibiotic antifungals
Antibiotic antineoplastics
Antibiotic antituberculous agents
Anticholinesterase parasympathomimetics
Antidepressants
Antidiarrhoeals
Antidiuretic hormones
Antidotes
Antiepileptics
Antifolate antineoplastics
Antifungals
Antimalarials
Antimony antiprotozoals
Antimuscarinics
Antineoplastics
Antiprotozoals
Antithyroid agents
Antituberculous agents
Antiulcer agents
Antivirals
Aromatics
Asparaginase antineoplastics
Aspartic acid
Benzimidazole anthelmintics
Benzodiazepine antagonists
Benzomorphan opioid analgesics
Beta blockers
Beta sympathomimetic vasodilators
Beta1 selective stimulants
Beta2 selective stimulants
Biguanide hypoglycaemics
Bile acid binding resins
Bismuth salts
Blood products
Borates
Calcitonin
Carbacephems
Carbapenems
Carbazepine antiepileptics
Cardiac glycosides
Cardiac inotropic agents
Catechol O-methyl transferase inhibitors
Central stimulants
Cephalosporins
Cephamycins
Chelating agents
Chloramphenicols
Class I antiarrhythmics
Class II antiarrhythmics
Class III antiarrhythmics
Class IV antiarrhythmics

Colchicum alkaloids
Colony stimulating factors
Contrast media
Coumarin anticoagulants
Cytoprotective agents
Diagnostic agents
Diamidine antiprotozoals
Dichloroacetamide antiprotozoals
Digitalis
Dopaminergic antiparkinsonian agents
E series prostaglandins
Edetates
Ergolines
Ergot alkaloids
Ergot compounds
Essential amino acids
Ethyleneimine antineoplastics
Expectorants
F series prostaglandins
Fat soluble vitamins
Fluorouracil
GABA related antiepileptics
Gastrointestinal agents
Glucose tests
Glycol and glycerol esters
Glycols
Gonad regulating hormones
Haemostatics
Histamine H2 antagonists
HMG CoA reductase inhibitors
Hydantoin antiepileptics
Hydrazide antituberculous agents
Hydroxynaphthoquinones
Imidazole antifungals
Immunosuppressants
Indanedione anticoagulants
Inhalation anaesthetics
Iron compounds
Laxatives
Leukotriene inhibitors
Lincomycins
Lipid regulating agents
Lithium
Macrolides
Medicinal enzymes
Methadone and analogues
Monobactams
Morphinan opioid analgesics
Neuroleptics
Nitrofuran antimicrobials
Nitrofuran antiprotozoals
Nitrogen mustards
Nitroimidazole antiprotozoals
Nitrosoureas

Oestrogen antagonist antineoplastics
Oestrogens
Opioid analgesics
Opioid antagonists
Opioid peptides
Opium alkaloid opioid analgesics
Opium poppy substances
Oral hypoglycaemics
Organic iodinated contrast media
Oxazolidinedione antiepileptics
Oxytetracyclines
Parasympathomimetics
Peripheral and cerebral vasodilators
Pethidine and analogues
Phenytoin
Pilocarpine
Platelet activating factor antagonists
Polyene antibiotics
Posterior pituitary hormones
Prophylactic antiasthmatics
Purine antagonist antineoplastics
Pyrimidine antagonist antineoplastics
Respiratory stimulants
Sedatives
Selective serotonin reuptake inhibiting
   antidepressants
Serotonin and analogues
Sex hormones
Somatotrophic hormones
Sulphonamides
Sulphone antileprotics
Sulphur mustards
Sympathomimetics
Tetracyclines
Thyrotrophic hormones
Triazene antineoplastics
Trimethoprim and derivatives
Trimethoprim sulphonamide
combinations
Typhoid vaccines
Uricosuric agents
Vasodilator antihypertensives
Vinca alkaloid antineoplastics
Vitamin B substances
Vitamin D substances
Vitamins

Water intoxication	Oxytocic hormones

MONITORING PATIENTS WITH RENAL DISEASE

17

S Dhillon

Clinical pharmacists need to understand the implications of renal disease on drug handling.

Clinically there are an increasing number of patients who present with renal disease. In addition the patient may have other medical problems which require drug treatment, hence a knowledge of drug handling and monitoring patients with renal disease is important.

Renal disease may present as acute renal failure which results in a sudden decrease in renal function and accumulation of nitrogenous waste. Others may present with chronic renal failure where there is a progressive decrease in renal failure.

CAUSES OF RENAL DISEASE

Renal disease may be due to:

- pre-renal causes, e.g. shock, hypotension
- renal causes, i.e. intrinsic renal disease, e.g. glomerular damage
- post-renal causes, e.g. obstruction.

Drug-induced renal disease may also be a problem; examples include: amphotericin B, benzylpenicillin, hydralazine, gold, penicillamine, phenylbutazone, sulphonamides.

Examples of specific drug-induced renal problems

- Vasculitis due to allopurinol, penicillins, phenytoin, sulphonamides and thiazides.
- Direct drug toxicity may be induced by aminoglycosides, frusemide, cephalosporins, paracetamol and salicylate overdose, tetracyclines, amphotericin B and iodinated contrast media.
- Renal obstruction, for example:

  — crystalluria induced by nitrofurantoin 6MP, methotrexate, sulphonamides (rare)
  — urate stone formation induced by cytotoxics
  — ureteric obstruction due to retroperitoneal fibrosis induced by methylsergide, methyldopa, hydralazine, ergotamine.

> ⚠ The most important consequence of renal disease is its influence on drug handling where drug excretion may be markedly affected.

Pharmacists should be aware that the uraemic state may result in a wide range of clinical problems and can use these clinical signs to identify patients who may have renal problems:

- Neurological
- Psychological
- Ocular
- Cardiovascular
- Gastrointestinal
- Peripheral neuropathy
- Dermatological
- Metabolic
- Haematological
- Endocrine.

KEY CHANGES IN PHARMACOKINETICS IN RENAL DISEASE

Absorption

Uraemic patients may show:

- an increase in gastric ammonia, i.e. increase in pH, resulting in a reduction in absorption of some drugs, e.g. iron, dextropropoxyphene, digoxin
- oedematous gut, this may result in a decrease in blood flow which reduces drug absorption, e.g. chlorpropamide, pindolol, frusemide.

Distribution

Plasma protein binding (PPB) changes may occur in renal patients resulting in changes in the volume of distribution (Vd). Patients may show:

- hypoalbuminaemia
- competitive drug displacement
- conformational changes in the albumin molecule resulting in decreased binding
- accumulation of drug metabolites which may act as displacing agents e.g. phenytoin PPB is reduced and Vd increased, digoxin Vd is reduced.

Interpretation of phenytoin levels in hypoalbuminaemia must be adjusted for the effect on protein binding. (*See* Phenytoin monograph p.313).

In general, a therapeutic range of 5–10 mg/L can be applied to unadjusted serum phenytoin levels.

Metabolism

Patients with renal impairment may have:

- accumulation of active metabolites. Examples include:

Drug	Metabolite
Allopurinol	Oxipurinol
Chlorpropamide	Hydroxy metabolites
Procainamide	n-Acetyl procainamide
Nitrofurantoin	Toxic metabolite

- increased rate of metabolic process:

Type of reaction	Effect
Oxidation	Mostly normal but antipyrine and phenytoin ↑ metabolism
Reduction	Reduced (slow) reactions
Glucuronide formation	No change

Pharmacodynamics

Patients with renal dysfunction may have increased drug sensitivity. This may be due to changes in the CNS distribution. Examples include:

- Thiopentone
- Catecholamines
- Cardioactive agents
- Antidepressants.

Other markers which may be useful in monitoring the renal dysfunction include:

- Urine microscopy

  — albumin
  — casts

- *p*-aminohipporate, amino acids, glucose
- proteinuria

  — β_2 microglobulin
  — α_2 microglobulin and retinol binding protein.

BOX 17.1 Assessment of renal function: parameters which can be used

---

Serum creatinine (SrCr)   6–15 mg/L
                               45–125 µmol/L
— Muscle breakdown product
— Produced at constant rate
— Dependent on muscle mass
— 10–15% lower in females

Creatinine clearance   90–120 mL/min
Commonly used as a measure of glomerular filtration rate
- Measured either by   — 24 h urine collection
                             — derived from equations, e.g.

Cockcroft Gault equation
Male

$$CrCl = \frac{1.23\,(140 - Age)\,wt}{Sr\ creatinine}$$

Female

$$CrCl = \frac{1.04\,(140 - Age)\,wt}{Sr\ creatinine}$$

    The assessment of creatinine clearance using Cockcroft and Gault needs to be interpreted with caution in patients who are:

- *Obese* — use IBW
- *Muscle wasting* — CrCl will be overestimated
- *Oedematous patients* — use IBW
- *Ascites* — use IBW, consider dilutional effect on SrCr
- *ARF* i.e. where two serum creatinine levels measured in 24 h vary by more than 20 µmol/L. This may represent non-steady state serum creatinine levels, therefore you may underestimate the degree of renal impairment. Use urea, this may be a better guide for deteriorating renal function.

Drug dosing in renal failure

Guide to Drug Dosage in Renal Failure *see* Avery's Drug Treatment Appendix D and BNF Appendix 2.

CLINICAL PHARMACY — RENAL CHECKLIST

You can assess whether you are dealing with a renal patient from the type of ward the patient is on; this may clearly suggest the patient has renal problems or this may be indicated by the consultant dealing with your patient.

However look out for specific prescription items:

- Aluminium hydroxide gel/capsules/tablets
- Frusemide
- Calcium resonium
- Chlorpheniramine
- Dialysis fluid
- Calcidol.

The patient may be on:

- Low sodium diet
- High protein diet.

The patient may show the following clinical or physical signs:

- Oedema
- Vomiting
- Mental confusion
- Scratch marks
- Fatigue.

The patient may have:

- Fluid balance chart
- Dialysis chart/bags
- 24 hour urine collection.

The following laboratory tests may be useful in monitoring:

- Creatinine
- Urea
- Electrolytes
- Other specific urine tests

   — Protein
   — Albumin
   — Microscopy

⚠ Remember clinical pharmacy implications:

- Gastrointestinal disturbances common: watch prescribing of antacids
- Plasma protein binding: caution with drugs that are highly plasma protein-bound
- Sodium and fluid retention: check for sodium content of drugs; check fluid requirements
- Renally excreted drugs/metabolites: caution with active metabolites
- Pharmacodynamics: caution with drugs where there is increased CNS sensitivity
- Dialysis: check if the drug is dialysed, you may need to titrate dosages.

REFERENCES

Bennett WM 1997 Guide to drug dosage in renal failure. In: Speight TM (ed) Avery's drug treatment: principles and practice of clinical pharmacology and therapeutics, 3rd edn. Adis International. pp. 1414–1443

Robinson DC, Baker DE 1988 Drug induced renal disorders. In: Koda-Kimble MA, Young LY (eds) Applied therapeutics – the clinical use of drugs, 4th edn. Applied Therapeutics Inc. pp.587–634

18

DRUG REMOVAL BY CONTINUOUS RENAL REPLACEMENT THERAPIES

G Davies

This chapter is intended to provide clinical pharmacists with a basic understanding of both the technology and principles which underpin the provision of renal replacement to patients in acute renal failure. The relationship between these relatively new techniques and drug removal is discussed in order to aid practitioners when selecting a dosing regimen.

Patients requiring intensive care often experience acute renal failure as a result of their underlying condition. The types of patients managed on an intensive care unit (ICU) form a diverse group, whose conditions are usually classified as medical emergencies. They may be admitted following:

- Severe trauma
- A cardiovascular event, e.g. a myocardial infarction
- Severe sepsis
- Elective surgery, e.g. repair of abdominal aortic aneurysm
- Haemorrhage
- A major burn.

The cause of the admission to the ICU coupled with its severity, the patient's age and any relevant past medical history leads to a number of pathophysiological events that often result in acute renal failure (ARF). Consequently ARF in the ICU patient is usually a direct result of their severe illness, particularly following failure of other major organ systems such as the heart or lungs. Therefore although the mortality in ICU patients who develop ARF is high (around 70%) it is, in the main, a reflection of the failure of other organs (Cameron 1990).

MANAGEMENT OF ARF

The management of ARF falls into three broad categories:

1. Preventive therapy
This often involves the aggressive treatment of infections, the use of inotropes to restore blood pressure and the rapid control of blood loss. The use of such interventions to treat conditions may often avoid ARF developing.

2. Corrective therapy

This is based on the theory that prompt intervention in patients with ARF may result in a reversal of the condition. Typical manoeuvres used are the restoration of circulating volume by correcting fluid and electrolyte deficits and the use of dopamine, frusemide or mannitol to promote or maintain urine production. It is also important to monitor and correct the patient's serum potassium value due to the potentially lethal consequences (cardiac arrest) associated with hyperkalaemia.

3. Supportive therapy

This aims to replace kidney function, by utilising artificial renal techniques, until the patient's own kidneys have adequately recovered. Traditionally peritoneal dialysis (PD) and intermittent haemodialysis (IHD) are used to support patients with chronic renal failure, however a number of factors make them less suitable for use in patients with ARF managed on the ICU (Table 18.1). These limitations have led to these traditional methods being superseded by a range of continuous techniques employing an extracorporeal circuit, housing a synthetic membrane, and using either the patient's own blood pressure or a pump to drive the system. Such techniques are referred to as the continuous renal replacement therapies.

Table 18.1   Disadvantages of conventional renal replacement therapies

Peritoneal Dialysis	Haemodialysis
Diaphragmatic splinting	Hypotension
Compromises ventilation	Requires highly trained personnel
Labour intensive	Requires specialised equipment
Inefficient removal of waste products	Hypoxaemia
Peritoneal sepsis	

CONTINUOUS RENAL REPLACEMENT THERAPIES (CRRT)

Continuous techniques, such as haemofiltration (CHF) and haemodialysis (CHD), sometimes referred to as haemodiafiltration, are now routinely used to manage ICU patients with ARF as they allow adequate fluid, waste metabolite and electrolyte removal without aggravating cardiovascular instability. Common to all these techniques is an extracorporeal circuit which serves as a conduit allowing passage of the patient's blood through a semipermeable membrane before returning it to the venous circulation. However, modification of these techniques by the addition of various pumps to maintain extracorporeal blood flow and to automate the process of fluid balance/replacement has led to the use of nomenclature which can sometimes be confusing (Ronco et al 1996). Nomenclature commonly used are shown in Box 18.1

BOX 8.1 CRRT nomenclature

CAVH: Continuous arterio-venous haemofiltration
A process of continuous ultrafiltration, removing a volume of between 10 and 20 litres of plasma water a day, most of which is replaced by a sterile isotonic solution. The technique employs an arterial access (usually femoral artery) to maintain the extracorporeal circuit.

CVVH: Continuous veno-venous haemofiltration
Similar in all aspects to CAVH except that a venous access is used and an external pump is employed to propel blood around the extracorporeal circuit. Ultrafiltration rates removing up to 50 litres of fluid a day can be achieved by increasing the speed of the blood pump.

CAVHD: Continuous arterio-venous haemodialysis (or haemodiafiltration)
A process employing both continuous ultrafiltration and diffusion to effect water and solute removal. CAVHD employs an arterial access to maintain the extracorporeal circuit to which the technique of continuous dialysis is added. Dialysis fluid is introduced, usually at a rate of 1 or 2 litres per hour, into the membrane in a countercurrent direction to the blood flow. Although the ultrafiltration rate achieved by this technique is less than with CAVH, the infusion of an isotonic replacement fluid to maintain circulating volume is still required.

CVVHD: Continuous veno-venous haemodialysis (or haemodiafiltration)
Similar in all aspects to CAVHD except that a venous access is used and an external pump is employed to propel blood around the extracorporeal circuit.

SCUF: Slow continuous ultrafiltration
Usually employing an arterial access this technique removes between 3 and 5 litres of ultrafiltrate a day and is intended to manage patients where fluid overload is a greater problem than the accumulation of nitrogenous waste (for example patients with heart failure). Consequently the ultrafiltration rate is adjusted to accommodate the fluid administered via parenteral nutrition or when giving intravenous antibiotics, inotropes or other drugs. The infusion of isotonic replacement fluid is usually not required.

Principles of CRRT

Haemofiltration removes solutes (waste products and drugs) by convective transport or ultrafiltration; that is movement of fluid across a semipermeable membrane when a pressure is applied to one side of that membrane. The rate of blood flow through the membrane generates the hydrostatic pressure which forces plasma water to move across the filter, 'dragging' various solutes, including many drugs, with it.

Continuous haemodialysis on the other hand combines the forces of convection with diffusion (the movement of solute along a concentration gradient between plasma and dialysate) to enhance the removal of these substances. The difference in flow rate which exists, within the membrane, between the dialysis fluid (17 to 34 ml/min) and the blood (75 to 150 ml/min) allows complete equilibration to occur resulting in the effective removal of solutes. As the solute clearance achieved by this technique is principally a result of diffusive and not convective forces it is not necessary to generate large volumes of ultrafiltrate and consequently the volume of replacement fluid required, compared with haemofiltration, is reduced.

Membranes used in CRRT

The membranes employed in the extracorporeal circuit to provide continuous renal replacement to the critically ill patient vary in two aspects. Firstly the materials used in their manufacture fall into three different groups:

- Cellulose
- Cellulose esters (usually acetate)
- Synthetic.

The majority of ICUs favour synthetic membranes due to the superior fluid and solute clearance achieved and their improved biocompatability properties when compared with the cellulose variety. A range of copolymers are used to manufacture these membranes, some of the most popular varieties used being made from polyacrylonitrile (PAN) [AN69S;Hospal®], polyamide [FH66, Gambro®] or polysulfone [Diafilter 20 Amicon®].

The membranes also vary according to their configuration, being either of hollow fibre or flat-plate design. The hollow fibre format packs thousands of individual membranes into a cylinder so that blood travels down the centre of each fibre with ultrafiltrate being formed by the pressure difference generated across the fibre wall. The flat-plate design arranges the membranes as a series of overlapping sheets with the blood flowing between them. Both configurations offer a similar surface area and internal volume (between 40 and 70 ml).

These membranes allow the passage of substances having a molecular weight of less than 20 000 Daltons, ensuring that most proteins and blood cells are retained within the circulation. However many proteins adsorb onto the surface of the membrane forming a 'second membrane' which may, depending on the properties of the filter used, result in further interactions with larger proteins, such as albumin, or encourage coagulation. These interactions are thought to limit the clinical life of the membrane, which is normally up to 3 days.

Drug removal by CRRT

Many factors influence the removal of drugs by these techniques, the most important of which can be classified into either drug or system variables (Table 18.2) (Golper & Bennett 1988).

Molecular size (weight and steric hindrance) is an important factor in the clearance of a drug by haemodialysis, but has less effect on clearance by haemofiltration. Convection (ultrafiltration) readily removes compounds with a molecular weight (MW) of up to 5000 Daltons (which includes most drugs; usually with an MW of between 200 and 2000 Daltons) so that those factors affecting either transmembrane pressure (e.g. filter blood flow) or filter permeability (e.g. build up of cells or protein on the filter surface) play a more important role in influencing drug clearance. Diffusion (dialysis) is the main driving force for drug removal during haemodialysis so that drugs with a low MW (approx. 500 Daltons) are favourably cleared by such a process, while the removal of larger solutes relies more on convection (Golper 1991).

The altered drug handling seen in critically ill patients further complicates the issue. Changes in the distribution volume of certain drugs correlates closely with the increased

Table 18.2 Factors affecting drug removal by continuous haemofiltration and haemodialysis

System variables	Drug variable
Systolic blood pressure	Protein binding
Blood flow to the filter	Volume of distribution
Site of vascular access	Steric hindrance
Protein-filter interactions	Drug concentration
Filter flux potential	Drug polarity
Membrane polarity	Molecular weight
Dialysis fluid rate*	
Ultrafiltration rate	

Applies to haemodialysis systems only.

extracellular volume and altered protein binding reported for such patients (Bodenham et al 1988). Such changes in pharmacokinetic parameters often result in a reduced clearance and an increase in the elimination half-life as observed for both ceftazidime and midazolam (van Dalen & Vree 1990).

Displacement of drugs from their protein binding sites by uraemic inhibitors, bilirubin, free fatty acids or other drugs, will increase the amount of unbound or active drug available for filtration, diffusion or binding to the membrane. For highly protein-bound drugs the increase in concentration of active drug could also result in deleterious effects on the patient. This has been documented for both phenytoin (Driscoll et al 1988) and midazolam (Shelly et al 1987), where the low serum albumin levels commonly seen in ICU patients are thought to be responsible for the toxicity reported.

Interactions between the membrane and drugs administered to the patient are highly complex but can have important implications for drug clearance (Kronfol et al 1987, Cigarran-Guldris et al 1991). As described earlier the majority of membranes used are synthetic copolymers possessing the ability to adsorb compounds onto their surface. The degree of adsorption reflects the drug used, its concentration, pH of the patient's blood and the type of membrane used (Kronfol et al 1986). For example, research has shown that approximately half of the first dose of tobramycin employed in patients with acute renal failure could bind to a polyacrylonitrile membrane (Kronfol et al 1987). This could potentially jeopardise the management of patients with severe infection by reducing the initial aminoglycoside plasma concentration. The majority of interactions involving drug-membrane binding appear to be complete within the first few hours of filter life so that consideration should be given, when selecting a drug, to the likely consequences of this effect on the patient's clinical condition (Rumpf et al 1977). In practice this effect is unlikely to be important for the majority of drugs commonly used on the ICU. Furthermore there is very little information available to assist the clinical pharmacist in identifying the drugs involved and the likely clinical significance.

Estimating a drug dose in patients receiving CRRT

Drug clearance from the body is the sum of the contributions made by a number of different routes of elimination. Removal by continuous haemodialysis or haemofiltration methods only appear to be clinically important when the clearance achieved by these routes exceeds 25% of the total body clearance of the drug. The dose administered, in such cases, may require modification.

> ⚠ Dosage adjustment is clinically important when the extracorporeal elimination exceeds 25% of the total body clearance for that drug.

Loading doses of drugs

Drugs that are principally cleared by the kidneys, such as gentamicin or digoxin, will accumulate if given in conventional doses to patients with renal failure so that either a reduced dose or an increased dosing interval should be employed. However, as the latter will delay the time taken for the drug to achieve the desired plasma steady state concentration (usually $4.5 \times$ the drug's elimination half-life), an initial loading dose may need to be given for certain drugs. The loading dose can be calculated from a knowledge of the drug's apparent volume of distribution (Vd), the patient's weight and the plasma level desired (Cp) using the following equation:

$$\text{Loading Dose (mg)} = [\text{Vd(litres/kg)} \times \text{weight (kg)}] \times \text{Cp (mg/L)}$$

[Equation 1 (Winter 1985)]

Although the reported changes in the volume of distribution of some drugs in critically ill patients limits the accuracy of this approach (Bodenham et al 1988), it is generally recommended that standard loading doses should be administered to patients receiving continuous renal replacement. The validity of doses calculated using Equation 1 depends on a close relationship existing between the plasma concentration measured and the therapeutic efficacy of the drug.

Administration of maintenance doses

A number of different approaches can be used to estimate the maintenance dose which should be administered to patients receiving either continuous haemofiltration or haemodialysis. The simplest method is to choose a dose based on an estimate of the creatinine clearance (Cl_{cr}) achieved by the extracorporeal system used. For haemofiltration systems the volume of ultra-filtrate (UFR) collected each hour can be used to represent the Cl_{cr} e.g. an UFR volume of 1800 ml per hour = Cl_{cr} of 30 ml/min (assuming for creatinine a sieving coefficient [S] of 1). When the UFR volume is greater than 15 ml per minute the dose selected should reflect that administered to patients with moderate renal failure; when the UFR is less than 15 ml per minute, the dose used should follow that recommended for patients with severe renal failure. Continuous haemodialysis systems, employing a dialysis flow rate of 1 litre per hour, normally achieve a Cl_{cr} of between 20 and 30 ml per minute, which can be used to select a dose either by following guidelines given for patients with moderate renal failure or by using standard references such as the Data Sheet Compendium or British National Formulary.

> ⚠️ A dose can be selected based on an estimate of the creatinine clearance achieved by the CRRT system employed.

A second approach is to use the sieving coefficient (S) value (or the fraction of non-protein-bound drug if S is unknown) of a drug to determine the extracorporeal clearance. The sieving coefficient of a drug is the proportion that will pass through the haemofiltration membrane during a period of pure ultrafiltration (Equation 2) and is largely dependent on its physiochemical properties (Lau et al 1986). The sieving coefficient is analogous to the partition coefficient of a compound and provides useful data on the likely removal of a drug by CHF. This relationship can be mathematically expressed as:

$$S = \frac{C_{(uf)}}{C_{(arterial)}}$$

where:

S is sieving coefficient;

$C_{(uf)}$ is concentration of drug in ultrafiltrate;

$C_{(arterial)}$ is concentration of drug in arterial circulation (i.e. pre-filter conc. of drug).

[Equation 2 (Colton et al 1975)]

A drug that freely passes through the membrane, during ultrafiltration alone will have a sieving coefficient of 1; whereas a drug that is not removed at all by the process will have an S value of 0. Examples of the sieving coefficients of a number of commonly prescribed drugs are shown in Table 18.3. More comprehensive data can be found in a number of recently published reviews (Bickley 1988, Bressolle et al 1994).

> ⚠️ The sieving coefficient (S) of a drug represents its ability to pass through the membrane used. Drugs with high S values are more likely to require supplemental doses.

Sieving coefficient values are unique to the filter system used to generate the data (Kronfol et al 1986). Extrapolating such values to other systems should ideally only be undertaken when an examination of the various filter characteristics and sampling details utilised in the original work has been completed. However, for practical purposes, such an approach is seldom possible so that S values are commonly used regardless of the system used to generate the results. The system variables most likely to influence clearance data are: the blood flow to the filter, the type of membrane used, the ultrafiltration rate and, in CHD, the dialysis fluid rate.

The extracorporeal clearance Cl_{hf} of a drug during continuous haemofiltration can then be calculated from a knowledge of the sieving coefficient and the ultrafiltration volume collected over a known period of time, as shown in Equation 3.

$$Cl_{hf} = S \times UFR \text{ (litres/hour)}$$

Where: UFR is average ultrafiltration rate recorded.

[Equation 3]

Sieving coefficients calculated during haemodialysis represent the proportion of a drug removed from the circulation by the combined forces of dialysis and ultrafiltration. As this will be influenced by the dialysate flow rate and the type of membrane used as well as those factors listed in Table 18.2, values may differ from those obtained during ultrafiltration alone, for the same drug.

Table 18.3 Sieving coefficients for drugs commonly prescribed in patients receiving continuous haemofiltration

Drug	Sieving coefficient*	Volume of distribution** (L/kg)	Normal route of elimination
Cefuroxime	0.9	0.25	Renal
Ceftazidime	0.9	0.25	Renal
Erythromycin	0.4	0.50	Hepatic
Gentamicin	0.8	0.25	Renal
Metronidazole	0.8	0.70	Hepatic
Theophylline	0.9	0.50	Hepatic
Phenytoin	0.4	0.80	Hepatic

*Compiled from Bickley 1988, Vos & Vincent 1991, Gravert et al 1983, Golper et al 1985
**Values obtained from standard references (calculated in people with normal renal function). Figures for patients with acute renal failure are not available.

Where the renal clearance of a drug for patients with normal kidney function is significant (i.e. greater than 25%) the extracorporeal clearance calculated (using Equation 3) can be used to determine the maintenance dose (MD) required, using Equation 4.

$$MD = D_{anuric} \times \frac{1}{\{1 - Fr_{(extra)}\}}$$

where:

D_{anuric} is recommended dose for anuric patients;

$Fr_{(extra)}$ is fraction of drug eliminated by extracorporeal route

$$= \frac{Cl_{hf}}{\text{Total body clearance}}$$

[Equation 4; Reetze-Bonorden et al 1993]

Irrespective of the dosing method employed, close monitoring of the plasma concentration of drugs possessing a narrow therapeutic range should, where available, be undertaken. Where the drug normally exhibits significant renal tubular secretion or reabsorption a change in dose may be necessary although currently no data are available in the literature to serve as a guide.

Utilising the results of clinical studies

Relatively few studies have investigated the clearance of drugs by continuous haemofiltration or haemodialysis. Although the information available is strictly only relevant to the particular dialysis membrane and the conditions used in those studies, extrapolation of these results is clearly useful. A brief review of some of the *in vivo* studies undertaken in continuous haemodialysis is shown in Table 18.4; these data have been extrapolated to offer dosing guidelines for patients receiving CAVHD to illustrate the problems associated with using such data to construct a dosing regimen. For example the variation in vancomycin clearance reported (ranging between 10.5 and 31 ml/min) by three different studies (Reetze-Bonorden et al 1991, Bellomo et al 1990, Davies et al 1992) could result in patients receiving three different dosing regimens. This highlights the importance of comparing the method or system used in the study with your own. Other variables, such as filter life, are rarely mentioned in published values of drug filter clearance. A new filter is more likely to bind 'free' drugs than one that has been in use for some time but few studies have investigated the change in drug

Table 18.4 Dosing guidelines for patients receiving CAVHD or CVVHD				
Drug (Reference)	Patient numbers	Total body drug clearance (mL/min)	Drug filter clearance* (mL/min)	Dosing guidelines
Ceftazidime (Davies et al 1991a)	5	24.8	13.1	1000 mg/24 h
Cefuroxime (Davies et al 1991a)	7	22.3	14	500–750 mg/12 h
Vancomycin (Reetze-Bonorden et al 1991)	7	17.1	8.1	1000 mg/60 h**
Vancomycin (Bellomo et al 1990)	3	10.5	N/R	1000 mg/96 h**
Vancomycin (Davies et al 1992)	8	31	12.1	1000 mg/48 h
Ciprofloxacin (Davies et al 1992)	10	264	16	200 mg/8 to 12 h
Gentamicin (Ernest & Cutler 1992)	5	20.5	5.2	80 mg/24 h**
Gentamicin (Davies et al 1991b)	4	N/R	20.5	80 mg/24 h
Tobramycin (Davies et al 1991b)	7	N/R	11.1	60 mg/24 h
Digoxin (Davies et al 1991b)	6	N/R	10.0	125 mcg/24 h

*All studies reported utilised a 0.43 m² polyacrylonitrile membrane (Hospal).
**Recommendations based on a 70 kg adult with normal protein binding.
Other values listed are as offered by the referenced authors. N/R = not reported.

clearance during the 'life' of a filter. Investigators should report details of the filter used, the ultrafiltrate rate, dialysate flow rate and mean blood pressure values so that others can utilise their findings. In addition most published *in vivo* studies of drug removal by these techniques involve small numbers of patients (rarely more than six and often just case reports). The critical nature of the illnesses of these patients is reflected in the diversity of their pharmacokinetic parameters, further diluting the usefulness of such studies. The provision of details relating to the variables known to influence drug clearance would at least enable the results of the various studies to be compared and correlated, so that more valid conclusions could be drawn.

Summary

Information presently available on the removal of drugs by CHF or CHD serves only as an approximate guide to the prescriber when deciding on a drug regimen for a particular patient. Where a loading dose is needed it can be estimated using the method described (Equation 1) or a standard dose given. Determining the maintenance doses of a drug can be carried out in a number of different ways.

A rough guide to drug dosage can be obtained, for haemofiltration systems, by assuming that the average UFR achieved by the patient represents their Cl_{cr}. Doses can then be based on the recommendations made by standard references. Where continuous haemodialysis is employed doses can be based on a Cl_{cr} of between 20 and 30 ml per minute. A more accurate prediction of drug clearance can be obtained from a knowledge of the drug's sieving coefficient. This data can then be used to design drug dosing regimens using standard pharmacokinetic approaches.

Although relatively few studies have examined the clearance of drugs by either continuous haemofiltration or dialysis, such information can be used to design a dosage regimen, provided an informed interpretation of the available literature, based on a knowledge of both system, patient and drug factors likely to influence clearance, is undertaken.

Until the results of further research work become available clinical pharmacists should adopt the approaches described above to guide the prescribing of drugs for patients receiving CHF/CHD, by evaluating the available literature and using, where applicable, plasma drug level monitoring in order to prevent drug toxicity or under dosage occurring.

REFERENCES

Bellomo R, Ernest D, Parkin G, Boyce N 1990 Clearance of vancomycin during continuous arteriovenous hemodiafiltration. Critical Care Medicine 18(2):181–183

Bickley SK 1988 Drug dosing during continuous arteriovenous hemofiltration. Clinical Pharmacy 7:198–206

Bodenham A, Shelly MP, Park GR 1988 Altered pharmacokinetics and pharmacodynamics of drugs commonly used in critically ill patients. Clinical Pharmacokinetics 14:347–373

Bressolle F, Kinowski JM, de la Coussaye JE, Wynn N, Eledjam JJ, Galtier M 1994 Clinical pharmacokinetics during continuous haemofiltration. Clinical Pharmacokinetics 26(6):457–471

Cameron JS 1990 Overview. In: Rainford D, Sweny P (eds) Acute renal failure. Farrand Press, London, p 11

Cigarran-Guldris S, Brier ME, Golper TA 1991 Tobramycin clearance during simulated continuous arteriovenous hemodialysis.

Contributions in Nephrology, Basel, Karger 93:120–123

Colton CK, Henderson LW, Ford CA, Lysaght MJ 1975 Kinetics of hemofiltration. 1. In vitro transport characteristics of a hollow-fiber blood ultrafilter. Journal of Laboratory and Clinical Medicine 85(3):355–371

Davies SP, Lacey LF, Kox WJ, Brown EA 1991a Pharmacokinetics of cefuroxime and ceftazidime in patients with acute renal failure treated by continuous arteriovenous haemodialysis. Nephrology, Dialysis, Transplantation 6:971–976

Davies SP, Kox WJ, Brown EA 1991b Clearance studies in patients with acute renal failure treated by continuous arteriovenous haemodialysis. Contributions in Nephrology, Basel, Karger 93:117–119

Davies SP, Azadian BS, Kox WJ, Brown EA 1992 Pharmacokinetics of ciprofloxacin and vancomycin in patients with acute renal failure treated by continuous haemodialysis. Nephrology, Dialysis, Transplantation 7:848–854

Driscoll DF, McMahon M, Blackburn GL, Bistrain BR 1988 Phenytoin toxicity in a critically ill, hypoalbuminemic patient with normal serum drug concentrations. Critical Care Medicine 16:1248–1249

Ernest D, Cutler DJ 1992 Gentamicin clearance during continuous arteriovenous hemodiafiltration. Critical Care Medicine 20(5):586–589

Golper TA 1991 Drug removal during continuous hemofiltration or hemodialysis. Contributions in Nephrology, Basel, Karger 93:110–116

Golper TA, Bennett WM 1988 Drug removal by continuous arteriovenous haemofiltration. Medical Toxicology 3:341–349

Golper TA, Wedel SK, Kaplan AA, Saad A-M, Donta ST, Paganini EP 1985 Drug removal during continuous arteriovenous hemofiltration: theory and clinical observations. International Journal of Artificial Organs 8(6):307–312

Gravert C, Schulz E, Sack K 1983 Ceftazidime in intensive care medicine and hemofiltration. Journal of Antimicrobial Chemotherapy 12(Suppl A): 177–180

Kronfol NO, Lau AH, Barakat MM 1987 Aminoglycoside binding to polyacrylonitrile hemofilter membranes during continuous hemofiltration. Transactions ASAIO 33:300–303

Kronfol NO, Lau AH, Colon-Rivera J, Libertin CL 1986 Effect of CAVH membrane types on drug-sieving coefficients and clearances. Transactions ASAIO 32:85–87

Lau A, Kronfol N, Jaber N, Libertin C 1986 Determinants of drug removal by continuous arteriovenous hemofiltration. Drug Intelligence and Clinical Pharmacology 20:467–468

Reetze-Bonorden P, Bohler J, Keller E 1993 Drug dosage in patients during continuous renal replacement therapy. Clinical Pharmacokinetics 24(5):362–379

Reetze-Bonorden P, Bohler J, Kohler C, Schollmeyer P, Keller E 1991 Elimination of vancomycin in patients on continuous arteriovenous hemodialysis. Contributions in Nephrology, Basel, Karger 93:135–139

Ronco C, Bellomo R, Wratten ML, Tetta C 1996 Today's technology for continuous renal replacement therapies. Clinical Intensive Care 7:198–205

Rumpf KW, Rieger J, Ansorg R, Dohl B, Scheler F 1977 Binding of antibiotics by dialysis membranes and its clinical relevance. Proceedings EDTA 14:677–688

Shelly MP, Mendel L, Park GR 1987 Failure of critically ill patients to metabolise midazolam. Anaesthesia 42:619–626

van Dalen R, Vree TB 1990 Pharmacokinetics of antibiotics in critically ill patients. International Care Medicine 16(Suppl 3):S235–S238

Vos MC, Vincent HH 1991 Continuous arteriovenous hemodiafiltration: predicting the clearance of drugs. Contributions in Nephrology, Basel, Karger 93:143–145

Winter ME 1985 Basic principles. In: Koda-Kimble MA, Young LY (eds) Basic clinical pharmacokinetics. Applied Therapeutics, Washington, pp 44–57

19

MONITORING PATIENTS WITH LIVER DISEASE

S Dhillon

The liver is a key organ for elimination and is responsible for the metabolism of many drugs. It is a principal organ for drug metabolism and pharmacists need to be aware of the influence of liver disease on pharmacokinetics and drug handling.

In liver disease the capacity, i.e. ability of the liver to metabolise drugs, may be impaired. Structural or functional abnormalities will influence the ability of the liver to handle drugs effectively. Functions of the liver and their degree of impairment in liver disease will assist the pharmacist in monitoring drug therapy.

DRUG-INDUCED LIVER DAMAGE

Many drugs may be implicated in drug-induced liver problems. Examples include those shown in Table 19.1

Table 19.1

Type of liver problem	Drug(s) implicated
Necrosis	Carbon tetrachloride, paracetamol, halothane
Fat	Sodium valproate
Hepatitis	Amiodarone, methyldopa, isoniazid
Hypersensitivity	Sulphonamides
Cholestasis	Sex hormones, erythromycin
Fibrosis	Methotrexate

BOX 19.1 Useful indices of liver dysfunction

- Bilirubin
- Enzymes
- Transaminases
- Alkaline phosphatase
- Gamma glutamyl transferase
- Albumin
- Coagulation factors

CHANGES IN PHARMACOKINETICS IN LIVER DISEASE

These are mainly related to metabolism.

Hepatic blood flow

The extent of impairment may be significant enough in cirrhosis, hepatic venous obstruction and portal vein thrombosis to affect the clearance of a number of drugs. At steady state the following equation gives the relationship between hepatic blood flow and the rate of elimination:

$$\text{Cl hepatic} = \frac{Q\,(C_i - C_o)}{C_i}$$

where:

Cl hepatic is hepatic clearance;
Q is hepatic blood flow;
C_i is concentration of drug presented to the liver;
C_o is concentration of drug leaving the liver.

Drugs which have a high extraction ratio will be affected by changes in the blood flow. The bioavailability of these drugs will be enhanced following oral administration with reduced hepatic blood flow. Clearance is hence affected by changes in hepatic blood flow. Examples include those shown in Box 19.2.

BOX 19.2 Drugs with a high extraction ratio E>0.7

- Propranolol
- Morphine
- Chlormethiazole
- GTN

Portal systemic shunting

The extent or presence of porto-systemic shunts in cirrhosis or portal vein thrombosis can affect drug metabolism. Blood may be deviated from the liver to the systemic circulation, thus increasing the bioavailability of drugs with high hepatic extraction.

Hepatocellular damage

A reduction in the functional ability of the liver to extract drugs may occur in acute liver failure. Extensive liver cell damage and necrosis and fibrosis can reduce the intrinsic clearance of a number of drugs. This will result in increased bioavailability of highly extracted drugs due to a reduction in first-pass metabolism. Low extraction ratio drugs will have reduced elimination and hence accumulation will occur. The dose may need to be reduced or the dosage interval extended. Examples include those shown in Box 19.3.

> **BOX 19.3 Drugs with a low extraction ratio E<0.3**
>
> - Diazepam
> - Phenytoin
> - Chloramphenicol
> - Paracetamol
> - Theophylline

Cholestasis

Cholestasis occurs when bile fails to pass from the hepatocyte to the duodenum resulting in accumulation in the blood. Absorption of lipid-soluble drugs may be reduced in cholestasis; in addition there may be displacement of highly protein-bound drugs by competition for the binding site.

Changes in plasma protein binding

Changes in protein binding will affect the clearance of those drugs which have a low extraction ratio and are binding sensitive. Changes in protein binding for drugs with a narrow therapeutic range which are highly plasma protein-bound will have a clinical effect. In general a lower total serum concentration is measured in the presence of the same free concentration.

Pharmacodynamic changes

There is an increased sensitivity to sedatives and/or hypnotics. Drugs such as benzodiazepines, hypnotics and opiates should be avoided or prescribed with caution due to the risk of encephalopathy. In addition diuretics and drugs which result in electrolyte disturbances, e.g. hypokalaemia and hypovolaemia, may contribute to hepatic encephalopathy.

CLINICAL PHARMACY — LIVER CHECKLIST

You can assess whether you are dealing with a liver patient from the type of ward the patient is on or the consultant dealing with your patient. Other clues are below.

Prescription items

- Lactulose high dose e.g. 30–40 ml qds
- Neomycin
- Spironolactone

- Magnesium salts
- Chlorpheniramine
- Cholestyramine
- Vitamin K
- Multivitamins
- Ranitidine
- Bile salts
- Chlormethiazole.

The patient may be on the following

- Low sodium diet
- Low protein diet
- Sedatives restricted.

The patient's physical appearance or clinical symptoms may be useful.

Look for:

- Girth measurements
- Skin sclera looks yellow
- Spider naevi
- Red palms
- Dupuytren's contracture
- Confusion
- Ascites.

The patient may be monitored

Look for:

- Liver function tests
- Haematology screen
- Specific markers.

Routine monitoring of laboratory tests

- Transaminases
- Gamma glutamyl transferase
- Alkaline phosphatase
- Bilirubin
- Serum albumin.

Remember clinical pharmacy implications:

- Gastrointestinal disturbances common: watch prescribing of antacids
- Plasma protein binding changes: caution with drugs that are highly plasma protein-bound
- Sodium and fluid retention: watch for sodium content of drugs, those causing electrolyte disturbances, watch fluid overload
- Metabolism: caution and reduce dose of drugs which are metabolised
- Pharmacodynamic changes: caution with CNS drugs, i.e. enhanced sensitivity, caution with drugs which may precipitate encephalopathy.

THERAPEUTIC DRUG LEVEL MONITORING

S Dhillon

20

Therapeutic drug monitoring (TDM) encompasses the measurement of serum drug levels and the application of clinical pharmacokinetics to improve patient care. The concept of clinical pharmacokinetics has developed over the last decade. TDM is defined as the use of drug levels, pharmacokinetic principles and pharmacodynamic factors to optimise drug therapy in individual patients. TDM has now developed successfully as an important area of clinical medicine. Advances in the development of sensitive and specific methods for the determination of drug and drug metabolite concentrations in biological fluids have advanced the implementation of TDM in routine clinical practice. Pharmacists should be able to apply pharmacokinetics in routine clinical practice on the wards.

The interpretation of serum drug concentrations requires a knowledge of:

- applied therapeutics
- clinical pharmacokinetics
- drug handling in organ dysfunction
- drug disposition and the influence of disease states
- interpretation of biochemistry and pathology
- factors which influence patient adherence to drug regimens.

The pharmacist has skills in some of these subject areas and through integrated practice and joint working with physicians, nurses and other members of the health care team can promote the rational and cost-effective use of TDM and improve patient care.

The ward pharmacist is in a unique position of being able to identify those patients who could benefit from drug level monitoring. The pharmacist should aim to:

- advise the physician on when to sample for drug level determinations
- apply pharmacokinetic principles to help interpret the drug level
- advise and follow up TDM requests to ensure appropriate action is taken.

TDM — WHICH DRUGS AND WHY?

Drugs where TDM is useful fulfil the following basic criteria.

- The intensity of the pharmacological effect is proportional to the drug concentration at the site of action.
- The drugs have an established therapeutic plasma concentration range.
- The relationship between plasma drug concentration and clinical effect is better than the relationship between the drug dose and its effect.
- Monitoring the drug levels enhances the ability of the clinician to maximise the clinical efficacy and minimise the toxicity of the drug.
- Drug toxicity and disease presentation are difficult to distinguish.

THERAPEUTIC RANGE

The therapeutic range can be defined as the range of drug concentration within which the drug exhibits maximum efficacy and minimum toxicity in the majority of patients. It is important to appreciate that the therapeutic range is a statistical concept and that for some patients the levels at which they respond or exhibit toxicity may fall outside of the most widely quoted ranges. Interpretation of the therapeutic range must take into account the age of the patient, the disease state for which the drug is prescribed and any implications for altered volume of distribution or protein binding. Several examples exist where these factors will alter the therapeutic range, e.g. theophyllines in neonatal apnoea and asthma, digoxin in the treatment of heart failure or atrial fibrillation.

Drugs that are commonly monitored include:

1. *Aminoglycosides* — gentamicin, tobramycin, netilmicin, amikacin, vancomycin
2. *Anticonvulsants* — phenytoin, carbamazepine, and occasionally phenobarbitone
3. *Cardioactive agents* — digoxin, procainamide, lignocaine, disopyramide, flecainide
4. *Others* — theophylline, lithium, methotrexate, cyclosporin.

TDM SERVICES — WHAT YOU NEED TO KNOW

- How is the service organised, by whom? What is the level of pharmacy involvement?
- TDM Service Document e.g. request form, TDM information guide.
- Role of pharmacy and clinical pharmacists on the wards.
- The drugs for which the service will operate.

- Types of assay techniques, sensitivity and specificity data and internal/external quality control procedures.
- The days and times of assay runs.
- The latest times by which the blood sample must arrive in the laboratory for inclusion in the scheduled run.
- Processing and reporting method for results.
- 'Out of hours' service arrangements

    a. clinical situations (such as overdose)
    b. availability of emergency assay techniques
    c. referral arrangements to other TDM services available (e.g. Poisons Units).

- Sample collection details — the volume of blood and the type of tube.
- Request form details and how the results will be reported to the physician (verbal and/or written report).

INTERPRETATION OF SERUM DRUG LEVELS

The interpretation of results requires:

- patient's physical details
- clinical and biochemical status
- the drug history, concurrent medication
- sampling details.

All this information together with the pharmacokinetics of the drug in question are needed for a valid interpretation of the serum level.

Based on this information, the patient's individualised pharmacokinetic parameters can be estimated: the clearance (Cl); volume of distribution (Vd); and elimination rate constant (k).

Individualisation of the pharmacokinetic parameters requires the information above together with population pharmacokinetic data. Using population data a set of initial pharmacokinetic parameters are calculated and a level is predicted for the time the blood sample was taken.

This value is compared with the assay result and the elimination rate constant or clearance is calculated from the measured serum level. The method of altering the elimination rate constant or clearance is done in a stepwise way e.g. iteration can be used until the predicted level approximates the measured level. This technique can only be used if the Vd of the drug does not vary widely.

Clearance is then calculated ($k \times Vd$) and this can be compared with the population clearance. Since population parameters are mean values, it is probable that the patient's actual parameters will lie within two standard deviations of the mean population value. If this is the case, the individualised pharmacokinetic parameters can then be used for dosage adjustments.

If the values for the individualised clearance vary widely, then the reason for this deviation should be sought and the following factors should be checked:

1. Patient's concurrent drug therapy
2. Patient compliance
3. Drug interactions
4. Medication error
5. Change in patient's clinical status
6. Malabsorption
7. Incorrect assay result
8. Timing of sample
9. Site of sampling
10. Storage of sample (degradation or haemolysis).

If no explanation can be discovered for the deviation and all the factors above have been examined, then it is likely that the patient's data do differ significantly from the population mean data.

It is only then that the observed level is used to make future dosage recommendations and predictions. Any advice on alterations in dosage must be made in view of the patient's clinical condition and the assumptions and limitations of therapeutic ranges.

Population pharmacokinetic data monographs are summarised on pp.311–315. Additional sources of population pharmacokinetic data include Avery's Drug Treatment, (Speight 1997) Appendix A.

USE OF CALCULATORS AND COMPUTER SOFTWARE PACKAGES

Pharmacokinetic interpretation of serum level data can be facilitated by using programmed calculators or computer software packages, however this is not essential and the application of basic clinical pharmacokinetics using a calculator can be used routinely.

A number of aids facilitating interpretation are now available and it is advisable to assess the individual package according to the needs of the service. Some available software packages are listed in Table 20.1. Pharmacists who intend to use a software package should ensure they understand the principles of the program, the pharmacokinetic model used, and the associated assumptions and limitations of the package.

Table 20.1 Some software packages available		
Program	**Hardware**	**Contact**
Computer programs		
OPT	IBM	Nodecrest Ltd Chertsey, Byfleet
Chrysellis	BBC/Sirius	Mr H Chrystyn Department of Pharmacy Bradford University
Heriot-Watt University	BBC	Mr S Hudson Pharmacy Department Strathclyde University 79 Grassmarket, Glasgow
Tobramycin (J Schentag)	Apple IBM	Eli Lilly Ltd
MWPharm Interactive curve fitting programme and patient simulations (180 drugs covered)	IBM Compatible	Mediware (MWPharm) Ltd Zenike Park 4, 9747 AN Groningen The Netherlands
Calculator programs		
American Society of Hospital Pharmacy	HP 41CV	ASHP 4630 Montgomery Avenue, Bethesda Maryland 20814, USA
Aminoglycosides Digoxin Theophylline	Texas 159	Mr D Crome Pharmacy Department Royal Liverpool Hospital Prescott St Liverpool L7 8XP

THERAPEUTIC DRUG MONITORING MONOGRAPHS

[From: Winter (1994), Evans et al (1992)]

Digoxin

- Therapeutic range: 1–2 ng/mL
- Bioavailability (F) — for tablets: 0.63
  — for Lanoxin syrup: 0.80
- Salt factor (S): 1.0
- Absorption rate constant (k_a) 1.5/h

The apparent volume of distribution (adults) can be described by the following equations:

$$Vd = 3.12 \times (Cl_{Cr}) + 3.84 \times (LBW) \text{ litres OR}$$
$$Vd = 6 \text{ L/kg}$$

LBW – lean body weight
Obesity > 15% use LBW.
Clearance (adults) — without heart failure:

$$Cl \text{ (L/h)} = 0.06 \times (Cl_{Cr}) + 0.05 \times (LBW) \text{ (Age} < 70 \text{ years)}$$
$$Cl \text{ (L/h)} = 0.06 \times (Cl_{Cr}) + 0.02 \times (LBW) \text{ (Age} > 70 \text{ years)}$$

— with heart failure (all adults):

$$Cl \text{ (L/h)} = 0.053 \times (Cl_{Cr}) + 0.02 \times (LBW)$$

Theophylline

- Therapeutic range: Asthma 10–20 mcg/mL; neonatal apnoea 5–15 mcg/mL
- Bioavailability (F): is assumed to equal 1.0
- Salt factor (S)   — 1.0 for theophylline
   — 0.79 for aminophylline

Absorption rate constants (Ka) for sustained release preparation (in Ka/h):

— Phyllocontin   0.35
— Nuelin S-A   0.27
— Theodur   0.18
— Slo-Phyllin   0.5
— Nuelin Liquid   2.0

Adult data

The apparent volume of distribution (Vd) can be described by the following equations:

    1. Vd = 0.5 litres/kg of total body weight
    2. Vd = 0.45 × (LBW) + 0.4 × (EBW) litre

EBW – excess body weight
EBW = total body weight – lean body weight
Estimated clearance values from population data:

$$\text{Clearance} = 0.04 \text{ litre/hour/kg} \times \text{disease factor}$$

It is likely that these factors may be applied to paediatric patients. Experience is limited as most children do not suffer from concurrent diseases.

Diseases	Factor
Non-smoker	1.0
Smoker	1.6
Congestive heart failure	0.4
Acute pulmonary oedema	0.5
Hepatic cirrhosis	0.5
Severe pulmonary obstruction	· 0.8

Paediatric population pharmacokinetic data (Table 20.2)

Table 20.2	Paediatric data		

Age	Clearance (L/h/kg)	Mean Vd (L/kg)
Neonates (premature to 6 weeks)	0.0229	0.63
Infants < 6 months Infants 6–11 months	0.048 0.12	0.50
Children 1–4 years Children 4–12 years	0.102 0.096	0.44 0.44

Carbamazepine

- Therapeutic range: 4–12 mcg/mL
- Bioavailability: assume F = 1
- Absorption rate constant: — Ka = 1.5/h (tablets)
  — Ka = 0.33/h (retard)

The apparent volume of distribution (adults) can be calculated from:

$$Vd = 1.12 \text{ L} \times (IBW) \text{ kg}$$

Clearance can be calculated from:

$$Cl = 0.056 \text{ L/h/kg}$$
$$Cl = 0.096 \text{ L/h/kg (paediatrics 4–12 years)}$$

Phenytoin

- Therapeutic range: 5 mcg/mL–20 mcg/mL
- Bioavailability (F): assumed to equal 1.0
- Salt factor (S): 0.92 (sodium salt)

Phenytoin shows non-linear pharmacokinetics. In practice, Michaelis-Menten pharmacokinetics are applied, and the equations are summarised below.

Population data:

$$Vd = 0.65 \text{ L/kg}$$
$$Km = 5.7 \text{ mg/L (adults)}$$
$$Km = 3.2 \text{ mg/L } (<15 \text{ years old})$$
$$Vm = 450 \times \left(\frac{wt}{70}\right)^{0.6} \text{mg/day}$$

To describe the relationship between the total daily dose [R(mg/day)] and the steady state serum concentration (Cp_{ss}), where $R = \dfrac{D}{\tau}$ (dose) (dosing interval)

1. $$RSF = \frac{Vm \times Cp_{ss}}{Km + Cp_{ss}}$$

    R = Total daily dose (mg/day)
    Vm = Maximum rate of metabolism (mg/day)
    Km = Plasma concentration (mg/L) at which rate of metabolism is 0.5 Vm
    Cp_{ss} = Steady state serum concentration (mg/L)

2. $$Cp_{ss} = \frac{Km \times RSF}{Vm - RSF}$$

3. $$RSF = Vm - \left(\frac{Km \times RSF}{Cp_{ss}}\right)$$

To decay a toxic plasma concentration Cp^1 to a desired plasma concentration Cp:

$$t_{decay} = \frac{\left[Km \times \ln\left(\dfrac{Cp^1}{Cp}\right)\right] + (Cp^1 - Cp)}{Vm/Vd}$$

t_{decay} = time (days) to allow Cp^1 to fall to Cp
ln = natural log

To calculate a 'corrected' Cp_{ss} for a patient with a low serum albumin:

$$Cp_{adjusted} = \frac{Cp^\star}{(1 - \alpha)\left(\dfrac{P^1}{P}\right) + \alpha}$$

$Cp_{adjusted}$ = Plasma concentration that would be expected if the patient had a normal serum albumin.

$Cp^{\star}$ = Steady state serum level observed
P^1 = Serum albumin concentration observed
P = 'Normal' serum albumin concentration 40 g/L
α = Phenytoin free fraction (0.1)

To calculate a 'corrected' Cp_{ss} for a patient with both uraemia and hypoalbuminaemia:

$$Cp_{adjusted} = \frac{Cp^{\star}}{(1 - \alpha)\, 0.44 \times \left(\dfrac{P^1}{P}\right) + \alpha}$$

0.44 = empirical adjustment factor
α = 0.2

BOX 20.1 Preparations	
Injection	Phenytoin sodium
Tablets	Phenytoin sodium
Capsules	Phenytoin sodium
Chewable tablets (Infatabs)	Phenytoin
Suspension	Phenytoin

REFERENCES

Speight TM(ed) Avery's drug treatment: principles and practice of clinical pharmacology and therapeutics, 3rd edn. Adis International.

Evans WE, Schentag JJ, Jusko WJ (eds) 1992 Applied pharmacokinetics: principles of therapeutic drug monitoring, 3rd edn. Applied Therapeutics.

Winter ME 1994 Basic clinical pharmacokinetics, 3rd ed. Applied Therapeutics Inc.

Reference

INTRAVENOUS DRUG ADMINISTRATION

B Langfield, A Mackeller

CALCULATION OF DOSE AND RATE OF ADMINISTRATION

Concentrations

Concentrations of drug in solution may be expressed in four different ways:

- *Percentage weight in volume (% w/v)*

Is expressed as the number of grams (g) of solute (dissolved substance) in a total final volume of 100 millilitres (ml) of solution.

A 55% w/v solution means 55 g in 100 ml of solution.

- *Percentage volume in volume (% v/v)*

Is expressed as the number of millilitres (ml) of the diluted liquid when made up to a total final volume of 100 millilitres (ml) of a second liquid.

A 40% v/v solution means 40 ml in a total volume of 100 ml of liquid.

- *Ratios*

These do not base the measurement on a fixed final volume of liquid or solvent.

1 in 1000 means 1 g in 1000 ml, i.e. 1 g/litre, which is equivalent to 1 mg/ml.

- *Molar solutions*

The 'mole' is a unit of mass which relates to the molecular weight or 'relative molecular mass' (RMM) of a compound, or to the 'relative atomic mass' (RAM) of an element.

Each molecule has a mass and its molecular weight or relative molecular mass (RMM) is calculated by adding up the relative atomic masses (RAMs) of all the atoms in the molecule.

A 'mole' is the RMM expressed in grams.

A molar solution of a compound contains 1 mole of the compound (measured in grams) dissolved in 1 litre of solvent, usually water.

The RMM of sulphuric acid (H_2SO_4) is 98, so a molar solution of sulphuric acid consists of 98 g of pure sulphuric acid dissolved in 1 litre of water.

The molarity of a solution is the number of moles (measured in grams) of solute in 1 litre of solvent.

The abbreviation M is usually used for a molar solution. A 5M sulphuric acid solution contains:

$$5 \times 98 = 490 \text{ g of sulphuric acid in 1 litre of water.}$$

Drip rate calculations

A standard 'giving' set or 'solution' set will administer 20 drops per ml of clear fluid.

A blood giving set will administer 15 drops per ml of blood (or 20 drops per ml of clear fluid).

Some burettes will administer 60 drops per ml.

> ⚠ It is important to check the number of drops per ml delivered by the giving set on the outer packaging as this may vary slightly between products.

The formula to calculate the drip rate required to deliver the correct volume to be administered is:

$$\text{Number of drops per minute} = \frac{\text{Volume to be given (ml)} \times \text{Number of drops/ml delivered by the set}}{\text{duration of the infusion (minutes)}}$$

Example
A drug is to be administered using a standard solution set at a rate of 50 mg/m^2/minute to a patient whose surface area is 1.6 m^2. The drug is a 4% w/v solution.

What drip rate should be used?

$$\text{The patient requires } 50 \times 1.6 = 80 \text{ mg/minute}$$
$$\begin{aligned} \text{A 4\% w/v solution} &= 4 \text{ g in 100 ml} \\ &= 4000 \text{ mg in 100 ml} \\ &= 40 \text{ mg in 1 ml} \end{aligned}$$

To obtain 80 mg divide the 1 ml by 40 mg and multiply by 80 mg:

$$= 80 \text{ mg in 2 ml}$$

The patient needs 2 ml/minute of the solution. Using the drip rate formula:

$$\begin{aligned} \text{Number of drops/minute} &= \frac{2(\text{ml}) \times 20}{1 \text{ (minute)}} \\ &= 40 \text{ drops/minute} \end{aligned}$$

Displacement values

When dry powder injections are reconstituted the powder displaces a certain volume of fluid — known as the 'displacement value' or 'displacement volume' of the drug. Errors will occur unless this displacement volume is considered when part vials are used to administer doses, as frequently occurs in neonates and children when the doses are small. Displacement values can be found in the relevant data sheets or paediatric dosage books.

The total final volume in the reconstituted vial is equal to the sum of the displacement value of the drug and the volume of diluent added. The volume of diluent added is generally reduced by a value equal to the displacement value.

Example
Dosage required: 50 mg/kg for a child weighing 8 kg.

The 500 mg vial has a displacement value of 0.3 ml, and 5 ml water for injection is generally used to reconstitute the drug.

What volume should be administered?

> Displacement value of the 500 mg vial = 0.3 ml
> Add 5 − 0.3 ml = 4.7 ml water to the vial to make a total volume = 5 ml
> Giving a final dilution of 500 mg in 5 ml
> Dosage required = 50 × 8 = 400 mg
> so 400 mg in $\dfrac{5}{500} \times 400 = 4$ ml

The difference if the displacement value is not considered is:

> Add 5 ml water to the 500 mg vial to make a total volume = 5.3 ml.

If 4 ml of this reconstituted drug is administered, the dose given to the patient will be:

$$\frac{500 \times 4}{5.3} = 377 \text{ mg}$$

23 mg less than prescribed.

RECONSTITUTION AND DILUTION

Awareness of possible interactions and knowledge of the basic steps to minimise or prevent these is essential. Interactions may occur between drugs, between the drug and diluent or the drug and container.

Drug stability

Problems can arise from three main areas: chemical breakdown or the influence of light; the precipitation of the drug out of solution; or incompatibilities or interaction of the drug with the plastic tubing used in the administration set or solution bag.

When several drugs interact with one another, a multi-lumen central venous cannula can be used. Each drug enters the vein separately from the others through its own lumen and the rapid blood flow dilutes the drugs to prevent harmful interactions.

1. Chemical breakdown
Chemical breakdown of a single drug can happen in any of several ways including:

- Hydrolysis
- Oxidation or reduction
- Photolysis or light degradation.

Hydrolysis. Invariably injectable drugs are made up in water or water based solutions like glucose or saline. In practice, degradation due to hydrolysis is not a significant problem. It may occur with drugs that are relatively unstable in aqueous solutions. These often need to be reconstituted immediately before use.

The pH of the solution is an important factor. Drugs that are not obviously acids or alkalis can have acidic or basic characteristics. For example, glucose 5% has a pH of approximately 4.0–4.2 (depending on the manufacturer).

Hydrolysis will often be accelerated by inappropriate pH changes which can occur if a diluent (or a second drug) causes the solution to become more acidic or more alkaline. Even the small difference in pH between sodium chloride 0.9% and glucose 5% injections, for example, can dramatically affect the stability of some drugs such as amphotericin. pH changes can often be controlled by adding a 'buffer solution' to the infusion fluid.

Temperature can also affect the rate at which hydrolysis occurs; usually the higher the temperature, the faster the reaction. But as with pH effects, this is not a serious problem under normal clinical conditions.

Oxidation/Reduction. Some drugs react with oxygen. Adrenaline, dopamine and ascorbic acid can react quite readily and, as with hydrolysis, the higher the temperature, the faster the reaction. Degradation can eventually occur over a period of time but under normal clinical conditions, oxidation is not a problem.

Slight colour changes (usually pink) may occur with some drugs, e.g. dopamine and noradrenaline. A minor discoloration usually represents minimal levels of oxidation. It is recommended that discoloured solutions are not used.

Reduction, or reaction with reducing agents is similar. Thiamine is particularly prone to attack by reducing agents and the effect is greater at higher temperatures.

Photolysis or degradation by light. Natural daylight, specifically UV radiation, is the main cause of light induced degradation. Examples of drugs prone to this are frusemide, nitroprusside, vitamin K, dacarbazine and amphotericin.

Fluorescent light is generally safe because it does not emit UV radiation. The exception is nitroprusside which is very sensitive and is degraded rapidly by both fluorescent light and natural daylight. Therefore, light protection of the infusion bag and administration set is essential for nitroprusside.

2. Precipitation

A precipitate can block tubing, filters, cannulae or catheters and may lead to coronary or pulmonary emboli if administered to the patient. The rate at which a precipitate forms depends on time and temperature. Where precipitation is thought possible, the infusion must be inspected carefully and frequently.

pH effects. Insoluble drugs are rendered soluble by conversion to a salt. This makes them more sensitive to pH changes. Injections formulated using the compound itself rather than the salt of the compound are not affected by changes in pH. Insulin is one such example.

Acid drugs (which are made into salts of sodium, calcium or potassium) generally have an alkaline pH in solution. When alkaline injections are diluted with solutions of a lower pH, the pH of the overall solution will decrease. If the fall is too great and the solubility of the original drug in its acid form is low, a precipitate may form. Hence, if phenytoin, which has a pH greater than 9, is diluted, the minimum volume of diluent should be used.

Similarly, basic drugs (formulated as an acid salt such as hydrochloride, sulphate or nitrate) are soluble in acidic solutions. Dilution of these acidic salts with solutions of a higher pH will raise the pH and a precipitate may form, e.g. gentamicin.

> As a general rule, salts of acidic drugs, in alkaline solutions, are more likely to precipitate on dilution than the salts of basic drugs.

Other dilution effects. Some drugs are very poorly soluble in water and have to be dissolved or solubilised using co-solvents. These solubilisers include ethanol, polysorbates and propylene glycol. If the injection is diluted the co-solvent is also diluted and the drug may precipitate, e.g. diazepam.

Drug–drug co-precipitation. If two oppositely charged ions are mixed in solution, they may react to form an insoluble ion-pair. Examples of drugs at risk of such an interaction are gentamicin with heparin; frusemide with aminoglycosides.

Formation of an insoluble salt. Metals like calcium, magnesium and iron will form an insoluble salt if allowed to mix with an acid drug.

> ⚠️ The commonest example of a calcium containing infusion is Hartmann's Solution (compound sodium lactate). This must not be mixed with an acid drug.

3. Interaction with plastic component

Almost all containers, administration sets and components are made from plastics. A few drugs may bind to these plastics and this may affect the dose delivered. Often these interactions can only be avoided by changing to polythene.

There are four types of process that can occur.

Adsorption. The drug binds to the surface of the plastic and does not penetrate any further.

The initial effect is a rapid and substantial drug loss from the solution. This occurs as the drug binds to the surface of the plastic. If this solution is run though a plastic/PVC line, initially the dose of drug is reduced due to adsorption. Subsequently the plastic surface becomes saturated and the delivery of the drug rapidly increases, e.g. insulin and interferons.

Insulin will adsorb onto any plastic, especially polyvinyl chloride (PVC) and also onto glass. To minimise the effect, insulin should not be added to an infusion bag but should be given by syringe pump and the line flushed with the drug prior to use.

Absorption. The drug migrates into the plastic. This is a more common occurrence than adsorption. It is a slower process but eventually an equilibrium is established between the drug within the plastic and the drug in solution.

PVC is made pliable and flexible by incorporating a 'plasticiser' during its manufacture. This presents a particular problem for lipid soluble drugs as they diffuse from the solution into the plasticiser within the plastic matrix. Examples of drugs affected are diazepam, chlorpromazine, nimodipine, carmustine.

Permeation. In this case, the drug migrates through the plastic to the outer surface where it evaporates. Losses from permeation can be substantial and they continue throughout the period of administration because the plastic never becomes saturated. PVC presents the biggest problem. Examples of drugs affected are nitrates (glyceryl trinitrate, isosorbide dinitrate) and chlormethiazole.

Many variables alter the magnitude of drug loss. These include drug concentration, flow rate, the surface area of the plastic, the type of plastic and the temperature.

Leaching. Leaching of the plasticiser into the solution can occur with PVC. The effect is not usually important except for cyclosporin infusions and storage of total parenteral nutrition regimens in PVC bags. Leaching from administration sets during infusion is relatively small but can occur from the rubber plungers of plastic syringes and may affect drug stability (e.g. asparaginase).

ADMINISTRATION

Methods

There are three methods:

1. *Bolus/i.v. push*
Usually given undiluted over three to five minutes.

2. *Intermittent infusion*
Usually given over 10 minutes and up to over 6–8 hours.

Used as an alternative to bolus administration for regular dosing, where slower administration of a more dilute solution is required to avoid toxicity, e.g. vancomycin must be given at a maximum rate of 10 mg per minute to avoid red man syndrome; erythromycin must be diluted to at least 5 mg in 1 ml to reduce the risk of thrombophlebitis.

3. *Continuous infusion*
The term is used when infusions are given continuously over 24 hours. The rate may be variable, e.g. dopamine and heparin. Continuous infusions are used where a continuous or controlled therapeutic response is required for drugs with a short half-life or a narrow therapeutic window. If a drug has a short half-life,

it will be eliminated from the body quickly. In most cases it can be assumed that no drug will remain in the body after a time interval of four half-lives. For example it is essential to maintain adequate levels of heparin in the plasma over a 24 hour period to treat a thrombosis. The half-life of heparin is approximately one hour. Therefore, it must be infused continuously to maintain its therapeutic effect.

If a drug has a narrow therapeutic window, e.g. aminophylline, there is a narrow range of plasma concentrations between which the drug exerts a therapeutic effect without toxicity. It is vital to maintain the drug concentration in the plasma within this range.

The administration set

The components that make up administration sets are shown in Figure 21.1. Manufacturers can provide any combination of components but if requirements are special, then the cost may be higher than for standard items. The components shown will vary from manufacturer to manufacturer and so this is not a comprehensive list.

A. Four-way lumen for central venous site which can infuse four drugs separately, each with its own lumen.
B. Three-way stopcocks, also known as 'traffic lights' so that additional drugs can be infused into a lumen or a peripheral line.
C. Cannula for peripheral site. The cannula has a steel inner needle that punctures the vein and is then withdrawn. The cannula has an extension line of its own and a three-way stopcock.
D. 150 ml burette for neonatal infusions with a volumetric pump shown with an extra injection port.
E. Air inlet port.
F. Roller clamp for closing off any administration line.
G. Silicone rubber insert in ordinary PVC tubing for use in neonatal infusions, because this rubber does not distort or 'creep' when compressed by the volumetric pump mechanism. Silicone rubber improves the accuracy of the administration rate.
H. Pressure disc for measuring pressure in the administration set during an infusion. Used in sets for volumetric and syringe pumps.
I. 'Y' connector (Y Site) for entry of another drug into the line.
J. Spike for insertion into the fluid bag, shown with its own injection port.

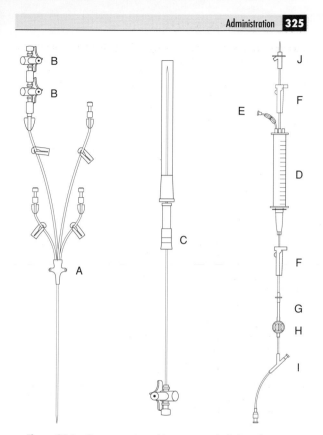

Figure 21.1 Components making up an administration set.

Infusion pumps

These can be grouped broadly into two types:

- Simple gravity drips
- Infusion pumps.

Simple gravity drips

These depend entirely on gravity to drive the infusion and generally use the cheapest administration sets. They comprise a drip chamber and use a roller clamp to control the flow rate which is measured by counting drops. They are suitable for infusing replacement fluids such as simple electrolytes which do not require any particular degree of accuracy. The delivery pressure developed for infusion depends entirely on the height of the liquid level in the container above the infusion site; at about one metre this pressure is 70 mmHg. The pressure in an adult peripheral vein is about 25 mmHg so provided there is not too much resistance to flow through the cannula, the infusion will run satisfactorily. The risk of extravasation is minimised by the use of low delivery pressures.

Limitations include the following:

1. The tubing can distort and flatten within the roller clamp over time.
2. The clamp position can be disturbed.
3. High fluctuations in venous pressure can reduce the flow rate.
4. The size of drops can vary with the fluid being infused.
5. The delivery pressures may be insufficient to provide arterial infusions and to deliver viscous fluids into a peripheral vein.
6. An open roller clamp may free flow without warning.

Infusion pumps

Infusion pumps are powered devices which provide the desired flow by a positive pumping action. They include:

Volumetric pumps.   The desired flow rate is set in millilitres (ml) per hour. A drop sensor may be present for the purpose of indicating an empty infusion bag, or for detecting inaccuracies in the flow rate.

Volumetric pumps achieve good delivery accuracies over a wide range of flow rates. They have safety features with alarms, for example to detect vascular occlusions and the presence of air bubbles in the infusion fluid. They can be used for both venous and arterial infusions and when the fluid reservoir is nearly empty they will automatically revert to a low delivery rate to keep the vein open. However, they are more expensive than other pumps and may require dedicated administration sets recommended by the manufacturers. It can sometimes be possible to insert the wrong set and the pump may still appear to work correctly.

Syringe pumps ('syringe drivers'). These are devices in which a syringe or cartridge containing the solution to be infused is secured in the pump and a plunger is driven forward at a predetermined rate to achieve the desired infusion rate. The flow rate may be set in millilitres (ml) per hour, millimetres (mm) per hour or millimetres (mm) per 24 hours.

Syringe pumps are used to administer drugs in concentrated solutions where fluid balance is important and/or when the rate of administration needs to be carefully controlled.

Modern syringe pumps have the same safety features as their volumetric counterparts and their administration sets are simple and relatively inexpensive. However, older models have insufficient safety features to minimise the possibility of free flow.

Mechanical backlash — the delay between starting the pump and achieving the constant infusion rate — is inherent in the pump mechanism. This delay can be therapeutically significant at very low infusion rates during the backlash period, hence, the need for the use of two pumps used concurrently for infusion of inotropes. The most modern designs incorporate mechanisms to compensate for backlash.

> Most syringe drivers require a specific brand or brands of syringe, due to the variation in the bore size of the syringes.

Patient controlled analgesia (PCA) pumps. These are devices in which the patient is able to initiate a bolus dose of the infusion solution for the relief of pain. Patients are prevented from altering the setting of the pump and pre-programmed restraints are placed on the parameters of the boluses. In addition, a basal rate delivery of solution outside the control of the patient may be provided.

Pumps for ambulatory use. These are small and light enough to be carried around by the patient without unduly interfering with everyday activities.

Anaesthesia pumps. These are syringe pumps suitable for the administration of anaesthetic agents. They are unsuitable for any other use.

Multi-purpose pumps. These pumps can be made to perform as one of the above pumps.

Other devices. These include non-electrically powered devices which do not have electrically generated alarm signals. Some of them are charged with a syringe and then deliver their output more or less continuously, with flow being controlled by a flow-regulating means, such as a capillary tube. This type of pumping device may use an elastomeric membrane which, once expanded, provides sufficient force to drive the infusion. Applications include PCA and emergency situations.

The performance of non-electrically powered devices is generally inferior to the devices mentioned above, but they may have other advantages, such as simplicity and the ability to operate in difficult environments.

Spring driven, clockwork and gas powered infusion devices are available but will not be discussed here.

Flow regulators. These are manually set, non-powered devices, which appear in a variety of forms and which clamp onto, or are inserted in the line. They usually have a rotary dial to give an indication of expected flow rate. Some of these devices claim to compensate for venous back pressure and maintain consistent flow.

Table 21.1	Advantages and disadvantages of pump types	
Pump Type	**Advantages**	**Disadvantages**
Simple gravity drip	Lowest cost Familiar to all staff Simple to set up Infusion of air less likely Minimises risk of extra-vascular infusion	Cannot be used for arterial infusions Requires frequent observation and adjustment Variability of drop size Infusion rates limited, especially with viscous fluids and small catheters Risk of free flow (open roller clamps) User may need to calculate drop rate
Volumetric pumps	Calibrated in ml/h Good volumetric accuracy Wide flow rate range Many features and facilities designed to ensure very safe operation	More expensive than most other pumps Some require dedicated sets* Some can be complicated to set up

(contd)

Table 21.1	Advantages and disadvantages of pump types (contd)	
Pump Type	Advantages	Disadvantages
	Comprehensive alarm systems Air-in-line detection Many have low occlusion alarm pressure settings Some have delivery pressure sensors Secondary infusion facility often available Can be used for both venous and arterial infusions Neonatal versions available	Incorrect set* can be loaded and pump appears to work
Syringe pumps	Usually calibrated in mm/h or mm/24 h Smooth and precise delivery at low flow rates Easy to operate	Free flow possible on older models without plunger clamps There can be problems with mechanical backlash Occlusion alarm pressure settings on earlier models are sometimes rather high which would result in a poor occlusion response Earlier models prone to incorrect fitting of syringe Danger of setting wrong rate. User must ensure whether pump is calibrated per hr or per 24 h

*Note: there are a number of volumetric pumps which use low-cost standard solution sets but it is important to note that the pump must be configured correctly for the specific set.

Risk classification of infusion pumps

The Department of Health has specified the performance and functions that an infusion pump must meet in order to be classified under one or more of the following risk categories (MDA 1995):

a. Neonatal risk
b. High risk
c. Lower risk
d. Ambulatory risk.

a. Neonatal risk infusion pumps. The first category, for infusions to neonates, requires equipment of high accuracy and consistency of flow with 0.1 ml/hour increments, low occlusion alarm times and very low bolus on release of occlusion. Comprehensive alarm displays which identify the precise problem and safety interlocks to prevent tampering while running are important.

b. High risk infusion pumps. This category of pumps is used for high risk infusions to adults, for drugs such as dopamine, dobutamine and cytotoxics. This category requires high accuracy and consistency of flow, good occlusion alarm response, comprehensive alarm displays which identify the precise problem and safety interlocks. Both neonatal and high risk pumps should have internal rechargeable battery back-up with a memory of parameters displayed so that vital data is not lost due to inadvertent switch off.

Neonatal and high risk infusion pumps must be accurate to within ± 5% of the set rate when measured over a 60 minute period. They must also satisfy short term minute to minute requirements which determine smoothness and consistency of flow rate. These pumps must not suck back during infusion, there should not be significant periods of zero flow and the flow rate should not have large fluctuations.

c. Lower risk infusion pumps. The third category, for lower risk infusion to adults but not to neonates, covers the infusion of simple electrolytes and antibiotics. The equipment does not need to be so accurate and consistent in output and need have only rudimentary alarm and safety systems. Battery back-up is not essential.

d. Ambulatory infusion pumps. The Department of Health has not yet assessed the risk associated with ambulatory infusion pumps. These pumps include all infusion equipment which may be worn on the person so that normal activities can be continued while the infusion is being given. The equipment will often be battery powered but clockwork mechanisms, elastomeric membranes or gas powered devices can also be used.

Drugs

To ensure safe administration of infusions, drugs can be classified into matching risk categories (Pickstone et al 1995). This classification is based on the perceived level of risk in the administration of that drug. This risk level may also be influenced by factors such as the environment in which the drug is being used. Once the risk level of a drug has been defined this can be matched to the performance and functions of the different categories of infusion pumps. Safe administration can then be ensured if the drug is administered using a pump of the same or higher risk level.

Filters

For a small selection of drugs, manufacturers recommend that in-line filters are used when administering the drug, e.g. flucytosine, mannitol, phenytoin and tetracycline. This is because there may be particulate deposits in the vial, e.g. tetracycline, or the solution is prone to precipitation, e.g. phenytoin.

The pore size of the filter required varies between products. Most standard solution administration sets contain a 15 micron filter. However, if a smaller pore size is required, a separate filter must be connected into the administration set e.g. phenytoin requires a 0.22–0.55 micron filter.

> ⚠️ In-line filters should only be used once.

REFERENCES

Medicines Devices Agency 1995 Device bulletin infusion systems. MDA DB 9503, May 1995

Pickstone M, Auty B, Jacklin A, Langfield B, Wootton R 1995 Intravenous infusion of drugs: part 2. A new safety protocol for intravenously infused drugs. BJIC 5:17–24

SODIUM CONTENT OF INJECTABLE DRUGS

22

B Langfield, C Walsh

Table 22.1 lists the sodium content (in mmol) of injectable drugs. Where there is more than one strength of ampoule/vial, the differing sodium contents have been given, whenever differences exist.

Table 22.1 Sodium content of injectable drugs	
Drug	**Sodium content**
Acetazolamide sodium	2.36 mmol/500 mg
Acetylcysteine	12.78 mmol/2 g
Aciclovir	1 mmol/250 mg
Adenosine	0.154 mmol/6 mg
Adrenaline (Evans product)	0.1–0.16 mmol/ml
	(1 in 1000 strength)
Alfentanil	No information available
Alprostadil	Nil
Alteplase	Nil
Amifostine	Nil
Amikacin	less than 0.5 mmol/500 mg
Aminophylline	Nil
Amiodarone	Nil
Amoxycillin	No information available
Amphotericin	
Fungizone®	less than 0.5 mmol/50 mg
Amphocil®	less than 0.5 mmol/50 mg
AmBisome®	0.4 mmol/50 mg
Ampicillin	0.73 mmol/250 mg
	1.47 mmol/500 mg
Aprotinin	7.70 mmol/70 mg
Ascorbic acid	3 mmol/500 mg
Atenolol	1.3–1.8 mmol/5 mg
Atracurium	Nil
Atropine	No information available
Azathioprine	0.2 mmol/50 mg
Azlocillin	10.48 mmol/5 g
	4.33 mmol/2 g
	2.17 mmol/1 g
Aztreonam	Nil
Benztropine	0.15 mmol/mg
Benzylpenicillin	1.68 mmol/600 mg
Betamethasone	No information available
Biperiden lactate	0.13 mmol/5 mg

(contd)

| Table 22.1   Sodium content of injectable drugs (contd) | |

Drug	Sodium content
Bretylium tosylate	Nil
Bumetanide	0.007 mmol/500 micrograms
Buprenorphine	Nil
Calcium gluconate	Nil
Cefotaxime	2.09 mmol/1 g
Ceftazidime	2.3 mmol/1 g
Cefuroxime	1.8 mmol/750 mg
Cephradine	less than 0.5 mmol/1 g
Chloramphenicol	0.7 mmol/300 mg
	3.1 mmol/1 g
Chlormethiazole	15–16 mmol/500 ml
Chloroquine	No information available
Chlorpheniramine	No information available
Cimetidine	0.154 mmol/100 mg
Ciprofloxacin	15.4 mmol/200 mg
Clonazepam	Nil
Clonidine hydrochloride	0.15 mmol/150 micrograms
Co-amoxiclav	1.6 mmol/600 mg
	3.1 mmol/1.2 g
Co-trimoxazole	1.64 mmol/480 mg
Cyclizine	Nil
Cyclosporin	Nil
Dantrolene	2 mmol/20 mg
Desmopressin	0.15 mmol/4 micrograms
Dexamethasone sodium phosphate	
Organon product	0.021 mmol/5 mg
MSD product	0.121 mmol/4 mg
Dexamethasone shock pak®	0.131 mmol/4 mg
Diamorphine hydrochloride	
Napp product	Nil
Evans product	Nil
Diazepam (Valium®)	0.66 mmol/10 mg
Diazepam (Diazemuls®)	Nil
Diazoxide	15 mmol/300 mg
Digoxin	
Wellcome product	No information available
Martindale paediatric product	No information available
Dipyridamole	Nil
Disodium etidronate	No information available
Disopyramide	No information available
Dobutamine	0.046 mmol/250 mg
Dopamine	0.526 mmol/5 ml for both strengths
	(200 mg/5 ml & 800 mg/5 ml)
Dopexamine	0.09 mmol/50 mg
Doxapram	No information available
Droperidol	No information available
Edrophonium	0.073 mmol/10 g
Enoximone	No information available

(contd)

Table 22.1	Sodium content of injectable drugs (contd)

Drug	Sodium content
Ephedrine	Nil
Epoprostenol	2 mmol in 50 ml buffer
Ergometrine	No information available
Erythromycin	Nil
Erythropoietin alpha (Eprex®)	No information available
Erythropoietin beta (Recormon®)	Negligible
Ethacrynic acid	No information available
Ethamsylate	Negligible
Ethanol	Nil
Etomidate	No information available
Fentanyl citrate	No information available
Filgrastim	Negligible
Flecainide	No information available
Flucloxacillin	
Floxapen®	0.57 mmol/250 mg
Ladropen®	1 mmol/500 mg
Fluconazole	15 mmol/200 mg
Flucytosine	34.44 mmol/2.5 g
Flumazenil	No information available
Folic acid	No information available
Folinic acid	1 mmol per ampoule (3 mg/ml)
	0.2 mmol/15 mg vial (powder)
	0.4 mmol/30 mg vial (powder)
	2.4 mmol/350 mg vial (powder)
	4.6 mmol/350 mg vial (solution)
Foscarnet	15.6 mmol/1 g
Frusemide	
Lasix®	0.28 mmol/20 mg
Lasix®	1.0 mmol/250 mg
Fusidic acid	14 mmol/500 mg
Gallamine	0.06 mmol/80 mg
Ganciclovir	2 mmol/500 mg
Gentamicin	
Roche product	Nil
Hoechst Roussel product	0.07 mmol/160 mg
	0.07 mmol/80 mg
	0.07 mmol/20 mg
David Bull product	0.02 mmol/40 mg
Glucagon	No information available
Glucose	Nil
Glyceryl trinitrate	
Tridil®	No information available
Nitronal®	Nil
Nitrocine®	Nil
Glycopyrrolate	0.15 mmol/200 micrograms
Gonadorelin	No information available
Granisetron	1.17 mmol/3 mg

(contd)

Table 22.1   Sodium content of injectable drugs (contd)

Drug	Sodium content
Heparin	
Unihep® (Leo)	0.21 mmol/ml in 1000 iu/ml
	0.13 mmol/ml in 5000 iu/ml
	0.625 mmol/ml in 25000 iu/ml
Monoparin® (CP)	0.025–0.032 mmol/ml in 1000 iu/ml
	0.125–0.16 mmol/ml in 5000 iu/ml
	0.625–0.8 mmol/ml in 25000 iu/ml
Human soluble insulin	
Actrapid®	No information available
Humulin S®	No information available
Velosulin®	No information available
Hydralazine hydrochloride	Nil
Hydrocortisone sodium phosphate	
Efcortesol®	0.66 mmol/100 mg
Hydrocortisone sodium succinate	
Efcortelan Soluble®	0.37 mmol/vial
Hyoscine N-butylbromide	No information available
Imipenem with Cilastatin	0.86 mmol/250 mg
	1.72 mmol/500 mg
Indomethacin	Negligible
Indomethacin (Indocid PDA®)	0.003 mmol/1 mg
Ketamine hydrochloride	2.26 mmol/200 mg for 200 mg/ 20 ml
	Other strengths negligible (500 mg/10 ml; 500 mg/5 ml)
Labetalol hydrochloride	Negligible
Lorazepam	No information available
Magnesium sulphate	Nil
Mannitol	No information available
Meptazinol	No information available
Metarminol	0.087 mmol/10 mg
Methohexitone sodium	4.652 mmol/1 g
Methotrimeprazine	0.037 mmol/25 mg
Methoxamine hydrochloride	4.43 mg/20 ml
Methyldopate hydrochloride	0.18 mmol/250 mg
Methylprednisolone	2.01 mmol/1 g
Metoclopramide	
Maxolon®	0.27 mmol/10 mg
Maxolon HD®	2.74 mmol/100 mg
Metoprolol tartrate	0.8 mmol/5 mg
Metronidazole	
Flagyl®	13 mmol/500 mg
Metrolyl®	14.55 mmol/500 mg
Midazolam	0.14 mmol/ml for both strengths (10 mg/5 ml: 10 mg/2 ml)
Milrinone	Nil
Morphine sulphate	Negligible
Nalbuphine hydrochloride	No information available

(contd)

Table 22.1 Sodium content of injectable drugs (contd)	
Drug	**Sodium content**
Naloxone	
Narcan®	0.15 mmol/ml
Narcan Neonatal®	0.15 mmol/ml
IMS product	0.15 mmol/ml
Neostigmine	0.143 mmol/ml in 0.5 mg/ml
	0.115 mmol/ml in 2.5 mg/ml
Octreotide	Negligible for vial (1 mg/5 ml)
	0.154 mmol/ml for ampoules
	(50 microgram/ml;
	100 microgram/ml;
	500 microgram/ml)
Ofloxacin	15.4 mmol/200 mg
Omeprazole	infusion: 0.15 mmol/40 mg
	IV injection: 0.13 mmol/40 mg
Ondansetron	0.16 mmol/2 mg
Oxytocin	No information available
Pancuronium bromide	No information available
Papaveretum B.P	0.004 mmol/15.4 mg
Paraldehyde	Nil
Pentamidine isethionate	Nil
Pentazocine	No information available
Pethidine	Nil
Phenobarbitone	
Rhone–Poulenc Rorer product	0.79 mmol for 200 mg/ml
Martindale product	0.11 mmol/ml for 15 mg/ml
	0.17 mmol/ml for 30 mg/ml
	0.29 mmol/ml for 60 mg/ml
	0.84 mmol/ml for 200 mg/ml
Phenoxybenzamine	Nil
Phentolamine mesylate	Negligible
Phenytoin	0.91 mmol/250 mg
Phytomenadione	
Konakian®	No information available
Konakian MM®	No information available
Piperacillin	1.84–1.94 mmol/1 g
Potassium chloride	Nil
Potassium phosphate	Nil
Prochlorperazine mesylate	No information available
Procyclidine	No information available
Promazine	No information available
Propofol	No information available
Propranolol hydrochloride	Nil
Protirelin	No information available
Quinine dihydrochloride	Negligible
Ranitidine	0.122 mmol/50 mg
Rifampicin	
Merrell product	Less than 0.5 mmol/300 mg
	and 600 mg

(contd)

Table 22.1 Sodium content of injectable drugs (contd)

Drug	Sodium content
Ciba product	Less than 0.5 mmol/300 mg and 600 mg
Ritodrine	No information available
Salbutamol	0.77 mmol/ml in 0.25 mg/5 ml
	0.15 mmol/ml in 0.5 mg/ml
	0.75 mmol/ml in 5 mg/5 ml
Salcatonin	No information available
Sodium Bicarbonate	150 mmol/1 litre (1.26% solution)
	500 mmol/1 litre (4.2%)
	1000 mmol/1 litre (8.4%)
Sodium chloride	150 mmol/1 litre (0.9% solution)
Sodium clodronate	2.1 mmol/300 mg
Sodium clodronate concentrate	0.2 mmol/60 mg
Sodium nitroprusside	0.34 mmol/50 mg
Sodium valproate	2.41 mmol/400 mg
Sotalol	0.5 mmol/40 mg
Sulphadiazine	4 mmol/1 g
Suxamethonium	
Anectine®	Nil
Scoline®	Negligible
Tazocin®	1.99 mmol/1 g
Teicoplanin	Less than 0.5 mmol/200 mg and 400 mg
Terbutaline sulphate	0.15 mmol/500 micrograms
Terlipressin	No information available
Tetracosactrin	0.14 mmol/250 micrograms
Tham	Nil
Theophylline	No information available
Thiamine hydrochloride	0.0124 mmol/100 mg
Thiopentone sodium	23.26 mmol/500 mg
Tobramycin	0.03 mmol/ml
Tolazoline	0.0357 mmol/ml for both strengths (10 mg/ml and 25 mg/ml)
Tranexamic Acid	Nil
Trimetaphan	Less than 0.01 mmol/250 mg
Trimethoprim lactate	Nil
Tubocurarine	Nil
Vasopressin	No information available
Vecuronium bromide	No information available
Verapamil	0.3 mmol/5 mg
Vitamins B and C	
Pabrinex IV High Potency®	No information available
Zidovudine	Nil

LABORATORY TESTS

23

A Kostrzewski, A Willson

In the tables that follow, we have quoted reference ranges for commonly performed tests. Many of these, for example serum potassium and sodium or red and white blood cell counts, vary little from hospital to hospital. Others may be affected by the characteristics of the indigenous population or by the test method used. The latter is particularly true of enzyme assays and so it is worth checking these tables against those used locally.

Typically, a reference range represents the mean result observed ±2 standard deviations, so a small percentage of the population will normally be outside this range even when healthy. The role of laboratory tests is therefore to screen for possible disease, to confirm a clinical diagnosis or to follow the course of a disease process. They can never be regarded as a diagnosis in themselves.

CLINICAL CHEMISTRY

Fluid balance (Table 23.1)

Water accounts for approximately 60% (approx. 42 L) of body weight. There is less water in women, 55% of body weight, owing to a higher body fat content — adipose tissue contains very little water. The metabolisms of sodium and water are closely linked both physiologically and clinically.

Table 23.1 Fluid balance over 24 hours in a healthy adult	Intake (ml)	Output (ml)
Oral fluids	1500	
Water in food	600	
Endogenous water production	400	
Losses		
Skin		500
Lungs		400
Faeces		100
Kidney		1500
Total	**2500**	**2500**

The osmolalities of the intracellular fluid (approx. 28 L) and extra cellular fluid (approx. 14 L) determine the distribution of water between compartments. In health the osmolality of plasma is approximately 285 mmol/kg.

Urea and electrolytes (Table 23.2)
The interpretation of the tests of urea and electrolytes is described in Table 23.2.

Acid-base balance (Tables 23.3 & 23.4)
The pH of blood is normally maintained between 7.35 and 7.45. It represents a balance between alkali (mainly bicarbonate, HCO_3^-) and acid (mainly carbonic acid, H_2CO_3), where the alkali is kept in excess. Hydrogen ions are generated by many of the metabolic reactions in the body and, in the presence of oxygen, removed from metabolic coenzymes to produce water. The dehydrogenated coenzymes are then able to participate in further reactions. When the blood pH is disturbed, metabolic reactions are impaired and death is likely to result when blood pH is outside the range 6.9–7.9. Tests of acid-base balance are in Table 23.3.

Other ion pairs are sometimes important. If tissue oxygenation is poor, for example after an infarct or in vascular insufficiency, hydrogen ions are not cleared in the usual way and pyruvate is reduced to lactate. Lactic acid builds up and is cleared only when oxygen is once again available.

Homeostasis
Balance is preserved by the interplay of several systems, most of which are capable of some adjustment in a disturbed environment. The lungs supply oxygen to tissues and expel carbon dioxide, so converting carbonic acid to water. In acidosis, or if there is an increase in carbon dioxide in the blood, respiratory rate increases. Erythrocytes mop up small amounts of carbon dioxide in exchange for bicarbonate and will rectify small acidotic disturbances, but their capacity is limited. They rely on regular 'rejuvenation' by healthy lungs and even then will make little contribution to correcting a severe imbalance.

The most potent mechanism for adjusting pH is in the kidney. Normally, bicarbonate is filtered in the glomerulus and an equal amount is put back into the blood from the tubular cells. In acidosis, bicarbonate continues to be secreted into the blood whilst hydrogen ions are lost in the urine. Hence there is a net gain in extracellular bicarbonate and loss of hydrogen ions. This mechanism is stimulated by a rise in blood carbon dioxide or carbonic acid.

Table 23.2 Urea and electrolytes

Test	Reference range	Interpretation
Bicarbonate	22–29 mmol/l	See Table 23.3 (Acid-base balance). Danger levels are <10 mmol/l or >40 mmol/l
Calcium	2.25–2.6 mmol/l	Adjust result for hypoproteinaemia: add 0.02 mmol/l for every g/l of serum albumin below 40 g/l. ⚠ Above 3.50 mmol/l = medical emergency, danger of cardiac arrest. 2.6–3.5 mmol/l, treat once diagnosis is made to avoid renal damage. Hydration plus other measures if needed. Below 2.25 usually symptom-free. Give oral vitamin D ± calcium if needed. Tetany usually only below 1.6 mmol/l. Low calcium levels are found in patients with hypomagnesaemia.
Chloride	95–105 mmol/l	Don't bother, it tells you very little.
Glucose	3.3–7.8 mmol/l (fasting)	Random venous plasma glucose ≥11.1 mmol/l or a venous plasma level above 7.8 mmol/l after overnight fast suggests diabetes mellitus. Equivocal results are clarified with glucose tolerance test. Level should return below 6.7 mmol/l 2 hours after 75 g challenge for venous or capillary whole blood.
Magnesium	0.7–1.2 mmol/l	Hypomagnesaemia has similar symptoms to hypocalcaemia. Especially likely with severe diarrhoea. Measurement indicated in normocalcaemic tetany. Hypermagnesaemia results in loss of muscle tone: occurs in renal failure especially if magnesium salts have been given. Symptoms above 2.5 mmol/l may cause cardiac arrhythmias.

(contd)

Table 23.2 Urea and electrolytes (contd)

Test	Reference range	Interpretation
Phosphate	0.8–1.4 mmol/l	Disturbed phosphate levels are rarely symptomatic in themselves but may affect calcium metabolism.
Potassium	3.5–5.3 mmol/l	⚠ Levels above 6.5 mmol/l may be dangerous and should be treated as an emergency: first with calcium and then with, for example, dextrose and insulin. This condition is often precipitated by acidosis which must be treated.
		Levels below 2.5 mmol/l usually result in muscle weakness and supplements are required. Alkalosis may also result. Mild hypokalaemia is rarely symptomatic.
Protein	50–70 g/l (total) 35–55 g/l (albumin)	Albumin exerts substantial osmotic pressure and levels below 20 g/l usually result in oedema. Hypoalbuminaemia may reflect haemodilution, nephropathy, cirrhosis or catabolism. Total protein is composed of albumin plus globulins. In cirrhosis, globulin levels may rise due to reticuloendothelial hyperplasia. Hyperalbuminaemia may occur with haemoconcentration but is not usually of clinical interest.
Sodium	133–149 mmol/l	Abnormal sodium levels should almost always be interpreted as water imbalance. Hence hypernatraemia usually reflects excess fluid loss or inadequate intake. Absolute sodium excess occurs with steroid therapy and in renal failure. Symptoms of confusion then coma occur 155–160 mmol/l. Give dextrose infusion (dialysis for absolute sodium excess). Hyponatraemia usually reflects haemodilution due to

(contd)

Table 23.2 Urea and electrolytes (contd)

Test	Reference range	Interpretation
Sodium (continued)		cardiac or renal failure and hypoalbuminaemia. Symptoms of weakness below 120 mmol/l; confusions likely below 100 mmol/l. Mild hyponatraemia usually symptom-free. Treat with water deprivation, mannitol or; for excess ADH, demeclocycline
Urea	2.5–6.5 mmol/l	Levels above 10 mmol/l may reflect renal failure, catabolic states, haemorrhage or high dietary protein. For pharmacists, indicates need to check other indicators of renal function (see appropriate table).
Zinc	10–23 μmol/l	May be low in hypoalbuminaemic state. Used to evaluate nutrition inadequacy in enteral or parenteral nutrition, diabetes and wound healing

Table 23.3 Tests of acid-base balance

Test	Reference range	Interpretation
Blood pH	7.35–7.45	This is the main indicator of immediate danger to life. Outside this range, metabolic function throughout the body is impaired. Blood pH reflects the ratio of acid to base and not absolute concentration. It may therefore mask a defect for which the body has compensated.
Base excess	−3 to + 3 mmol/l	Reflects the amount of acid required to titrate blood back to pH 7.4 It therefore adds little more than knowledge of pH.
Bicarbonate	22–29 mmol/l	This is the absolute amount of bicarbonate present in the blood and reflects renal and metabolic function.
$p\mathrm{CO_2}$	4.5–6.0 kPa or 34–45 mmHg	This is the partial pressure of carbon dioxide in blood and, since it is in equilibrium with carbonic acid, reflects the absolute amount of acid in the blood (except where there is a significant amount of lactic acid). It is the indicator of respiratory function (carbonic acid is not measured directly as it is volatile and present only in small concentrations).
Standard bicarbonate	22–27 mmol/l	This is a measurement of bicarbonate plus related alkalis conducted at $p\mathrm{CO_2}$ of 40 mmHg. Comparison with the actual bicarbonate level permits assessment of the relative contributions of the erythrocytes and kidneys.

Potassium

Sodium conservation by the kidney and the sodium pump at cell walls exchange sodium ions for potassium or hydrogen ions. There is free competition between these two species and balance may be disturbed if there is a lack or preponderance of one or the other. For example, metabolic acidosis will increase the concentration of hydrogen ions and hence the amount cleared from the blood at these two sites. Since the amount of sodium exchanged is unaltered, clearance of potassium will be diminished and hyperkalaemia results. Conversely, alkalosis can produce a relative hypokalaemia.

This may lead to a problem of interpretation. If hydrogen and potassium ion concentrations are both abnormal, which was the primary disturbance? In the absence of a known cause, it is reasonable to assume that an acidosis with hyperkalaemia has been set up by a primary acidosis, since primary hyperkalaemia is relatively uncommon. On the other hand, hypokalaemia is more likely than primary alkalosis.

Acidosis

Respiratory acidosis is a result of accumulation of carbon dioxide: a raised carbonic acid concentration is caused by depressed respiration. The disturbed acid/alkali ratio is a result of increased acid. Metabolic acidosis, on the other hand, occurs due to a net fall in bicarbonate ions. These may be lost by poorly functioning kidneys or be used up in buffering excessive hydrogen ions from the tissues. The imbalance here is due to a decrease in alkali.

When pH is disturbed by a malfunction of one system, other mechanisms attempt to compensate. A respiratory alkalosis will cause the kidneys to excrete hydrogen ions and so a rise in pH is achieved by a net increase in bicarbonate ions. Conversely, when plasma bicarbonate is diminished by a metabolic acidosis, the lungs will attempt to restore normal pH by exhaling more carbon dioxide. In general, the kidneys are more effective in compensating for acid-base defects than are the lungs.

Ketoacidosis

This is distinguished from other types of metabolic acidosis by its cause and several concurrent electrolyte disturbances. Insulin lack leads to hyperglycaemia and thus osmotic diuresis and profound dehydration. Also, intracellular metabolism switches to fat with ketones and acid by-products. Acidosis produces secondary hyperkalaemia. Treatment is with insulin and rehydration, plus careful attention to potassium levels.

Alkalosis

Over-breathing may precipitate alkalosis by reducing the carbon dioxide level of the blood and hence the carbonic acid concentration. Production of bicarbonate by the kidneys will be slowed and the pH corrected.

Rarely, metabolic alkalosis can occur, for example in severe potassium depletion or pyloric stenosis. The lungs do not compensate for this state.

The inter-relation of acid-base disturbances and the ability of the body to compensate for primary imbalances make the interpretation of results exceedingly difficult. Nonetheless, it is important to identify the primary disturbance so that the correct diagnosis and therapy can be found.

Acid-base disturbances

The common disturbances of acid-base balance, both acutely and after compensation, are described in Table 23.4.

Liver function tests (Table 23.5)

On a simplified level, abnormal liver function can be divided into three types:

Acute cellular damage

This occurs with acute hepatitis or toxicity to the liver. The main effect is that enzymes, normally present in large amounts in liver cells and in relatively small amounts in serum, leach out of the now permeable liver cell walls. These are mainly alanine and aspartate transaminase (ALT and AST), and they appear in massively increased quantities in the blood. A second effect is that the liver fails to clear bilirubin from the blood and so it builds up in its unconjugated form.

Chronic cellular damage

After long-term insults to the liver, as with alcohol-induced cirrhosis, cells pass through the stage described above and eventually die. They are replaced by fibrous tissue. Hence, transaminase levels are often normal but the elements of the blood which the liver is responsible for producing occur in small concentrations. Cirrhosis is thus characterised by hypoalbuminaemia and an increased prothrombin time, resulting from a reduction of clotting factors.

Cholestasis

Blockage of the bile duct may be mechanical or due to chemical action. Many drugs produce this effect. The result is that many substances normally excreted in the bile build up in

Table 23.4 Acid-base disturbances

Disturbance		Acute change	After compensation
Respiratory acidosis CO_2 not cleared by the lungs. Chronic obstructive airways or barbiturate or opiate poisoning.	pH	↓	↓
	$p\text{CO}_2$	↑	↑
	HCO_3^-		↑
	Standard HCO_3^-	↑	↑
	K^+		↑
Respiratory alkalosis Excessive CO_2 clearance by lungs. Hysterical over-breathing, CNS lesion or salicylate poisoning.	pH	↑	↓
	$p\text{CO}_2$	↓	↓
	HCO_3^-		↓
	Standard HCO_3^-	↓	↓
	K^+		
Metabolic acidosis Excessive lactic acid production or base loss. Anaerobic metabolism, e.g. circulatory failure, renal disease, ketoacidosis.	pH	↓	↓ or →
	$p\text{CO}_2$	↓	↓
	HCO_3^-		↓
	Standard HCO_3^-	↓	↓
	K^+	↑	↑
Metabolic alkalosis Secondary to potassium depletion or loss of gastric acid. Chronic diuretic therapy or pyloric stenosis.	pH	↑	↑
	$p\text{CO}_2$	—	—
	HCO_3^-	↑	↑
	Standard HCO_3^-	↑	↑
	K^+	↓	↓

the liver and appear in the blood. Conjugated bilirubin and alkaline phosphatase (ALP) are the most useful to measure. Another enzyme, gamma-glutamyl transferase (GGT) behaves similarly but is a less reliable indicator of disease since it is subject to induction. It will, for example, show increased serum levels after exposure to several drugs or a significant alcohol load.

The differential diagnosis of liver disease relies on the relative disturbance of each of these indicators, as well as on other tests. Bilirubin is usually measured as total (free plus conjugated) and is differentiated only if other tests are equivocal.

Kidney function tests (Table 23.6)

Tests of renal function attempt to estimate the glomerular filtration rate (GFR) which is normally in the range of 100–140 ml/min. A reduction implies that a proportion of nephrons have closed down and so clearance of nitrogenous waste, drug metabolites and other mainly polar substances is similarly diminished.

A reliable estimate of GFR is extremely useful for the adjustment of drug therapy if this relies on renal excretion. Methods usually rely on observing a substance which is totally cleared by the glomerulus and not subject to reabsorption. An intravenous dose of insulin can be administered and serum and urinary concentrations measured to calculate clearance. Although the answer is likely to be very accurate, this method is too inconvenient for routine use.

An endogenous substance which is produced by the body at a constant rate should exhibit a constant plasma concentration unless its elimination is altered. Therefore, urea and creatinine levels are often monitored. They are cleared by the glomerulus, and an elevated concentration implies a diminished excretion.

Urea

This is a breakdown product of protein metabolism and raised levels (uraemia) are an important sign of renal failure. However, a constant production rate cannot be assumed and levels may also be elevated by high protein meals, tissue damage and catabolism. Although urea levels are of utmost interest to the clinician, they are poor quantitative indicators for pharmacokinetic estimations.

Table 23.5 Liver function tests

Test	Reference range*	Interpretation
Alanine transaminase (ALT or SGPT)	5–30 i.u./l	Markedly raised in hepatocellular damage. Mildly raised in cholestasis and sometimes in cirrhosis. Also raised after circulatory failure with hypoxia.
Albumin	35–55 g/l	Levels below 20 g/l usually result in oedema. Also decreased in haemodilution, nephropathy and catabolism. Hypoalbuminaemia of hepatic origin indicates chronic damage, e.g. cirrhosis.
Alkaline phosphatase (ALP)	20–100 i.u./l	Markedly raised in cholestasis. Mildly raised in hepatocellular damage. Also raised in diseases of bone, e.g. osteomalacia, Paget's disease and carcinoma. Also present in placenta and so raised in third trimester of pregnancy.
Aspartate transaminase (AST or SGOT)	5–40 i.u./l	Markedly raised in hepatocellular damage. Mildly raised in cholestasis and sometimes in cirrhosis. Also raised after circulatory failure with hypoxia. Present in cardiac and skeletal muscle and so raised after infarction and muscle trauma.
Bilirubin (total bilirubin)	2–20 mmol/l	Raised in cellular damage of the liver and cholestasis. Also raised in haemolytic states.
Bilirubin (direct)	<3 μmol/l	Measures conjugated bilirubin. Raised level can indicate source of hepatic failure.

(contd)

Table 23.5 Liver function tests (contd)

Test	Reference range*	Interpretation
Gamma-glutamyl transferase (GGT)	5–45 i.u./l	Markedly raised in cholestasis. Raised in cellular damage, during therapy with enzyme inducers such as phenobarbitone and phenytoin and after substantial alcohol intake.
Prothrombin ratio	1–1.2	Coagulation factors normally made in hepatic parenchyma. Prothrombin ratio will be raised in severe, usually chronic, liver damage. This change is resistant to vitamin K supplements. Also raised in cholestasis when absorption of vitamin K is impaired. In this case, prothrombin time can be shortened with intravenous vitamin K or an oral water-soluble analogue.

Reference ranges are particularly variable for most of these tests depending on the method and conditions of assay.

Table 23.6 Kidney function tests

Test	Reference range	Interpretation
Creatinine clearance	97–140 ml/min (Males) 85–125 ml/min (Females)	This is the best quantitative estimate of GFR using an endogenous indicator. It is not susceptible to theoretical errors but accuracy of 24-hour urine collection and urinary creatinine assay are limiting factors.
Creatinine concentration	50–120 μmol/l (Males) 40–100 μmol/l (Females)	Levels elevated in catabolism and pregnancy. Otherwise, should be adjusted according to age, sex and weight (see text). For example, a level of 100 μmol/l would reflect healthy kidneys in a young male adult but severe renal impairment in the elderly.
Urea (BUN)	1–5 mmol/l	Levels above 10 mmol/l probably reflect renal impairment although trends within an individual are more instructive than isolated measurements. For the clinician, urea remains an invaluable index of disease state.

Creatinine

This is a product of muscle breakdown and in normal anabolic states is produced at a constant and reliable rate. It is, therefore, more useful than urea. Several investigators have noted that muscle turnover is variable according to age, sex and body weight and many nomograms and formulae have been produced to improve estimates of GFR based on serum creatinine concentrations. The following formula is often used:

$$\text{Creatinine clearance (ml/min)} = \frac{\begin{matrix}1.23\ (\text{males}) \\ 1.04\ (\text{females})\end{matrix} \times (140 - \text{age in years}) \times (\text{weight in kg}^*)}{[\text{Serum creatinine in micromoles/l}]}$$

= approx. GFR

*If obese use ideal body weight (IBW). Obese patients are >20% of IBW. To calculate IBW in kg: Males = 50+(2.3h), Females = 45.5+(2.3 h) where h is the number of inches the patient is over five feet high.

> The creatinine clearance formula does not apply to children, in pregnancy, when there is marked catabolism or when renal function is rapidly changing.
> Where a more accurate determination is required, creatinine clearance can be measured directly by taking a serum creatinine level in conjunction with measurement of creatinine in a 24-hour urine sample.

Heart (Table 23.7)

Diagnosis of myocardial infarction depends upon three main elements: an appropriate history, ECG changes and elevation of certain serum enzyme levels. The absence of one sign does not exclude infarction since, for example, a history is not always available and ECG and enzyme changes do not always take place. Most clinicians would therefore accept two out of three signs.

Creatinine kinase and aspartate transaminase are both present in cardiac muscle and, following damage, appear in the blood in greatly elevated concentrations. The degree of elevation is a rough index of the extent of damage. Because neither enzyme is tissue-specific (CK also occurs in skeletal muscle and AST in the liver, erythrocytes, skeletal muscle and kidney) most laboratories monitor a further enzyme known as hydroxybutyrate dehydrogenase (HBD or LD_1). This is a coenzyme of lactate dehydrogenase and is a specific monitor of cardiac damage. Measurement of the enzyme lactate dehydrogenase contributes little since it is distributed around the body in a similar pattern to AST.

A sustained elevation of AST plus a rise in ALT following infarction usually indicates a secondary involvement of the liver.

Cardiac enzymes are usually measured as soon as possible after the suspected infarct and their course is followed during the recovery phase. In the absence of re-infarction, levels should subside in the times indicated in Table 23.7.

Table 23.7 Enzyme elevation after myocardial infarction			
	CK	AST	HBD
Onset of rise (hours)	4–12	6–12	8–24
Peak (hours)	20–40	20–40	30–70
Duration of rise (days)	2–5	2–6	5–12
Extent of rise	up to 10×	up to 8×	up to 6×

CK has two subunits, M and B, this gives three isoenzymes: BB–from brain, MM–from skeletal muscle, and MB–from the heart (CK–MB). CK–MB starts to rise 4–6 hours post infarct and peaks at 24 hours. CK–MB = <25 u/l and <6% of total CK.

Miscellaneous laboratory tests (Table 23.8)

Some notes on the interpretation of selected laboratory tests are given in Table 23.8.

Drugs which interfere with laboratory tests (Table 23.9)

Certain drugs may interfere with the results of laboratory tests. These are listed in Table 23.9.

Drugs which cause electrolyte disturbances (Table 23.10)

These are listed in Table 23.10.

Table 23.8 Miscellaneous laboratory tests

Test	Reference range	Interpretation
Alpha-1-antitrypsin	2–4 g/l	Phenotyping done on those with low levels. Can be useful in some cases of cirrhosis and emphysema.
Amylase (serum)	60–300 U/l*	Derived from the pancreas and usually raised in acute pancreatitis or in abdominal trauma. Sometimes raised in renal failure when clearance is impaired. *Large variation between labs.
Cortisol suppression test	200 nmol/l	Measured on the morning following a 2 mg dexamethasone dose. Failure to suppress cortisol usually indicates adrenal hyperplasia or tumour. Assay cross reacts with prednisolone.
CSF (glucose) CSF (protein)	2.8–4 mmol/l 0.2–0.5 g/l	Infections of CSF are often characterised by raised protein and reduced glucose. Both may be raised after haemorrhage. Visual and microbiological examination are essential.
Folate (serum) Folate (RBC)	5–15 µg/l 150–600 µg/l	Depressed serum folate should not be used as an absolute diagnosis of folate deficiency since it is determined by recent dietary history. Body stores of folate are sufficient for 3 to 4 months and RBC levels are the best guide to these store levels.
Iron (serum)	10–30 µmol/l (men) 7–25 µmol/l (women)	True iron deficiency produces a low serum iron and raised iron binding capacity (IBC or TIBC). Both indices are lowered in, for example, rheumatoid arthritis.
Iron binding capacity (serum)	45–72 µmol/l	

(cont.)

Table 23.8 Miscellaneous laboratory tests (contd)

Test	Reference range	Interpretation
Lipids: cholesterol (total) cholesterol (HDL)	<5.2 mmol/l Male 0.9–2.0 mmol/l Female 1.0–2.3 mmol/l	Triglyceride levels must be taken after a fast of at least 12 hours since the level is dependent on diet. Apart from the primary hyperlipidaemias and their cardiovascular sequelae, hypercholesterolaemia can be caused by diabetes, nephrotic syndrome and biliary obstruction; hypertriglyceridaemia can accompany diabetes, nephrotic syndrome pancreatitis, alcohol and oral contraceptives. Low levels of HDL are associated with a high risk of an MI.
triglycerides (fasting)	<2.0 mmol/l	Triglyceride values increase with aging.
Osmolality serum	285–295 mOsm/kg	↑ fluid depletion ↓ fluid excess
Thyroxine (total) Free T_4 Free T_3	60–140 mmol/l 10–25 pmol/l 5–10.2 pmol/l	↑ Hyperthyroidism (Graves' disease) can be confirmed with TRH challenge. ↓ Hypothyroidism should be confirmed with TSH measurement and possibly a TRH challenge. Thyroxine levels may be decreased by salicylates and phenytoin through binding displacement.
Urate (serum)	Male 0.24–0.48 mmol/l Female 0.16–0.36 mmol/l	↑ may lead to gout. May be due to increased production, e.g. from hereditary purine metabolic defect and carcinoma, or from diminished excretion, e.g. in glomerular failure, acidosis and with diuretics.
Vitamin B12 (serum)	160–900 ng/l	↓ leads to macrocytic anaemia and to peripheral neuropathy. May be due to diet deficiency, pernicious anaemia, ileitis or short bowel syndrome. Stores normally last for 2 to 4 years. Cause can be verified by the Schilling test.

Table 23.9 Drugs which interfere with laboratory tests

Test	Effect	Drug	in vivo (V) or in vitro (T)
Alanine transaminase	+	Amitriptyline	V
	+	Amphotericin B	V
	+	Erythromycin	V
	+	Halothane	V
	+	Isoniazid	V
	+	Levodopa	V
	+	Nalidixic acid	V
	+	Nitrofurantoin	V
	+	Phenytoin	V
	+	Rifampicin	V
	+	Salicylate	V
	+	Streptokinase	V
	+	Sulphonamides	V
	+	Valproate	V
Alkaline phosphatase	−	Acetylcysteine	T
	+	Carbamazepine	V
	−	Clofibrate	V
	+	Disulfiram	V
	−	EDTA	V
	+	Erythromycin	V
	+	Methyldopa	V
	+	Nitrofurantoin	V
	−	Nitrofurantoin	T
	+	Phenytoin	V
	+	Rifampicin	V
	+	Sulphonamides	V
	−	Zinc salts	T
Amylase	+	Asparaginase	V
	+	Corticosteroids	V
	+	Fat emulsions	T
	+	Frusemide	V
	+	Metformin	V
	+	Morphine	V
	+	Pancreatic enzymes	T
	+	Valproate	V
Aspartate transaminase	+	Cimetidine	V
	+	Erythromycin	V
	+	Halothane	V
	+	Isoniazid	V
	+	Levodopa	V
	+	Mercaptopurine	V
	+	Methyldopa	V
	−	Metronidazole	V

(contd)

Table 23.9 Drugs which interfere with laboratory tests (contd)

Test	Effect	Drug	in vivo (V) or in vitro (T)
Aspartate transaminase (continued)	+	Nitrofurantoin	V
	+	Paracetamol	T
	+	Paracetamol	V
	+	Phenytoin	V
	+	Rifampicin	V
	+	Salicylate	V
	+	Streptokinase	V
	+	Sulphonamides	V
	+	Valproate	V
Bilirubin	+	Carbamazepine	V
	+	Chlordiazepoxide	V
	+	Cimetidine	V
	+	Disulfiram	V
	+	Erythromycin	V
	+	Fluphenazine	V
	+	Fusidic acid	V
	+	Halothane	V
	+	Ibuprofen	V
	+	Imipramine	V
	+	Mercaptopurine	V
	+	Methyldopa	T
	+	Methyldopa	V
	+	Nitrofurantoin	V
	+	Oral contraceptives	V
	+	Phenothiazines	V
	+	Phenytoin	V
	−	Pindolol	T
	+	Quinidine	V
	+	Rifampicin	T
	+	Rifampicin	V
	+	Sulphamethoxazole	V
	+	Sulphasalazine	V
	+	Theophylline	T
Calcium (See also Table 23.10)	+	Hydrallazine	T
Cholesterol	+	Chenodeoxycholic acid	V
	+	Chlorpromazine	T
	+	Chlorthalidone	V
	−	Cholestyramine	V
	+	Corticosteroids	T
	+	Corticosteroids	V
	+	Hydrochlorothiazide	V
	+	Iodides	T

(contd)

Table 23.9 Drugs which interfere with laboratory tests (contd)			
Test	**Effect**	**Drug**	**in vivo (V) or in vitro (T)**
Cholesterol	+	Levodopa	V
(continued)	–	Neomycin	V
	–	Nitrates	T
	+	Oral contraceptives	V
	+	Phenytoin	V
	–	Prazosin	V
	+	Vitamin C	T
Glucose (blood)	–	Aspirin	V
(see also Table 23.10)	+	Chlorpromazine	V
	+	Chlorthalidone	V
	–	Clofibrate	V
	+	Corticosteroids	V
	–	Cyproheptadine	V
	+	Fructose	T
	–	Guanethidine	V
	+	Isoprenaline	V
	+/–	Levodopa	T
	+	Levodopa	V
	+	Lithium	V
	+	Metoprolol	V
	+	Oral contraceptives	V
	+	Phenytoin	V
	+/–	Propranolol	V
	–	Tetracycline	T
	+	Thiazides	V
Glucose (urine)	+	Acetazolamide	V
	+	Aspirin	T
	+	Cephalosporins	T
	+	Chloral	T
	+	Corticosteroids	V
	+	Fructose	T
	+	Glucagon	V
	+	Hydrallazine	T
	+	Isoniazid	T
	+/–	Levodopa	T
	+	Methyldopa	T
	+	Nalidixic acid	T
	+	Oxazepam	T
	+	Penicillin (large dose)	T
	+	Probenecid	T
	+	Streptomycin	T
	+/–	Tetracycline	T
	+	Thiazide	V
	+/–	Vitamin C	T

(contd)

Table 23.9 Drugs which interfere with laboratory tests (contd)			
Test	Effect	Drug	in vivo (V) or in vitro (T)
Urea	+	Acetohexamide	T
(see also Table 23.10)	+	Methoxyflurane	V
	−	Streptomycin	T
	+	Sulphonylureas	T
	+	Tetracycline	V
	+	Thiazides	V
	+	Trimethoprim	V
Uric acid	+	Acetazolamide	V
	+	Acetylcysteine	T
	+	Aspirin	V
	+/−	Clofibrate	V
	+	Ethambutol	V
	+	Frusemide	V
	+	Hydrallazine	T
	+	Levodopa	T
	+	Levodopa	V
	+	Methyldopa	T
	+	Propranolol	V
	+	Thiazides	V
	+	Vitamin C	T

HAEMATOLOGY

Automated blood counts are virtually routine for patients coming into hospital. These results, and the results of more specialised tests, may be useful for pharmacists. They may form the basis for drug therapy, e.g. iron and vitamin supplements, or they may be an index of disease progress, e.g. leukaemia. Alternatively, they may demonstrate drug toxicity.

Blood screening

Erythrocytes

Routine screening of erythrocytes is often performed using a Coulter Counter technique combined with microscopy. These tests demonstrate the size, number and colour of red blood cells, whether they are of normal shape and the percentage of young cells (reticulocytes).

Iron deficiency results in pale or hypochromic cells and these are normally smaller than usual. Deficiency of vitamin B12 or folate does not affect the nature of cytoplasm but reduces the frequency of cell division in the marrow. The red cells are therefore larger (macrocytic), but have a normal colour. A marrow biopsy demonstrates that red cell precursors are also larger than normal (megaloblasts). When folate and iron deficiencies combine, red cells are both macrocytic and hypochromic.

Conditions such as the thalassaemias, where abnormal haemoglobin chains are incorporated into erythrocytes, result in an abnormal shape of the cell as well as deficiencies in oxygen transport.

Erythrocytes normally have a life of 100–120 days and are eventually destroyed by the macrophages. For the first day or so they contain the remnants of a cell nucleus and after staining can be recognised as reticulocytes. Hence, normal production and destruction of erythrocytes are characterised by a reticulocyte count around 1%. If there is marrow aplasia and production is suppressed, the count will often be low. Alternatively, if erythrocytes are prematurely destroyed by macrophages, for example in macrocytosis or a haemoglobinopathy, the proportion of reticulocytes in the circulation will increase. There may be an accompanying increase in serum bilirubin as a result of increased haemoglobin breakdown. Similar changes, but to a more dramatic extent, are seen in haemolytic anaemias.

Anaemia

Anaemias are conditions of the blood where there are quantitative or qualitative changes of the erythrocytes.

Leucocytes

White blood cells (leucocytes) may be classified microscopically into two groups according to whether they contain granules in the cytoplasm. The granulocytes are further subdivided according to the staining characteristics of the granules (hence neutrophils, basophils and eosinophils). Two distinct types of cell comprise the agranulocytes, these being the monocytes (macrophages) and lymphocytes. The latter is the only class of leucocyte which does not exhibit phagocytic activity. The functions of the various types of cell are summarised in Table 23.11.

Coagulation tests

The most common test performed is the prothrombin time (PTT) which tests the extrinsic and common coagulation pathways. A normal result is 10–14 seconds. It may be expressed with reference to a standard preparation and a normal prothrombin ratio is in the range 1–1.2. When a patient is anticoagulated, the aim is to achieve a ratio of around 2. Most laboratories will accept a value between 1.5 and 4.

An alternative — the Thrombotest — has a normal range of 60–100% while the target range for anticoagulation is 5–17%.

Table 23.10 Drugs which cause electrolyte disturbances

Electrolyte	Drug	Effect	Mechanism
Calcium	Acetazolamide	→	↓ renal reabsorption
	Aminoglycosides	→	↓ renal reabsorption (rare)
	Calcitonin	→	↓ resorption of bone
	Calcium salts	←	•
	Corticosteroids	→	↓ GI absorption, resorption of bone and renal absorption
	Lithium	←	↑ Parathyroid hormone (rare)
	Magnesium salts	→	↓ GI absorption
	Mithramycin	→	Parathyroid hormone antagonism
	Oestrogens	→	?
	Oral contraceptives	←	↓ Albumin synthesis
	Parathyroid hormone	←	↑ GI absorption, resorption of bone and renal reabsorption
	Phenobarbitone/phenytoin	→	↑ Vitamin D metabolism
	Phosphates	→	↓ GI absorption
	Tamoxifen	←	? (rare)
	Thyroid hormones	←	↑ resorption of bone
	Vitamin D	←	↑ GI absorption, resorption of bone and renal reabsorption
Glucose	Alcohol	→ ↑ (less often)	↓ Gluconeogenesis ↑ Glycogenolysis
	Clonidine	→	↓ Insulin secretion
	Corticosteroids	←	↑ Gluconeogenesis + antagonise insulin

(contd)

Table 23.10 Drugs which cause electrolyte disturbances (contd)

Electrolyte	Drug	Effect	Mechanism
Glucose (continued)	Diuretics (not spironolactone)	↑	↓ Glucose tolerance
	Isoniazid	↑	↓ Gluconeogenesis
	Levodopa	↑	↑ Glucagon secretion
	Oral contraceptives	↑	↓ Glucose tolerance
	Phenytoin	↑	↓ Insulin secretion (rare)
	Propranolol	↑ (less often)	↓ Glycogenolysis
			↓ Insulin secretion
	Salicylates	↓	↑ Glucose uptake (high doses)
	Theophylline	↑	↑ Glycogenolysis and gluconeogenesis
		↓	↑ Insulin secretion
Magnesium	Aminoglycosides	↓	Toxic tubular damage
	Amphotericin B	↓	Toxic tubular damage
	Cisplatin	↓	Toxic tubular damage
	Digoxin	↓	↑ Renal loss
	Frusemide	↓	↑ Renal loss
	Lithium	↑	? (rare)
	Magnesium salts	↑	•
	Thiazides	↓	↑ Renal loss (less than with frusemide)

(contd)

Table 23.10 Drugs which cause electrolyte disturbances (contd)

Electrolyte	Drug	Effect	Mechanism
Phosphate	Aluminium salts	↓	↓ Absorption
	Corticosteroids	↓	↑ Resorption of bone
	Nutrition in malnourished subjects	↓	↑ Cellular uptake
	Thiazides	↓	?
Potassium	Aminoglycosides	↓	Toxic tubular damage
	Amphotericin B	↓	Toxic tubular damage
	Bicarbonates	↓	↑ Cell uptake + renal loss
	Captopril	↑	↓ Renal loss (aldosterone production)
	Carbenoxolone	↓	↑ Renal loss (aldosterone-like)
	Corticosteroids	↓	↑ Renal loss (aldosterone-like)
	Cytotoxics	↑	Rapid cell lysis
	Dinoprost	↓	↑ Renal loss (prostaglandin agonist)
	Fludrocortisone	↓	↑ Renal loss (aldosterone-like)
	Frusemide	↓	↑ Renal loss
	Indomethacin	↑	↓ Renal loss (prostaglandin antagonist)
	Insulin + glucose	↓	↑ Cell uptake
	Laxatives	↓	↓ Reabsorption from GI tract
	Levodopa	↓	↑ Renal loss (reduced by carbidopa and benserazide)
	Penicillins (large dose)	↓	Secondary to renal excretion of large amounts of anionic penicillin

(contd)

Table 23.10 Drugs which cause electrolyte disturbances (contd)

Electrolyte	Drug	Effect	Mechanism
Potassium (continued)	Salbutamol (i.v.)	↑	↑ Cell uptake + ↑ renin secretion
	Spironolactone	↑	↑ Renal uptake (aldosterone antagonist)
	Succinylcholine	↑	Transient loss of intracellular potassium
	Thiazides	↓	↑ Renal loss
Sodium	Carbamazepine	↓	May ↑ ADH production
	Chlorpropamide	↓	Augmentation of ADH
	Corticosteroids	↑	↑ Renal reabsorption
	Cyclophosphamide	↓	↓ Water excretion
	Demeclocycline	↑	Inhibition of ADH
	Indomethacin	↓	↓ Renal loss (prostaglandin antagonist)
	Laxatives	↓	↑ GI water loss in excess of sodium
	Lithium	↑	↑ Renal water loss in excess of sodium
		↓	↑ Renal sodium loss
	Oxytocin	↓	ADH-like action
	Phenytoin	↑	Inhibition of ADH
	Thiazides	↓	↑ Renal loss in excess of water
	Tolbutamide	↓	Augmentation of ADH (less than with chlorpropamide)
	Vincristine	↓	↑ ADH production

(contd)

Table 23.10 Drugs which cause electrolyte disturbances (contd)

Electrolyte	Drug	Effect	Mechanism
Urea	Allopurinol Aminoglycosides Amphotericin B Busulphan Carbamazepine Cephalosporin Colistin Frusemide Gold Methotrexate Methyldopa Mithramycin Mitomycin C Penicillamine Phenindione Phenylbutazone Phenytoin Probenecid Radio-contrast media Salicylates Stibophen Sulphonamides Tetracyclines Vancomycin		These drugs have all been reported to be nephrotoxic and are therefore capable of producing uraemia. Cytotoxic agents may also produce uraemia through rapid tissue breakdown.

Table 23.11 Function of blood cells

Test or cell name	Reference range	Description or function	Interpretation
Basophils	$0.01-0.1 \times 10^9$/l (0.1% of WBC)	Identical to mast cells which they eventually become.	↑ (Basophil leucocytosis) in granulocytic leukaemia or sometimes in ulcerative colitis.
Eosinophils	$0.04-0.4 \times 10^9$/l (1–4% of WBC)	Appear similar to neutrophils but feature in allergic response and defence against parasites.	↑ (Eosinophilia) in atopic asthma, hay fever etc., amoebiasis and worm infestation, some lymphomas and skin disease.
ESR	0–9 mm/h (men) 0–20 mm/h (women)	Erythrocyte sedimentation rate (rate of all of red cells in anticoagulated specimen)	It should be slow. ↑ in infections and some inflammatory diseases. Like pyrexia, it is a non-specific indicator but can be used to discover or follow a disease process.
Ferritin	Male 15–300 μg/l Female 15–200 μg/l		May be normal in presence of iron deficiency due to acute phase reaction. Useful in differential diagnosis of hypochromic, microcytic anaemias. Decreased in iron deficiency anaemia and increased in iron overload.
Hb	14–18 g/dl (men) 12–16 g/dl (women)	Haemoglobin concentration	Symptomatic below 9–10 g/dl. If chronic, may lead to cardiomegaly: decreased by haemorrhage, iron deficiency, marrow depression or increased haemolysis (e.g. macrocytic or haemolytic anaemia, haemoglobinopathies).

(contd)

Table 23.11 Function of blood cells (contd)

Test or cell name	Reference range	Description or function	Interpretation
HbAlc	< 6%		Indicator of glycaemic control over the preceding 2 months.
Carboxy-Hb	< 1.5 %		Can be up to 10% in smokers. Toxic levels > 20%, can be lethal if > 50%.
Hct (haematocrit)	39–54% (men) 36–47% (women)	Packed cell volume of anticoagulated blood	Crude indicator of red cell volume. More specific information is derived from RBC and MCV.
Lymphocytes	$1.3–3.55 \times 10^9/l$ (20–35% of WBC)	B-cells responsible for immunity against foreign (mainly bacterial) cells through production of immunoglobulins. T-cells act as helpers to B-cells and provide cell-mediated immunity against intracellular organisms (e.g. viruses, fungi and protozoa) and foreign cells (e.g. grafts).	↑ (Lymphocytosis) mononucleosis, viral infections, tuberculosis, toxoplasmosis, some leukaemias and autoimmune diseases. ↓ (Lymphopenia) in marrow failure or with, for example, corticosteroids and azathioprine.
MCH	27–32 pg		Mean cell haemoglobin: indicates weight in each cell. Determined by MCV and MCHC, which give more useful information.

(contd)

Table 23.11 Function of blood cells (contd)

Test or cell name	Reference range	Description or function	Interpretation
MCHC	32–36 g/dl	Mean cell haemoglobin concentration indicates quality of the cytoplasm regardless of cell size.	↓ (hypochromic) especially in iron deficiency but also in inflammatory disease (e.g. rheumatoid arthritis, thalassaemia, sideroblastic anaemia).
MCV	82–95 fl	Mean cell volume	↓ (microcytic) in iron deficiency ↑ (macrocytic) in folate or B12 deficiency, liver disease, after alcohol and some cytotoxics.
Monocytes (macrophages)	$0.1–0.8 × 10^9$/l (1.8% of WBC)	Large phagocytes	↑ (Monocytosis) in tuberculosis, endocartis and typhoid fever. Also in lymphoma and leukaemia.
Neutrophils	$2.2–7 × 10^9$/l (45–75% of WBC)	Attracted to sites of inflammation and infection; phagocytosis of foreign cells or defective host cells and killing of bacterial cells.	↑ (neutrophil leucocytosis) especially in bacterial infections and inflammation but also in carcinoma, leukaemia and metabolic disorders such as gout and acidosis. ↓ (neutropenia) in viral infections, autoimmune disease, in marrow failure, or after many drugs (phenylbutazone, chlorpromazine, chloramphenicol, phenytoin, etc.).

(contd)

Table 23.11 Function of blood cells (contd)

Test or cell name	Reference range	Description or function	Interpretation
Platelets (thrombocytes)	$100-400 \times 10^9/l$	Mechanical plugging of haemorrhage and initiation of coagulation.	↓ (thrombocytopenia) in marrow failure or toxicity, leukaemia, splenomegaly or if destruction is increased in immune thrombocytopenic purpura.
RBC	$4.5-6 \times 10^{12}/l$ (men) $4.3-5.5 \times 10^{12}/l$ (women)	Red blood cell (count)	↑ in fluid depletion, polycythaemia ↓ in fluid overload, macrocytic anaemia, marrow aplasia, haemolytic anaemia.
Retics	$0.5-1.5\%$	Proportion of young red cells (reticulocytes)	Should be raised as a response to blood loss or anaemia. May remain low in iron, folate or B12 deficiency, carcinoma, marrow hypoplasia or malnutrition.
WBC	$4-11 \times 10^9/l$	White blood cell (count)	↑ (leucocytosis) usually indicates infection. Marked increase may indicate malignancy. ↓ (leucopenia) may be due to drugs, some infections and hypersensitivity reactions. Differential counts essential.

The activated partial thromboplastin time or kaolin-cephalin time (APTT, PTTK or KCT) is a test of intrinsic clotting pathways with a normal range of 30–40 seconds. Prolongation of this time is usually due to clotting factor deficiency. The test is used to monitor heparin therapy when it should achieve between 1.5 and 2.5 times the normal value.

SI UNITS FOR CLINICAL CHEMISTRY

Table 24.1 Conversion from Traditional to SI Units

Test	Unit	To SI Unit
Acid phosphatase (King-Armstrong)	0.56 KA	= 1 iu/l
Amylase		1 iu/l
Aspartate transaminase (Asp-T or SGOT)		iu/l
Blood gases $p\mathrm{CO_2}$ $p\mathrm{O_2}$	mmHg × 0.133 mmHg × 0.133	= 1 kPa = 1 kPa
Blood hydrogen ion concentration	pH is a log unit so no easy conversion	nmol/l
Serum albumin	10 × g/100 ml	= 1 g/l
Serum bicarbonate	1 mEq/l	= 1 mmol/l
Serum bilirubin	mg/100 ml × 17.1	= 1 mmol/l
Serum calcium	mg/100 ml × 0.25	= 1 mmol/l
Serum chloride	1 mEq/l	= 1 mmol/l
Serum creatinine	mg/100 ml × 88.4	= 1 μmol/l
Serum globulin	g/100 ml × 10	= g/l
Serum glucose	mg/100 ml × 0.055	= mmol/l
Serum iron	mg/100 ml × 0.18	= μmol/l
Serum magnesium	mEq/l × 0.5	= mmol/l
Serum phosphate (inorganic)	mg/100 ml × 0.32	= mmol/l

(contd)

Table 24.1 Conversion from Traditional to SI Units (contd)		
Test	**Unit**	**To SI Unit**
Serum potassium	mEq/l	= mmol/l
Serum sodium	mEq/l	= mmol/l
Serum triglycerides	mg/100 ml × 0.011	= mmol/l
Serum urate	mg/100 ml × 0.17	= mmol/l
Serum urea	mg/100 ml × 0.17	= mmol/l
Total iron-binding capacity	mg/100 ml × 0.18	= μmol/l
Urinary calcium	mg/24 h × 0.025	= mmol/24 h
Urinary creatinine	mg/24 h × 0.0088	= mmol/24 h
Urinary phosphate	mg/24 h × 0.032	= mmol/24 h
Urinary urea	g/24 h × 16.6	= mmol/24 h

(Reproduced with permission from Hyde J, Willson A 1989 The SK&F Clinical Pharmacy Handbook, 2nd edn. Smith Kline and French Laboratories Ltd, Welwyn Garden City)

PHARMACOKINETICS IN CLINICAL PRACTICE

S Dhillon

Basic skills and knowledge of applied pharmacokinetics are required by clinical pharmacists in routine practice. Pharmacists should be able to:

- apply one compartment pharmacokinetics to single and multiple dosing following the intravenous and oral administration of drugs
- state the rationale for using TDM to optimise drug therapy
- identify drugs which should be routinely monitored
- apply the basic principles of interpretation of serum drug concentrations in practice
- apply one compartment pharmacokinetics to describe steady state serum drug concentrations following oral dosing.

Pharmacokinetics provides a mathematical basis to assess the time course of drugs and their effects in the body. It enables the following processes to be quantified:

Absorption
Distribution
Metabolism
Excretion

It is these pharmacokinetic processes, often referred to as **ADME**, that determine the drug concentration in the body.

Ideally the drug concentration of a drug should be measured at the site of drug action, i.e. at the receptor. However, due to inaccessibility, drug concentrations are normally measured in whole blood from which serum or plasma is generated. Other body fluids such as saliva, urine and cerebrospinal fluid are sometimes used. It is assumed that drug concentrations in these fluids are in equilibrium with the drug concentration at the receptor. Drug concentrations refer to total drug concentration, i.e. a combination of bound and free which are in equilibrium with each other. In clinical practice the drug concentration is measured in serum or plasma.

For most drugs routinely monitored in practice one assumes a first-order rate for the processes of ADME, i.e. the amount of a drug A is decreasing at a rate that is proportional to the amount of drug A remaining in the body; thus the rate of elimination of drug A can be described as:

$$\frac{dA}{dt} = -kA \text{ where k is first order rate constant}$$

The reaction proceeds at a rate which is dependent on the concentration of drug A present in the body. Most drugs when used in clinical practice at therapeutic doses follow first-order elimination processes. However in overdose situations they may show saturation and follow zero-order elimination. Some drugs in therapeutic doses will show zero-order elimination processes and this requires the application of Michaelis-Menten kinetics to interpret these drugs in clinical practice. Examples include phenytoin, high-dose salicylates and high-dose theophyllines (mainly reported in paediatrics)

PHARMACOKINETIC MODELS

Pharmacokinetic models are hypothetical structures which are used to describe the fate of a drug in a biological system following its administration.

One compartment model

Following drug administration, the body is depicted as a kinetically homogeneous unit. This assumes that the drug achieves instantaneous distribution throughout the body and that the drug equilibrates instantaneously between tissues. Thus the drug concentration time profile shows a monoexponential decline and can be described using the equation below. It is important to note that this does not imply that the drug concentration in plasma is equal to the drug concentration in the tissues. However, changes in the plasma concentration quantitatively reflect changes in the tissues.

The equation to describe the change in Cp_t (drug concentration at any time t) describes monoexponential decay.

$$Cp_t = Cp^o\, e^{-kt}$$

where:

Cp^o is initial concentration at time 0 h;
k is first-order elimination rate constant.

Two compartment model

This model resolves the body into central and peripheral compartments. These compartments have no physiological or anatomical meaning; however it is assumed that the central compartment comprises tissues which are highly perfused such as heart, lungs, kidneys, liver and brain. The peripheral compartment comprises less well-perfused tissues such as muscle, fat and skin. Drugs such as gentamicin, theophylline and digoxin show a two compartment model. However in practice one compartment kinetics can be used to describe the serum concentration time profile providing the samples are taken after the distribution phase is complete.

PHARMACOKINETIC PARAMETERS

The following section will describe the basic pharmacokinetic parameters for a one compartment model and their application in clinical practice.

Elimination rate constant

The elimination rate constant can be used to calculate the fraction of a dose eliminated per unit of time. For a one compartment model the elimination of the drug is described by a first-order process.

Volume of distribution

The volume of distribution is defined as the volume of plasma in which the total amount of drug in the body would be required to be dissolved, to reflect the drug concentration attained in plasma. The volume of distribution (Vd) has no direct physiological meaning; it is not a 'real' volume and is usually referred to as the apparent volume of distribution. Some drugs may have limited tissue distribution hence their Vd reflects total plasma volume, e.g. gentamicin Vd 15 litres, whereas other drugs show intensive distribution, e.g. amiodarone Vd 2000 litres.

Half-life

The time required to reduce the plasma concentration to one half its initial value is defined as the half-life ($t_{1/2}$) i.e. $t_{1/2}$ = 0.693/k. The time taken to reach steady state serum concentrations, i.e. when the rate of administration is equal to the rate of elimination, is approximately equal to $5 \times t_{1/2}$. At steady state the change in serum concentrations within a dosing interval are the same.

Clearance

Drug clearance can be defined as the volume of plasma in the vascular compartment cleared of drug per unit of time by the processes of metabolism and excretion. Clearance is constant for all drugs that are eliminated by first-order kinetics. Drugs can be cleared by renal excretion or metabolism or both. With respect to the kidney and liver etc, clearances, are additive, i.e.

$$Cl_{(total)} = Cl_{renal} + Cl_{non-renal}$$

Mathematically, clearance is the product of the first-order elimination rate constant (k) and the apparent volume of distribution (Vd).

Thus:

$$Cl_{(total)} = k \times Vd$$

Relationship with half-life ($t_{1/2}$):

$$t_{1/2} = \frac{0.693 \times Vd}{Cl}$$

PHARMACOKINETIC APPLICATIONS

Table 25.1 summarises the basic pharmacokinetic equations which can be applied on the wards.

Table 25.1 Basic pharmacokinetic equations	
Pharmacokinetic equation	Comments on the clinical use of the equations
Single i.v. bolus injection $Cp_t = Cp^o\, e^{-kt}$	This equation describes the serum concentration at any time (t) after a single intravenous dose. This equation can be used to calculate monoexponential decay. If you have a toxic serum concentration use this equation to estimate the time for decay of a toxic level to a desired serum concentration (see below).
e^{-kt} $1 - e^{-kt}$	Fraction of a dose remaining Fraction of a dose eliminated

(contd)

Table 25.1 Basic pharmacokinetic equations (contd)	
Pharmacokinetic equation	Comments on the clinical use of the equations
$Cp^o = \dfrac{SFD}{Vd}$	Loading dose. Let Cp^o equal the desired serum concentration
$t_{1/2} = \dfrac{0.693}{k}$	The half-life can be estimated using this equation. Times to reach steady state serum concentrations are 4–5 times the half-life
$Cl = kVd$	The total body clearance can be calculated using this equation
Single oral dose $Cp_t = Cp^o \dfrac{ka}{(ka-k)} (e^{-kt} - e^{-kat})$	This equation is used to calculate the serum concentration at any time (t) after a single oral dose.
Multiple i.v. bolus injections (a) $Cpss_t = Cp^o \dfrac{(e^{-kt})}{(1 - e^{-k\tau})}$	This equation is used to calculate the serum concentration at any time (t) within a dosing interval at steady state following multiple bolus intravenous dosing.
(b) $Cpss_{max} = Cp^o \dfrac{1}{(1 - e^{-k\tau})}$	This equation is used to calculate the maximum serum concentration at steady state i.e. t = 0. To estimate the peak serum concentration then (t) must be selected: e.g. for gentamicin t peak = 1 hour
(c) $Cpss_{min} = Cp^o \dfrac{(e^{-k\tau})}{(1 - e^{-k\tau})}$	This equation is used to calculate the minimum trough serum concentration at steady state following multiple intravenous bolus dosing
i.v. infusion prior to steady state $Cp_t = \dfrac{DS}{\tau Cl} (1 - e^{-kt})$	This equation can be used to calculate a serum concentration at any time (t) after starting an intravenous infusion
i.v. infusion at steady state $Cpss = \dfrac{DS}{\tau Cl}$	This equation can be used to calculate the steady state serum concentration during an intravenous infusion

(contd)

Table 25.1 Basic pharmacokinetic equations (contd)

Pharmacokinetic equation	Comments on the clinical use of the equations
Multiple oral dosing at steady state $$Cpss = \frac{Cp^0\ ka}{(ka-k)}\left[\frac{e^{-kt}}{(1-e^{-k\tau})} - \frac{e^{-kat}}{(1-e^{-ka\tau})}\right]$$	This equation is used to calculate a concentration at any time (t) within a dosing interval, at steady state following oral dosing.
The maximum concentration is given by: $$Cpss_{max} = \frac{Cp^0\ ka}{(ka-k)}\left[\frac{e^{-k\ tss_{max}}}{(1-e^{-k\tau})} - \frac{e^{-ka\ tss_{max}}}{(1-e^{-ka\tau})}\right]$$	This equation calculates the peak concentration at steady state following oral dosing
The time at which the maximum concentration occurs: $$tss_{max} = \frac{1}{(ka-k)}\ \ln\left[\frac{ka\ (1-e^{-k\tau})}{k\ (1-e^{-ka\tau})}\right]$$	This equation calculates the time to reach a peak concentration at steady state following oral dosing
The minimum concentration is given by: $$Cpss_{min} = \frac{Cp^0\ ka}{(ka-k)}\left[\frac{e^{-k\tau}}{(1-e^{-k\tau})} - \frac{e^{-ka\tau}}{(1-e^{-ka\tau})}\right]$$	The minimum or trough concentration at steady state i.e. at the beginning of a dosage interval
Loading doses $$Ld = \frac{Vd\ Cp}{SF}$$ $$Ld = \frac{Vd\ (Cp_{desired} - Cp_{observed})}{SF}$$	This equation can be used to calculate loading doses following oral or intravenous administration. Select the target serum concentration usually in the middle of the therapeutic range
The average steady state concentration (Cpss) $$Cpss = \frac{SF\ dose}{Cl\tau}$$	This equation can be used to calculate maintenance doses (dose/τ) following oral or intravenous administration
$$\text{Time for decay} = \frac{\ln Cp_1 - \ln Cp_2}{k}$$	Toxic level decay equation which assumes first-order elimination, complete absorption and distribution.

Cp_t is serum drug concentration at any time (t).
Cp^o is initial serum concentration at time 0 h.
k is first-order elimination rate concentration.
ka is first-order absorption rate constant.
Vd is volume of distribution.
Cl is total body clearance.
S is salt factor.
F is bioavailability.
$Cpss_t$ is steady state serum concentration at any time (t).
$Cpss$ is average steady state serum concentration.
$Cpss_{min}$ is trough or minimum serum concentration at steady state.
$Cpss_{max}$ is peak or maximum serum concentration at steady state.
tss_{max} is time of peak serum concentration at steady state.
D is dose.
Ld is loading dose.
τ is dosing interval.
ln is natural log.

COMPARATIVE DOSES OF CORTICOSTEROIDS

26

Apart from the dose differences of corticosteroids there are qualitative differences in their actions. Consequently, side-effects may occur when one steroid is substituted for another. For further details see Table 26.1.

Table 26.1 Comparative doses of corticosteroids for systemic use based on glucocorticoid properties	
Corticosteroid	Dose (mg)
Betamethasone	0.7
Cortisone	25
Dexamethasone	0.75
Hydrocortisone	20
Methylprednisolone	4
Prednisolone	5
Prednisone	5
Triamcinolone	4

(Reproduced with permission from Hyde J, Willson A 1989 The SK&F Clinical Pharmacy Handbook, 2nd edn. Smith Kline and French Laboratories Ltd, Welwyn Garden City)

CALCULATING BODY SURFACE AREA FROM WEIGHT AND HEIGHT

27

The nomogram shown in Figure 27.1 may be used to calculate the body surface area from the weight and height of the patient. Mark on the patient's weight and height, and then draw a line between the two points. Read off the surface area from the point where this line crosses the middle line.

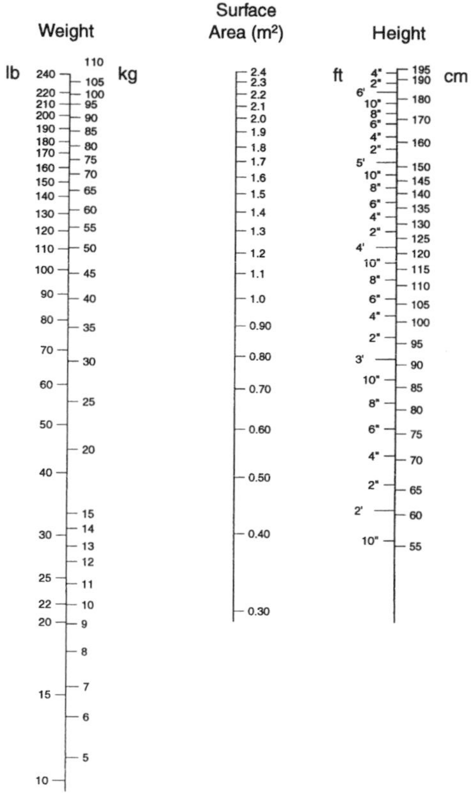

Figure 27.1 A nomogram for calculating body surface area from weight and height. (Reproduced with permission from Hyde J, Willson A 1989 The SK&F Clinical Pharmacy Handbook, 2nd edn. Smith Kline and French Laboratories Ltd, Welwyn Garden City.)

A & E	accident and emergency
ABG	arterial blood gases
ACE	angiotensin converting enzyme
ACTH	adrenocorticotrophic hormone
ADH	antidiuretic hormone
AF	atrial fibrillation
AIDS	acquired immunodeficiency syndrome
ALL	acute lymphoblastic leukaemia
AML	acuyte myeloid leukaemia
ANF	antinuclear factor
APTT	activated partial thromboplastin time
ARDS	adult respiratory distress syndrome
ARF	acute renal failure
ASD	atrial septal defect
ASO	antistreptolysin O
AST	aspartate transaminase
ATN	acute tubular necrosis
AXR	abdominal X-ray
BBB	bundle branch block
BD	bis diurnale (twice a day)
BMT	bone marrow transplant
BNF	British National Formulary
BP	blood pressure
BTS	blood transfusion service
CABG	coronary artery bypass graft
CAH	chronic active hepatitis
CAPD	chronic ambulatory peritoneal dialysis
CCF	congestive cardiac failure
CCU	coronary care unit
CLL	chronic lymphatic leukaemia
CML	chronic myeloid leukaemia
CMV	cytomegalovirus
CNS	central nervous system
COLD	chronic obstructive lung disease
COP	colloid osmotic pressure
CSF	cerebrospinal fluid
CSU	catheter specimen of urine
CT	computerised tomography
CVA	cerebrovascular accident
CVP	central venous pressure

CVS	cardiovascular system
CXR	chest X-ray
DIC	disseminated intravascular coagulation
DIP	distal interphalangeal
DM	diabetes mellitus
DVT	deep venous thrombosis
EBV	Epstein-Barr virus
ECF	extracellular fluid
ECG	electrocardiogram
EEG	electroencephalogram
ELISA	enzyme-linked immunosorbent assay
EMG	electromyography
ERCP	endoscopic retrograde cholangiopancreatography
ESR	erythrocyte sedimentation rate
FBC	full blood count
FEV1	forced expiratory volume in 1 sec
FFP	fresh frozen plasma
FSH	follicle stimulating hormone
FVC	forced vital capacity
GABA	gamma-aminobutyric acid
GFR	glomerular filtration rate
GGTP	gamma glutamyl transpeptidase
GH	growth hormone
GI	gastrointestinal
GIT	gastrointestinal tract
GKI	glucose/potassium/insulin
GN	glomerulonephritis
GVH	graft versus host disease
HBV	hepatitis B virus
HIV	human immunodeficiency virus
HLA	human leucocyte antigen
HSV	herpes simplex virus
IBD	inflammatory bowel disease
IBW	ideal body weight
ICF	intracellular fluid
ICP	intracranial pressure
IHD	ischaemic heart disease
IM	infectious mononucleosis
IMHP	intramuscular high potency
INR	international normalised ratio
ISQ	idem status quo (i.e. unchanged)
ITP	idiopathic thrombocytopenic purpura
IVC	inferior vena cava
IVHP	intravenous high potency
IVU	intravenous urography
JVP	jugular venous pressure
KCCT	kaolin cephalin clotting time
LA	left atrium

LBBB	left bundle branch block
LFTs	liver function tests
LH	luteinising hormone
LIF	left iliac fossa
LV	left ventricle
LVF	left ventricular failure
MCHC	mean corpuscular haemoglobin concentration
MCV	mean corpuscular volume
MEN	multiple endocrine neoplasia
MI	myocardial infarction
MIBG	meta-iodo benzyl guanidine
NSAID	non-steroidal anti-inflammatory drugs
OGTT	oral glucose tolerance test
OM	olim mane (once daily in the morning)
PA	pulmonary artery, pernicious anaemia
PCV	packed cell volume
PDA	patent ductus arteriosus
PE	pulmonary embolism
PEEP	positive end-expiratory pressure
PEFR	peak expiratory flow rate
PFTs	pulmonary function tests
PIP	proximal interphalangeal
PR	per rectum
PRN	pro re nata (as required)
PRV	polycythaemia rubra vera
PT	prothrombin time
PTC	percutaneous transhepatic cholangiogram
PTH	parathyroid hormone
PTT	partial thromboplastin time
PUO	pyrexia of unknown origin
QDS	quater diurnale summensum (four times a day)
RA	rheumatoid arthritis
RAST	radio-allergosorbent test
RBBB	right bundle branch block
RCC	red cell count
RIF	right iliac fossa
RVF	right ventricular failure
SLE	systemic lupus erythematosus
ST	sinus tachycardia
SVC	superior vena cava
SVT	supraventricular tachycardia
TB	tuberculosis
TBG	thyroid binding globulin
TDS	ter diurnale summensum (three times a day)
TIA	transient ischaemic attack
TIBC	total iron-binding capacity
TIP	terminal interphalangeal
TPN	total parenteral nutrition

TRH	thyrotrophin-releasing hormone
TSH	thyroid stimulating hormone
U&E	urea and electrolytes
URTI	upper respiratory tract infection
US	ultrasound
UTI	urinary tract infection
VF	ventricular fibrillation
VSD	ventricular septal defect
VT	ventricular tachycardia
VWF	von Willebrand factor
WBC	white blood count
WPW	Wolff-Parkinson-White

INDEX